Compassion-Based Practices for Secondary Traumatic Stress

Compassion-Based Practices for Secondary Traumatic Stress is a comprehensive guide that merges profound theoretical insights with practical compassion-based practices. Tailored for helping professionals working with survivors of trauma, this resource illuminates a path toward addressing secondary traumatic stress and promoting vicarious posttraumatic growth through a compassionate lens. Distinguished by its in-depth and hands-on creative approach, inclusion of East Asian philosophical principles, and harmonization of self- and other-oriented compassion, this resource guide provides empowering tools for helping professionals from diverse fields of practice and their host organizations.

Ruth Gottfried, PhD, serves as head of the David Yellin Academic College Dance Movement Therapy Master's Degree Program and is an ambassador of applied compassion, certified through the flagship program at Stanford University's Center for Compassion and Altruism Research and Education. As an academic researcher, Dr. Gottfried's work focuses primarily on trauma, secondary traumatic stress, and compassion.

Compassion-Based Practices for Secondary Traumatic Stress

A Resource Guide for Helping Professionals

Ruth Gottfried

Illustrated by Vicky Alvarez

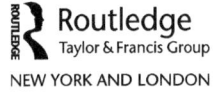
Routledge
Taylor & Francis Group

NEW YORK AND LONDON

Designed cover image "The Compassionate Path": © Vicky Alvarez

First published 2025
by Routledge
605 Third Avenue, New York, NY 10158

and by Routledge
4 Park Square, Milton Park, Abingdon, Oxon, OX14 4RN

Routledge is an imprint of the Taylor & Francis Group, an informa business

ISBN: 978-1-032-44472-7 (hbk)
ISBN: 978-1-032-44471-0 (pbk)
ISBN: 978-1-003-38174-7 (ebk)

DOI: 10.4324/9781003381747

Typeset in Times New Roman
by Apex CoVantage, LLC

The information in this volume is not intended as a substitute for consultation with healthcare professionals. Each individual's health concerns should be evaluated by a qualified professional.

Praise for Compassion-Based Practices for Secondary Traumatic Stress

"Compassion-Based Practices for Secondary Traumatic Stress is a welcome contribution to the fields of secondary traumatic stress and compassion, and a helpful and hopeful gift for all those who care for survivors of trauma. As a graduate of the Applied Compassion Training (ACT) at Stanford University and an expert on secondary traumatic stress – Ruth Gottfried compassionately bridges state-of-the-art science and practical insights with the mindset, heart set, and skillset of benefiting survivors of trauma and the professionals caring for them. The effects of her brilliant resource guide will, without doubt, lead to a more compassionate world for us all."

Robert Cusick, Co-Founder and Director,
Applied Compassion Training™ CCARE at Stanford University

"This is an exemplary work grounded in the fields of trauma, secondary traumatic stress, mindfulness, vicarious posttraumatic growth, and compassion. Ruth Gottfried's comprehensive resource guide brings forward theoretical and practical wisdom which will serve as an essential resource for helping professionals dealing with secondary traumatic stress. Highly recommended for all professionals working in the field of trauma."

Asher Ben-Arieh, PhD, Professor of Social Work,
The Haruv Chair for the Study of Child Maltreatment & Dean
of the Paul Baerwald School of Social Work and Social Welfare,
The Hebrew University of Jerusalem

"With this resource guide, Ruth Gottfried has made a substantial contribution to the health and wellbeing of all of us who work in the field of traumatic stress. In her unique way, Ruth gently and methodically helps us gain an evidence-based understanding of secondary traumatic stress and how compassion-based practices can help reconnect us to our minds, our bodies, and to each other. *Compassion-Based Practices for Secondary Traumatic Stress* is an invaluable resource for all who care for others while trying to balance care of self."

Jessica G. Eslinger, PhD, Assistant Professor,
University of Kentucky Center on Trauma and Children

"*Compassion-Based Practices for Secondary Traumatic Stress* is a wonderful, timely toolbox, and a must-read for helping professionals caring for individuals who have experienced trauma. Thank you, Ruth, for providing a creative, user-friendly, and healing bridge between the fields of compassion and secondary traumatic stress, and for being such an inspiring ambassador of applied compassion."

Neelama Eyres, Co-Founder and Director,
Applied Compassion Training™ CCARE at Stanford University

"Ruth Gottfried's resource guide is practical, research-supported, comprehensive, and widely applicable to all manner of helping professions and their host organizations. It is essential reading for every helping professional."

Hal A. Lawson, PhD, Professor of Social Welfare & Professor of
Education Leadership & Policy, University of Albany, SUNY

"Having first learned about secondary trauma as a clinical social worker and experiencing it first hand, then in my role as a social scientist, I can say that Ruth Gottfried's work is truly cutting edge. Starting with a very comprehensive and well thought out description of secondary traumatic stress and related concepts, this resource guide is rooted in sound science. From this evidence base, Ruth then offers a comprehensive approach to compassionately addressing secondary traumatic stress in many settings. I wish I had this book when I was a practicing social worker and will recommend it to my students and colleagues working in the field of trauma."

James Caringi, PhD, MSW, LCSW, Professor, University of Montana
School of Public and Community Health Sciences/ Co-Director
of the Developmental Adversity, Resilience and
Transformation Lab (DART) Lab

"*Compassion-Based Practices for Secondary Traumatic Stress* is a beautifully written and illustrated resource guide that serves as a compassionate compass for professionals caring for survivors of trauma. The enriching blend of theory and practical knowledge and the inspiring integration of Buddhist principles is highly commendable. Effortlessly engaging readers with its readability, this comprehensive guide can be revisited time and again, offering fresh insights with each encounter."

Dafna Tener, PhD, Associate Professor, Head of the BSW and MSW
for graduates in fields other than social work programs, The Paul
Baerwald School of Social Work and Social Welfare, The Hebrew
University of Jerusalem

"*Compassion-Based Practices for Secondary Traumatic Stress* is a must-read for helping professionals and organizational leaders in the field of trauma. Ruth Gottfried guides readers through a wealth of scientific knowledge in the fields of secondary traumatic stress, vicarious posttraumatic growth, and compassion, offering detailed and practical recommendations that bridge extensive realms of expertise. As a dance movement therapist, Ruth's profound knowledge shines through, and the integration of the body, movement, and creativity into her practical recommendations make her work both unique and incredibly valuable."

Einat Shuper Engelhard, PhD, Head, Dance Movement Therapy program, Graduate School of Creative Art Therapies, University of Haifa

"The compassionate path offered by Ruth Gottfried elegantly integrates research and practice to provide a much-needed review of where the fields of secondary traumatic stress and compassion are today. It likewise offers concrete compassion-based practices that can be used by all professionals in trauma-exposed fields. This book should become an essential resource for all."

Françoise Mathieu, MEd, RP, Author of
The Compassion Fatigue Workbook

"*Compassion-Based Practices for Secondary Traumatic Stress* is a distinct and valuable offering to the secondary traumatic stress community and field of compassion. Ruth Gottfried's writing, selection of content, and citations are accessible, relevant, and profound – a rare and special combination of characteristics by an expert. I am recommending this resource guide to participants in my program at Stanford and to you, too."

Monica Hanson, Co-Founder and Director,
Applied Compassion Training™ CCARE at Stanford University

"*Compassion-Based Practices for Secondary Traumatic Stress* offers a wide variety of creative solutions, grounded in empirical evidence, for addressing and coping with secondary traumatic stress. The inclusion of individual and group variations of all practices makes this a great resource for individuals, supervisors, or team leaders."

Stephanie K. Gusler, PhD, Assistant Professor,
University of Kentucky Center on Trauma and Children

FOR FORBES

when we meet teardrops,
compassion with outstretched arms,
raindrops and redwoods

Contents

TABLES

ILLUSTRATIONS

Note. The illustrations were created using watercolors and pencil on water-color paper.

HAIKUS

Acronyms

American Psychiatric Association **(APA)**
Applied Compassion Training **(ACT)**
Center for Compassion and Altruism Research and Education **(CCARE)**
Center on Trauma and Children **(CTAC)**
Compassion for Secondary Traumatic Stress **(CSTS)**
Diagnostic and Statistical Manual of Mental Disorders, Fifth Edition, Text Revision **(DSM-5-TR)**
Posttraumatic Growth **(PTG)**
Posttraumatic Growth Inventory **(PTGI)**
Posttraumatic Stress Disorder **(PTSD)**
Secondary Traumatic Stress **(STS)**
Secondary Traumatic Stress Domain Scale **(STS-DS)**
Secondary Traumatic Stress-Informed Organizational Assessment **(STSI-OA)**
Secondary Traumatic Stress Innovations and Solutions Center **(STS-ISC)**
Secondary Traumatic Stress Policy Analysis Tool **(STS-PAT)**
Secondary Traumatic Stress Scale **(STSS)**
Self-Compassion Scale **(SCS)**
Self-Compassion Scale Short Form **(SCS-SF)**
Substance Abuse and Mental Health Services Administration **(SAMHSA)**
Vicarious Posttraumatic Growth **(VPTG)**

Note. To enhance readability, most acronyms' full terms are repeated at the beginning of each section as well as in each practice, ensuring clarity and aiding in the comprehension of terminology throughout.

ABOUT THE AUTHOR AND THE ILLUSTRATOR

About the Author

Ruth Gottfried, PhD, is a dance movement therapist, supervisor, and senior lecturer at the David Yellin Academic College in Jerusalem, Israel, where she serves as Head of the Master's Degree Program in Dance Movement Therapy. Additionally, Ruth teaches at the School of Social Work and Social Welfare at the Hebrew University of Jerusalem. Along with her work in Israel, Ruth is a consultant for the Secondary Traumatic Stress Innovations and Solutions Center (STS-ISC) at the University of Kentucky's Center on Trauma and Children (CTAC).

Ruth's professional journey showcases her commitment to continuous growth and expertise. Having successfully completed her graduate studies in dance movement therapy at the University of Haifa, Ruth carried out two postdoctoral appointments focusing on STS at Tel Aviv and Georgia State Universities – with the latter appointment supported by a Haruv Institute postdoctoral fellowship. Moreover, Ruth is currently pursuing a second PhD at Tel Aviv University's Department of East Asian Studies, focusing on compassion from a Buddhist perspective.

As an Ambassador of Applied Compassion, certified through the flagship program at Stanford University's Center for Compassion and Altruism Research and Education (CCARE), Ruth facilitates the *Compassion for STS* (CSTS) training program, featured in this resource guide, for helping professionals across diverse fields of practice caring for survivors of trauma. She likewise conducts teacher trainings for group leaders wishing to facilitate the CSTS program within their professional networks.

Examples of testimonials shared by participants who attended CSTS training sessions at the University of Kentucky's CTAC STS-ISC include:

- "Dr. Gottfried was very knowledgeable and effective. The way she wove together information about STS and how to practice self-compassion and compassion for others was excellent."
- "Feeling focused, energized, grounded, and at peace. The training was wonderful and extremely useful. Dr. Gottfried has an amazing calming voice, and her calm, connected presence was felt and appreciated throughout the training. So relaxing and helpful to be walked through ways we can teach ourselves to compassionately handle STS."
- "I am so happy I attended Dr. Gottfried's training. It was fantastic. She addressed so much, so well, and in such a relaxed way. The training provided great useful, practical information and practices while also planting seeds for further practice and organizational change."

To access Ruth's full CV and receive more information on scheduling a CSTS training or an invited lecture, please visit https://csts.care or contact info@csts.care

About the Illustrator

Vicky Alvarez is a visual artist and illustrator based in the United Kingdom and Spain. She finds joy in the introspective and meditative nature of art-making and draws inspiration from nature and her inner world, embracing moments of simplicity, innocence, and vulnerability. Most recently, Vicky's creative exploration has led her to study art therapy, and she is currently working as an art therapist in training with adolescents. To learn more about Vicky and her inspiring artwork, please visit https://vickyalvarez.com

ACKNOWLEDGMENTS

This resource guide, encompassing the *Compassion for Secondary Traumatic Stress* (CSTS) training program, is offered under the auspices of the Applied Compassion Training (ACT) at Stanford University's Center for Compassion and Altruism Research and Education (CCARE); and the Secondary Traumatic Stress (STS) Practice Laboratory and STS Innovations and Solutions Center (STS-ISC) at the University of Kentucky's Center on Trauma and Children (CTAC).

With deep appreciation, I wish to express my gratitude to James R. Doty, Founder and Director of CCARE and Professor of Neurosurgery at Stanford University, as well as to ACT's outstanding co-founders, directors, and teachers Monica Hanson, Neelama Eyres, and Robert Cusick. Your unwavering commitment to cultivating a more compassionate world has had a profound impact on the lives of countless individuals, myself included. Thank you for ACT, which has been pivotal in shaping this resource guide into a compassionate response to STS.

My heartfelt appreciation and gratitude are likewise extended to Ginny Sprang, Professor of Psychiatry and Executive Director of the University of Kentucky's CTAC. Thank you, Ginny, for being both an inspiring mentor and friend and for gifting this resource guide, and me, with such an insightful Foreword. Thank you also to CTAC's exceptionally skilled and dedicated staff – with special thanks to Jessica G. Eslinger and Stephanie K. Gusler for their thoughtful suggestions and warm and enthusiastic support of this resource guide.

Furthermore, I am deeply honored by Lama Tsering Everest's willingness to review the manuscript and meet to discuss the topic of self-compassion from a Buddhist perspective. For knowledgeable feedback that further helped me refine the final draft, my appreciation is conveyed to Charles R. Figley, Brian E. Bride, Hal Lawson, James Caringi, Françoise Mathieu, Tara Brach, Asher Ben-Arieh, Dafna Tener, Valters Negribs, Einat Shuper Engelhard, Chava Weiss, Ili Margalit, and Merav Cohen-Shalev. Thank you all for the time you invested and for your kind and supportive guidance. Your contributions are truly appreciated.

It is with wholehearted appreciation that I also wish to thank Vicky Alvarez for her artistic contributions that so gracefully illuminate these pages. Thank you, Vicky, for sharing your talent, for your intuitive alignment, and for imbuing this resource guide with the translucent beauty of watercolors. Relatedly, I wish to thank my dear friend and colleague Melissa Bar-Ilan, trauma therapist, and mindfulness teacher, for insightful recommendations, including the wonderful suggestion that Vicky Alvarez illustrate this work.

Additionally, I offer my sincere gratitude to Routledge publisher Anna Moore for believing in the initial manuscript, for motivating me to expand it to its current scope, and for valuable guidance throughout the publishing process. Thank you, Anna, for championing the dissemination of the topics addressed in this resource guide to a wider audience. Your expertise, support, and pleasant collaboration are greatly valued.

Moreover, I wish to acknowledge the dedicated team at Routledge Publishing, whose professionalism and commitment to excellence have been evident at every stage of the publishing process. Your collective efforts have made this journey both smooth and rewarding. A warm thank you is likewise extended to Maureen E. Angell for providing first-class copyediting services that contributed to the quality and clarity of this work.

And within and among it all, I thank my beloved family for their patience and encouragement throughout the writing journey, with special thanks extended to my parents, Murray and Susan Moinester. First, for blessing me with the name "Ruth" – rooted in the Hebrew word *re'ut* for "companion" and defined as "compassion" (Collins, 2023) – and second, for their generosity of time and wisdom in multiple reviews along the way. Your love and support are a true blessing.

Last yet foremost, a deep bow of gratitude to Forbes Ellis, Director of Volunteer Services at Hospice of Santa Cruz County. Your presence has been central in my decision to study dance movement therapy, join ACT, and embark on a second PhD in Buddhist studies focusing on compassion. Thank you for gracing my path and for being such an ongoing source of inspiration. May your compassionate heart, dear Forbes, shine through these pages like the compassionate path itself – so beautifully illuminated within this resource guide.

thank you, guiding light –
you are my inspiration:
glow of gratitude

Warm Embrace

An illuminated candle

FOREWORD

Almost 20 years ago, an employee of mine, I will call her Kate, came to my office to tender her resignation. She sat before me, lips trembling, and explained that her work as a trauma therapist needed to end if she was ever to be happy again. She described intrusive thoughts associated with the trauma experienced by the individuals in her care, difficulties experiencing positive emotions, and interpersonal irritability related to her work, which was negatively affecting her family life, job satisfaction, and ability to concentrate and sleep. "I have to face it that I am not strong enough to do this work," she said, tearfully adding, "I worked so hard to be a therapist, and now it brings me no joy." Despite my efforts to affirm, validate, and normalize, Kate remained despondent and resolved. Kate was experiencing symptoms of secondary traumatic stress (STS) and a profound sense of professional failure.

Kate left my office that day facing an uncertain professional future, but even as she moved on to a less stressful job, her story became intertwined with my own. I, too, had experienced similar thoughts and feelings about my work as the center's director. Kate's resignation felt like evidence of my own failure to respond to a suffering that I should have recognized. I felt as if I had let Kate down and wondered if there were others like her. Clearly, Kate and I could have benefited from self-compassion during that time.

Since that day, I have learned that these shared experiences are far too common. "Self-compassion involves recognizing that suffering and personal inadequacy are part of the shared human experience – something that we all go through rather than being something that happens to 'me' alone" (Neff et al., 2007, p. 140). Furthermore, Neff and Germer (2018) posited that if we are to respond to challenging situations with self-compassion, we need to counter suffering with kindness and a nonjudgmental stance. Moreover, we need to accept our suffering as part of the human condition and pay mindful attention to our difficulties as part of a shared professional experience.

The compassionate approach offered here by Dr. Ruth Gottfried for addressing STS is likened to other "third-wave" interventions that aim to decrease psychological distress by changing the person's relation to their problems (e.g., Acceptance and Commitment Therapy, Dialectical Behavioral Therapy, Mindfulness-Based Cognitive Therapy; e.g., Karatzias et al., 2019). A promising aspect of this compassionate approach is that it disputes stigmatizing perspectives (e.g., "I am not strong enough to do this work") that can discourage helping professionals from acknowledging STS-related reactions associated with their work.

Fortunately, there is emerging evidence that self-compassion may be skillfully applied to reduce traumatic stress symptoms. A systematic review summarizing knowledge on the association between trauma, self-compassion, and posttraumatic stress disorder (PTSD) by Winders et al. (2020) suggested that higher levels of self-compassion may reduce the impact of trauma exposure and attenuate PTSD symptoms. Additionally, Rushforth et al.'s (2023) systematic review provided preliminary evidence that self-compassion may be beneficial in reducing STS. Such findings add to a growing body of literature that demonstrates that as self-compassion increases, one can also expect decreases in negative outcomes such as stress, fear of failure, anxiety, depression, shame, rumination, and self-criticism (Diedrich et al., 2016; Johnson & O'Brien, 2013; Mosewich et al., 2013; Neff & Germer, 2013; Odou & Brinker, 2015; Smeets et al., 2014).

Luckily, Dr. Gottfried has put together an inspiring toolbox of methods to apply self-compassion skillfully in a mindful, present-centered manner; one that is straightforward, practical, and likely to provide a more direct line to happiness and wellbeing than other methods such as distraction, avoidance, or withdrawal. Supporting this idea, Odou and Brinker (2015) found that in the face of a negative experience, while self-compassion and distraction similarly decrease negative affect, self-compassion is more effective at improving overall positive affect. This may be because self-compassion acts on positive and negative affect simultaneously by mindfully focusing on kindness and connectedness, which can lead to more self-agency and hope during painful encounters. Distraction (or avoidance and withdrawal), on the other hand, may reduce negativity but does not necessarily lead to positive emotion.

This is important as research in positive psychology demonstrates a causal link between positive emotions and success, countering the notion that achievement is first in temporal order (Lyubomirsky et al., 2005). For my former employee Kate, it is unlikely that a reduction of negative affect alone would have been salient enough to overcome her STS symptoms; rather, she needed effective trauma treatment and a compassionate approach to enhance her ability to experience a positive transformation.

A compassionate approach within workplaces extends to compassion among the workforce. This is exemplified by Dr. Gottfried's skillful approach that harmonizes self- and other-oriented compassion in line with East Asian philosophical insights. Instrumental in this regard are the STS-related personal practices that emphasize extending compassion to colleagues, the compassion-based group practices, and the self- and other-oriented recommendations for compassionate leadership. Creating compassionate STS-informed organizations requires a commitment to a three-pronged approach that combines individual, team, and organization-wide efforts (e.g., Sprang et al., 2021).

When compassion exists as part of the organizational culture, it helps staff feel valued, listened to, and less alone (e.g., Kanov et al., 2004). Moreover, a compassionate organizational culture may enhance vicarious posttraumatic growth (VPTG; e.g., Cleary et al., 2023) and create an environment of staff buy-in that can increase retention, staff morale, and effectiveness as well as the likelihood of staff fulfilling the organizational mission (Barclay & Barclay, 2011; Lown et al., 2019). Stemming from the preceding points, organizations that wish to thrive in this respect need to be led by STS-informed and compassionate leaders, with a caring and compassionate culture permeating the entire organization (Friedman & Gerstein, 2017; Sprang, 2018a).

Throughout this resource guide, the phenomenon of exchange is likewise evident and leads one to understand and accept that we can improve our ability to be effective in our work by compassionately nurturing our professional selves. Jon Conte reminded us of this mandate when he wrote, "We are stewards not just of those who allow us into their lives, but of our own capacity to be helpful" (as cited in van Dernoot Lipsky & Burk, 2010, p. xii). Indeed, the promise of compassionate trauma-informed care requires that those implementing the approach have the internal capacity to create such an experience for those served.

It is thereby empowering to have this compendium of resources, anchored in scientific research, that helping professionals from a wide range of fields can use to enhance their self- and other-oriented compassion. Imagine if all members of an organization (senior leaders, too) were to embody STS-related compassion toward themselves and others – the benefits would no doubt compound and transform the organizational culture toward a more successful and humane approach to working with survivors of trauma; and create a ripple effect that could positively impact communities as well. Well-grounded in a wide-ranging body of relevant theory and practical expertise, Dr. Gottfried's resource guide has given us the tools to take on this challenge.

Ginny Sprang, PhD, Professor,
College of Medicine, Department of Psychiatry,
Executive Director of the University of Kentucky Center on Trauma and
Children (CTAC), Principal Investigator: Secondary Traumatic Stress
Innovations and Solutions Center (STS-ISC) & STS Practice Laboratory.

Preface

"My belly was black and blue," she recounted, revealing the extent of the severe domestic abuse she had suffered throughout her pregnancy. After empathically listening to this courageous mother who had sought my care for her child – a child who had thankfully been born healthy and was now 10 years old – I began experiencing secondary traumatic stress (STS) reactions as a result of my indirect exposure to the trauma they had endured. I have since come to realize that although I was unfamiliar with the concept of STS at the time, this experience marked the beginning of my journey toward creating this resource guide.[1]

It is widely accepted that helping professionals working with individuals who have experienced trauma are at high risk of developing STS, recognized as traumatic stress originating from indirect exposure to trauma (Molnar et al., 2017). Focusing on mindful, compassion-based practices for addressing STS as well as the connections between these practices and the science of recovery and wellbeing,[2] this resource guide is directed toward helping professionals from diverse fields of practice. These include but are not limited to physicians, nurses, psychologists, social workers, creative arts therapists, counselors, educators, and their host organizations.

By incorporating more compassion into their personal and professional lives, helping professionals can use their "passion for compassion" to address STS and to promote vicarious posttraumatic growth (VPTG; i.e., "the experience of growth as a result of indirect trauma exposure;" Arnold et al., 2005, as cited in Deaton et al., 2023, p. 17). This is important, as the wellbeing of helping professionals can have a positive reciprocal effect on the individuals for whom they care, the colleagues with whom they work, their organizations as a whole, and the communities in which they live (e.g., Brend & Sprang, 2020; Gottfried & Bride, 2018).

The comprehensive literature review provided in the first part of this resource guide serves as a valuable foundation for engaging in the personal and group practices featured in the second part. This is because a thorough understanding of the theoretical concepts can lead to a more nuanced comprehension of the practices. Alternatively, it is possible to begin practicing prior to reading the literature review – as the embodied learning may enhance helping professionals' curiosity to consider the interface between practice and theory. Either way, completing the STS-Domain Scale (STS-DS) before and after engaging with this resource guide is recommended (see Appendix A).

Inspired by leading researchers in the fields of trauma, STS, VPTG, and compassion, as well as traditional Buddhist compassion-based meditative techniques – the practices included herein are carefully crafted original practices or have been thoughtfully adapted from existing ones to offer fresh insights. These practices incorporate a wide range of approaches, predominantly contemplative in nature, alongside creative, arts-based activities. The latter, as the arts can assist in the expression of indirect trauma-related experiences in a reparative way (e.g., Deaton et al., 2021; Malchiodi, 2020; Perry, 2014; Perryman et al., 2019).

Notably, this resource guide is presented using an invitational approach and inclusive, trauma-informed language, aiming to establish a safe and welcoming environment for learning, reflection, and engagement. It serves as both a starting point and an ongoing resource that helping professionals can revisit and tailor according to their individual needs, preferences, circumstances, and worldviews. Besides, this guide is not only valuable for helping professionals currently experiencing STS but also for those seeking to replenish the compassion they extend to themselves and others proactively as a protective measure.

May you recognize that YOU are a conduit of compassion. In the beginning, it may feel challenging to create the compassionate change that you are hoping for. However, by embracing patience, continuity of practice, and the cultivation of a beginner's mind,[3] you can enhance your ability to address STS and promote VPTG compassionately. In doing so, you will also be creating a compassionate ripple effect, extending its positive influence to survivors of trauma, the compassionate caregivers caring for them, and a more compassionate world for us all.

across the river –
a path with dancing colors:
pink petals and gold

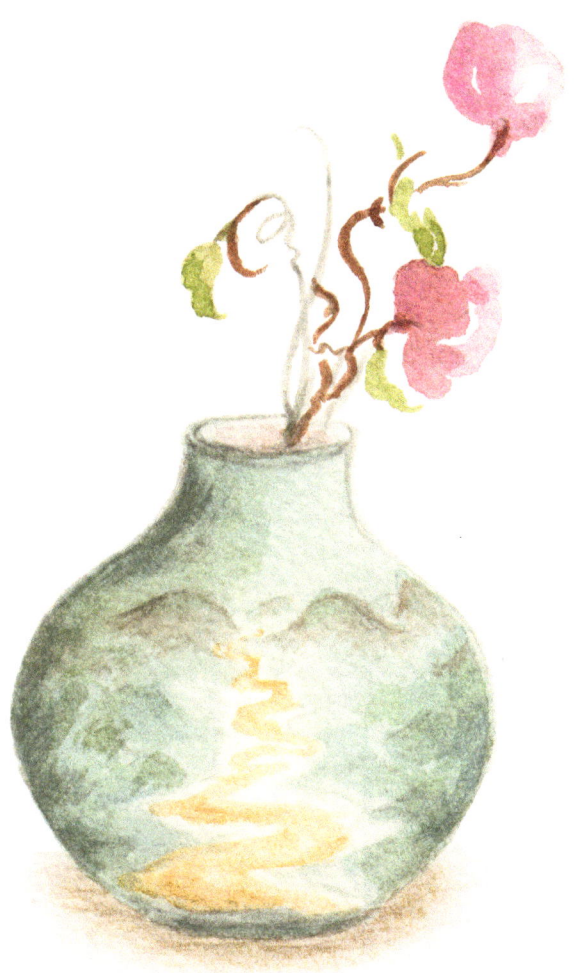

Invitation to the Path

A vase with a golden path and flowers

Part I

THE SCIENCE OF TRAUMA, SECONDARY TRAUMATIC STRESS, AND COMPASSION

Establishing Pure-Hearted Motivation[1]

May compassion become your compass and passion:
A guiding light for you and yours and all creation.[2]

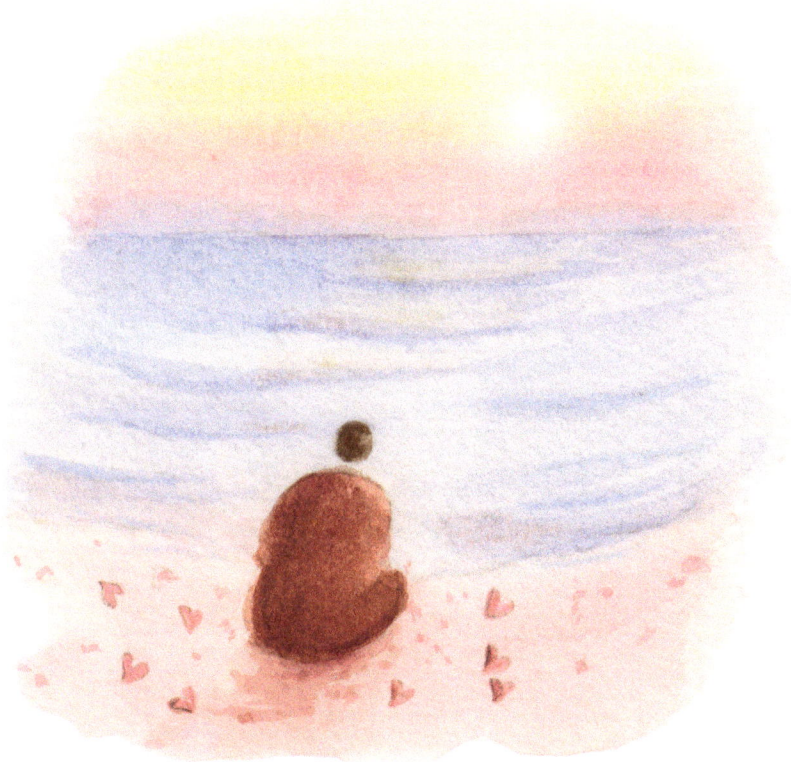

Pure-Hearted Motivation

Figure sitting on a shore with heart-shaped seashells

Overview of the Literature Review

This literature review highlights selected topics organized in four sections focusing on: (a) trauma, (b) secondary traumatic stress (STS), (c) compassion for self and others, and (d) compassion within and beyond organizational contexts. A concise overview of the main themes encompassed within this review follows:

- *Section I – Trauma:* This section defines the terms *trauma* and *posttraumatic stress disorder* (PTSD) and explores trauma types, triggers, and retraumatization. Additionally, it examines stress responses and introduces a mindful response to perceived threat from a Buddhist perspective. Furthermore, this section presents key principles and guidance recommendations for trauma-informed care as well as an exploration of the term *posttraumatic growth* (PTG) and PTG-related elements.
- *Section II – STS:* Moving forward, this section delves into the term *STS* as well as related concepts (i.e., *compassion fatigue, vicarious traumatization*, and *burnout*) and addresses indirect trauma exposure pathways. In addition, it provides information on STS symptoms, risk factors, and recommendations, along with a concise overview of STS prevalence and best practice principles. Moreover, key organizational foci and efforts for addressing STS are highlighted. This section concludes with a focus on the concept of *vicarious posttraumatic growth* (VPTG).
- *Section III – Compassion for self and others:* Continuing the exploration, this section begins by exploring the connection between wisdom and compassion, delving into how these concepts, along with indirect trauma exposure, are viewed through a Buddhist lens. It also reviews definitions and conceptualizations of both self- and other-oriented compassion while exploring their intricate connections with relevant additional terms. For example, this section offers a Buddhist perspective on self-compassion as a skillful means, outlines the dynamics of generous vs. judgmental interpretations associated with compassion, and describes the flourishing that can occur naturally and reciprocally when care recipients are in the presence of compassionate caregivers. Brief references to topics associated with compassion within the workplace are likewise provided, setting the stage for the upcoming section.
- *Section IV – Compassion within and beyond organizations*: Shifting focus more prominently toward the workplace, this section investigates self- and other-oriented compassion within organizational contexts. It examines the concepts of *compassion competence* and self- and other-oriented *compassionate leadership* and presents leadership recommendations for compassionately addressing STS via the COMPASSION acronym. It likewise explores links between compassion and social

action while examining the broader topic of indirect trauma exposure from a public health perspective.

For further exploration and enrichment, each of these four sections includes endnotes that offer enhanced explanations and reading recommendations. While endnotes are often overlooked, they are filled with extra insights and bonus content (see the "Hidden Gems" section). Significantly, this resource guide's comprehensive bibliography inherently provides additional reading suggestions. This extensive collection of resources serves as a valuable companion for those seeking to expand further their knowledge of the topics addressed within these pages.

Section I

TRAUMA

Trauma – Definition

The term *trauma* has its origins in ancient Greek, where it literally translates to "wound" (Winders et al., 2020). In the Diagnostic and Statistical Manual of Mental Disorders, Fifth Edition, Text Revision (DSM-5-TR; American Psychiatric Association [APA], 2022), trauma is defined as stemming from exposure to actual or threatened death, serious injury, or sexual violence. A broader definition of the term states that *trauma* can result from "an *event*, series of *events*, or set of circumstances that is *experienced* by an individual as physically or emotionally harmful or life threatening; and that has adverse *effects* on the individual's functioning and mental, physical, social, emotional, or spiritual wellbeing." (Substance Abuse and Mental Health Services Administration [SAMHSA], 2014, p. 7)[1]

Notice the three **E**s in the aforementioned definition of the term *trauma* (Papa & Robinson, 2023; SAMHSA, 2014):

- *Event* – This may include an actual or extreme threat of physical or psychological harm or severe neglect that hinders healthy development.[2] Such an event or circumstance may occur once or repeatedly over time.
- *Experience* – This signifies that subjective perception plays a role in determining whether an event or circumstance is experienced as traumatic.

DOI: 10.4324/9781003381747-2

As such, what may be experienced as traumatic for one individual may not be traumatic for another.
• *Effects* – This means that the adverse effects of the event or circumstance are a component of the definition of trauma. The duration of said effects can vary from short-term to long-term and manifest either immediately or have a delayed onset.

When considering the concept of *trauma*, it is also important to remember that, like their clients,[3] helping professionals may directly experience traumatic events. This includes helping professionals' personal history of direct trauma as well as work-related direct exposure to trauma (e.g., experiencing or witnessing physical and/or verbal violence directed toward them by clients or clients' family members; Mathieu, 2012).

Relatedly, *shared trauma* is a term signifying the same traumatic event, series of events, or set of circumstances collectively experienced by both helping professionals and those in their care. Shared trauma, therefore, contains aspects of both direct and indirect trauma since helping professionals are exposed to the same traumatic events as their clients (e.g., wars, global pandemics, and natural disasters; Hensel et al., 2015; Tosone, 2012; Tosone et al., 2021).[4] Of note is that compassion-based practices may attenuate both trauma and shared trauma symptoms (e.g., Kaiser Permanente, 2021; Winders et al., 2020).

Trauma Types

The term *trauma types* typically encompasses two broad categories: (a) *acute trauma*, characterized by single-incident traumatic events like experiencing a car crash or robbery, and (b) *chronic trauma*, characterized by prolonged and repeated traumatic events such as neglect or homelessness.[5] Trauma types can likewise exist along a continuum, such as the continuum ranging from *impersonal trauma* (e.g., natural disasters) to *interpersonal trauma* (e.g., abuse by a stranger) and *attachment trauma* (e.g., abuse by a caregiver; Luyten & Fonagy, 2019).

Extensive global research conducted across multiple disciplines has identified numerous additional types of trauma, further enhancing the understanding of the diverse manifestations of the term (e.g., Scott et al., 2023). For example, Scott et al. described 11 trauma types. These categories are not necessarily mutually exclusive, and their presentation order does not imply the significance or prevalence of any particular category:[6]

• *Individual trauma* – This type of trauma typically results from a single adverse event/circumstance that occurs to an individual (e.g., physical assault).
• *Developmental trauma* – This type of trauma refers to experiences that occur during a particular period in life that can negatively impact development (e.g., housing or food insecurity during childhood or old age).

- *Indirect trauma* – This type of trauma may develop after being indirectly exposed to a traumatic event experienced by a significant other (e.g., hearing/learning that a relative or friend was sexually abused).
- *Interpersonal trauma* – This type of trauma typically occurs within relationships where the individuals involved share a degree of familiarity with each other, such as between family members or spouses (e.g., intimate partner violence).[7]
- *Group, community, or collective trauma* – This type of trauma denotes instances where a specific group or community of people experiences trauma (e.g., first responders who lose teammates in a natural disaster).
- *Racial trauma* – This type of trauma occurs when individuals experience racial discrimination, threats of injury, or events that are shaming/humiliating due to their race. Such experiences may involve individual or systemic racial trauma and range from microaggressions to overt acts of racism (e.g., anti-Asian racism following the COVID-19 outbreak).
- *Cultural trauma* – This type of trauma signifies occurrences that undermine the heritage of a society/culture through biased treatment, marginalization, or disparities (e.g., forced migration).
- *Historical trauma* – This type of trauma happens when a significant historical event negatively impacts an entire society/culture (e.g., slavery).[8]
- *Naturally caused trauma* – This type of trauma generally indicates inevitable adverse events that occur naturally (e.g., earthquakes).
- *Human-caused trauma* – This type of trauma implies incidents stemming from human errors such as accidents or technological disasters (e.g., an aircraft crash) as well as the intentional perpetration of trauma (e.g., terrorism).
- *Mass trauma* – This type of trauma involves large-scale intentional or unintentional, human-caused or natural disasters that adversely impact a large number of individuals within a shared time span (i.e., the individuals are not necessarily associated with the same group/community; e.g., pandemics).

Relatedly, the term *cumulative trauma* encompasses the impact of all the trauma types an individual has experienced throughout their lifetime (Kira et al., 2013). Meanwhile, the term *complex trauma* pertains to the experience of enduring multiple forms of severe and pervasive traumatic events as well as the subsequent immediate and enduring adverse effects stemming from such exposure (National Child Traumatic Stress Network, 2018).

Posttraumatic Stress Disorder (PTSD) – Definition

PTSD is defined as a stress-related mental health disorder that can develop following exposure to one or more traumatic events (APA, 2022). In order to meet PTSD diagnostic criteria as outlined in the DSM-5-TR (APA, 2022; First et al., 2022), an individual must meet several criteria,[9] of which the first (i.e., Criterion A) is exposure to trauma. Namely, exposure to trauma can occur in the following ways: (a) direct exposure to trauma, (b) witnessing trauma, (c) learning that trauma was experienced by a significant other, and/or (d) indirect exposure to negative details of the trauma experienced by others.

In line with DSM-5-TR (APA, 2022) guidelines, PTSD is further characterized by the presence of four hallmark symptom clusters that began or worsened after exposure to the traumatic event: (a) intrusion and re-experiencing, (b) avoidance, (c) negative alterations in cognition and mood,[10] and (d) hyperarousal and reactivity symptoms. These trauma-related reactions can manifest in different ways. They can either be stable and persistently present or unstable/intermittent and triggered by stress. Alternatively, they can be concealed for many years and resurface abruptly (Levine, 2010).

Specifically, DSM-5-TR (APA, 2022) guidelines state that:[11]

- The cluster of *intrusion and re-experiencing* (i.e., Criterion B) comprises the following symptoms associated with the traumatic event: unwanted intrusive and upsetting thoughts that range from mild unwanted memories, distressing nightmares, to full dissociative flashbacks, and/or physical reactivity following exposure to traumatic reminders (e.g., dizziness, increased heart rate, and/or trembling).
- The cluster of *avoidance* of reminder cues (i.e., Criterion C) involves the following symptoms associated with the traumatic event: avoidance of internal trauma-related thoughts and/or feelings, and/or avoidance of external reminders of the trauma, such as certain people, places, and/or activities/circumstances.
- The cluster of *negative alterations in cognition and mood* (i.e., Criterion D) involves a broad cluster of symptoms associated with the traumatic event, including the following: inability to remember key features of the traumatic event, negative thoughts/assumptions regarding oneself, others, and/or the world, exaggerated/unrealistic blame of oneself and/or others, decreased interest in previously enjoyable activities, feelings of isolation, negative affect, and/or difficulty experiencing positive emotions.
- The cluster of *hyperarousal and reactivity* (i.e., Criterion E) constitutes the following symptoms associated with the traumatic event: irritability, aggression, risky or destructive behavior, hypervigilance, a heightened startle reaction, difficulties concentrating, and/or difficulties sleeping.

During the first month following exposure to a potentially traumatizing event, it is natural to experience stress-related reactions, and in many individuals, such reactions naturally resolve after the initial upheaval. However, when symptoms persist for more than one month (i.e., Criterion F), a

PTSD diagnosis may be considered. Of note is that the DSM-5-TR lists two additional core criteria (i.e., Criteria G and H), which respectively signify that in order to qualify for a PTSD diagnosis, symptoms need to create significant personal distress or functional impairment and not be due to substance use, medication, and/or other types of illnesses (APA, 2022).

The term *subthreshold PTSD* denotes symptoms that compromise individuals' functioning yet do not meet the full criteria for a diagnosable PTSD disorder (Hruska et al., 2023; Marshall et al., 2001). This implies that there is a spectrum from: (a) normal stress, (b) traumatic stress, (c) posttraumatic stress, to (d) PTSD. The related term *comorbid PTSD* refers to co-occurring disorders (e.g., PTSD coupled with substance abuse issues; Cloitre et al., 2019; Condon et al., 2023; Herman, 1992a; Karatzias & Cloitre, 2019; Roberts et al., 2022).[12]

Significantly, the DSM-5-TR (APA, 2022) includes a cultural formulation interview that consists of a set of inquiries/prompts designed to delve into individuals' own cultural definitions of the trauma-related clinical challenges they are experiencing. Moreover, the cultural formulation interview covers a range of aspects, including individuals' perspectives on the origins, contexts, available sources of support, service expectations, and potential obstacles to seeking assistance and accessing treatment – with the aim of facilitating culturally competent care.

Trauma Triggers and Retraumatization

Following a traumatic event, various cues, such as specific people, places, and/or circumstances, can serve as reminders of the trauma. These reminders, referred to as *trauma triggers*, are unique to each individual and can involve anything that elicits a recollection of the traumatic event (e.g., sights, sounds, and/or smells; Gerdes, 2019; Grabbe & Miller-Karas, 2018). When such multisensory cues, often embedded in implicit memory,[13] are activated, the whole neural network in which the traumatic memory is stored can become stimulated, leading the individual to recall the traumatizing event (van der Kolk, 2002).

Relatedly, *trigger warnings* are textual, verbal, or image-based cues that are intended to caution individuals regarding potentially distressing forthcoming content that might trigger trauma-associated memories. Trigger warnings, as such, highlight particular contents that may reasonably elicit trauma responses (Jones et al., 2020). It is important to recognize, however, that trigger warnings are not intended to assist individuals in avoiding triggering content but rather to help them prepare for said content (Lockhart, 2016). Notably, trigger warnings can also function as a considerate gesture, allowing individuals who may not be clinically traumatized yet may still find certain topics uncomfortable to prepare themselves and avoid being caught off guard (Gerdes, 2019).[14]

Regarding *retraumatization*, this term refers to the resurfacing of trauma-related symptoms that can occur either because of an associated new traumatic experience or as a result of otherwise-related triggering stimuli (e.g., Schippert et al., 2023). The severity and persistence of traumatic stress reactions that arise from retraumatization can vary depending on the potential triggers involved and how survivors of trauma reacted to the previous traumatic event(s) they experienced (e.g., Watson, 2016).

Retraumatization can negatively impact individuals' wellbeing and overall recovery processes. Trauma-informed care that addresses retraumatization aims to support individuals in navigating and healing from the complex interactions between past traumas and current triggers, thereby fostering resilience.[15] By understanding the multifaceted nature of retraumatization, helping professionals can provide clients with tailored support and empower healing (e.g., Grossman et al., 2021; Schippert et al., 2023).

Trauma-Informed Care

The pioneering work of researchers such as Herman (1992b) and van der Kolk (1994) on trauma and recovery has paved the way for trauma-informed care (Harris & Fallot, 2001). Trauma-informed care is "grounded in an understanding of and responsiveness to the impact of trauma, that emphasizes physical, psychological, and emotional safety for both providers and survivors" (Hopper et al., 2010, p. 82). Accordingly, helping professionals are encouraged to be sensitive to the possibility that both the individuals in their care and the colleagues with whom they work may have experienced trauma – regardless of whether or not clients or colleagues present themselves as such or are even aware of it themselves (Knight, 2015; Spence, 2021).

The terms *trauma-informed care* and *trauma-specific services* are sometimes used interchangeably. However, there is a distinction between them. Trauma-informed care emphasizes a supportive organizational culture where all staff have the awareness, knowledge, and skills to support survivors of trauma.[16] On the other hand, trauma-specific services refer to the actual prevention, intervention, or treatment services that directly address traumatic stress reactions as well as any ensuing co-occurring disorders (DeCandia et al., 2014).

Subsequently, in line with the four **R**s associated with trauma-informed care (SAMHSA, 2014), helping professionals are encouraged to prioritize: (a) **R**esisting retraumatization as it can interfere with the healing process, (b) **R**ealizing the pervasive impact of trauma exposure, (c) **R**ecognizing the signs and symptoms associated with trauma exposure, and (d) **R**esponding by incorporating knowledge about trauma exposure into their service delivery and peer interactions. These recommendations are applicable to direct and/or indirect trauma-related reactions – as both PTSD and secondary traumatic stress (STS) are core components of a trauma-informed approach.

Notably, these recommendations can be expanded to include **R**esourcing, which signifies the importance of professionals being well-informed about the available community resources and support services specifically tailored for addressing traumatic stress reactions. With respect to survivors of trauma, resourcing also involves actively collaborating with survivors to determine which resources align best with their needs and preferences, as well as helping them identify solutions to relevant financial, geographic, cultural, or linguistic issues that may be impacting their access to resources (e.g., Raja et al., 2021).

Key Principles and Guidance Recommendations

According to SAMHSA (2014), and further cited by researchers such as Levenson (2017), Henshaw (2022), and Mahood et al. (2023), there is an overarching six-step approach to providing trauma-informed care. These steps involve the following interconnected principles, which build upon each other and are not necessarily meant to be applied in a linear fashion:[17]

- S*afety* – This principle ensures that helping professionals and the clients in their care feel secure both physically and psychologically. Specifically, it encompasses the provision of care in a physically safe environment and fosters interpersonal interactions that consistently prioritize a sense of security.
- *Transparency and trustworthiness* – These fundamental principles highlight the importance of professional decisions being made with honesty and openness. By conducting decision-making processes in a transparent manner, helping professionals can establish and nurture trust among the individuals affected by these decisions, including clients, clients' family members, and staff.
- *Peer support* – This principle encourages solidarity among colleagues with lived experiences of trauma since a supportive network and mutual self-help are key to recovery. Peer support provides a valuable space for colleagues to connect, learn from one another, and offer mutual assistance and encouragement that can foster healing and growth.
- *Collaboration and mutuality* – These principles emphasize the importance of reducing power imbalances and promoting mutual respect within the workplace. This entails acknowledging that every individual, irrespective of their position within the organization, plays a pivotal role in delivering trauma-informed care.[18]
- *Empowerment, voice, and choice* – These principles prioritize providing strength-based and skill-building care that empowers individuals to play an active role in shaping their healing process. By amplifying individuals' voices, their needs and preferences can guide the care they receive, encompassing their involvement in both the evaluation and

design of services. Moreover, these principles prioritize safeguarding informed choice and thereby promote shared decision-making and goal-setting.
• *Cultural, historical, and gender issues* – These principles denote a proactive approach to transcending biases and stereotypes, specifically in relation to topics such as ethnicity, religion, sexual orientation, and gender identity. Furthermore, they represent a commitment to an organizational culture that is sensitive to the cultural requirements and potential historical traumas experienced by the individuals being served and those delivering the services.

Organizations across service-sectors and systems are likewise encouraged to follow SAMHSA's (2014) widely cited ten guidance recommendations, presented here briefly, for implementing a trauma-informed approach (e.g., Mahood et al., 2023):

• *Governance and leadership* – The organization's governance and leadership are committed to both funding and fostering a trauma-informed approach, ensuring its effective implementation and long-term maintenance.
• *Policies* – The organization has written policies and protocols that ensure an approach that is trauma-informed, reflecting a foundational component of the organization's mission.
• *Physical setting* – The organization offers trauma-informed care within a physical environment that promotes a sense of safety.
• *Engagement and involvement* – The organization provides relevant trauma-informed engagement and involvement opportunities for all individuals offering or receiving services.
• *Collaboration across sectors* – The organization values and supports cross-sector collaborations that are based on trauma-informed key principles and guidance recommendations.
• *Screening, assessment, and treatment* – The organization offers empirically based screening, assessment, and treatment services that reflect a trauma-informed approach.[19]
• *Workforce training and development* – The organization provides ongoing trauma-informed professional training and development to its workforce.
• *Quality assurance and progress monitoring* – The organization incorporates ongoing trauma-informed monitoring designs for quality assurance, utilizing validated trauma-oriented research measures.
• *Evaluation* – The organization utilizes measures and evaluation frameworks for assessing the implementation and effectiveness of its services. These frameworks are informed by an understanding of trauma, incorporating appropriate trauma-focused research tools.

• *Financing* – The organization has financial structures in place to support trauma-informed care that encompasses all the preceding recommended items.

Implementing trauma-informed care principles and guidance recommendations into practice reduces the chances of dysfunctional dynamics within helping relationships. Moreover, it presents opportunities for corrective experiences both for those receiving and offering care (Harris & Fallot, 2001; Levenson, 2017). Importantly, adopting a trauma-informed approach necessitates more than a single or specific technique. It requires a sustained commitment to trauma-informed organization-wide transformation (Scott et al., 2023).

Stress Responses

Understanding stress responses provides insight into the complex range of responses individuals may exhibit when faced with perceived threat and is an integral component of trauma-informed care. Examples of stress expressions include: (a) *flock* – looking to others to help interpret a perceived threat, (b) *flight* – running away/fleeing from a perceived threat, (c) *fight* – confronting a perceived threat aggressively, (d) *freeze* – becoming immobilized or "stuck" when faced with a perceived threat, and (e) *flop or faint* – collapsing when faced with a perceived threat (Price, 2018; Winfrey & Perry, 2021).[20]

These natural "bottom-up" responses are essential for our safety and survival in instances of imminent threat.[21] However, they shut down the part of our brain responsible for executive functions like critical thinking, problem-solving, reasoning, decision making, and impulse control. In other words, when a perceived threat activates a stress response, our higher-order thinking tends to shut down, we temporarily lose the ability to "think," and we oftentimes react automatically rather than respond mindfully (Matto et al., 2013; Price, 2018).[22]

Significantly, there is growing empirical evidence to support the idea that negative feelings (e.g., feeling stressed) can limit our thinking. This constriction is believed to be an evolved adaptation that helped our ancestors survive in dangerous situations by focusing their cognition on specific action urges such as flight or fight (e.g., Price, 2018). Winfrey and Perry (2021) likewise explained that "all experience is processed from the bottom-up, meaning, to get to the top, 'smart' part of our brain, we have to go through the lower, 'not-so-smart part.' This sequential processing means that the most primitive, reactive part of our brain is the first to interpret and act on the information coming in from our senses" (p. 29).

A Mindful Response to Trauma Triggers –
A Buddhist Perspective

Mindfulness, which originates from ancient Buddhist teachings and has been referred to as the heart of Buddhist meditation (Thera, 1962), is "the awareness that emerges through paying attention on purpose, in the present moment, and nonjudgmentally to the unfolding of experience moment by moment" (Kabat-Zinn, 2003, p. 145).[23] While not specifically addressing trauma as a distinct concept, Buddhist teachings offer valuable mindful approaches that can contribute to healing in the face of suffering, including experiences that are traumatic (e.g., Gethin, 2015).

Significantly, Mitra and Greenberg (2016, p. 412), based on Bodhi (2011), expanded the understanding of the term *mindfulness* to encompass the "extension of mindfulness practice via ethical action to the enactment of compassion at the interpersonal level." Mitra and Greenberg further stated that "the argument for an extension of mindfulness-based practice to broader interpersonal applications necessarily rests on the cultivation of insight and wisdom" (p. 412). This aligns with Varela et al.'s (1991) concept of *non-naïve compassion,* which is expressed in ethical action that stems from the realization of our interconnectedness with others.[24]

A contemporary Buddhist approach to trauma processing involves mindfully facing or "leaning into" suffering in a trauma-sensitive way (Brach, 2004; Treleaven, 2018). The objective of trauma-informed mindfulness is to help survivors of trauma practice mindfulness in a way that ensures that they can safely observe and tolerate the range of their traumatic experiences. It is also worth noting that trauma-informed mindfulness has been recommended for affect regulation by the polyvagal theory, which legitimizes the study of age-old practices that lead to positive shifts in autonomic state (D'Angelo, 2022; Porges, 2011).[25]

Referring back to the notion of "leaning into" suffering, the term *face* which can signify mindfully facing trauma triggers rather than automatically reacting to them, is in line with the primary stress expressions' nomenclature (i.e., *flock, flight, fight,*[26] *freeze, and flop/faint*). This transformative possibility, characterized by continuous conscious awareness of the body's internal states while experiencing a trigger, can empower individuals to respond mindfully rather than automatically react in a defensive manner when trauma is triggered (e.g., Haase et al., 2016; Szoke et al., 2022).

The *pain paradox* is another example of an approach that integrates Buddhist conceptualizations with Western research regarding mindfulness and trauma (Briere, 2015). According to this approach, survivors of trauma often engage in distress-sustaining behaviors that involve withdrawing, suppressing, numbing, or distracting themselves from upsetting trauma-related internal states. In line with Briere, while these strategies may initially support psychological wellbeing, they also hinder awareness that can be achieved by mindfully facing distressing internal states associated with the trauma. Maté (2022) addressed this paradox by emphasizing that "pain is inherently compassionate, as it tries to alert us to what is amiss" (p. 387) and that "healing, in a sense, is about unlearning the notion that we need to protect ourselves from our own pain" (p. 387).

As pertaining to trauma, this is important as trauma can lead individuals to perceive somatic sensations as threatening,[27] which can override their ability to consider their current context and reactivate autonomic defensive reactions linked with previously experienced traumatic events (Porges, 2021). By mindfully acknowledging such implicit experiences – to which the autonomic nervous system, which operates without conscious awareness, is continually responsive – habitual, automatic response patterns can be interrupted. This, in turn, allows the inherent flexibility and capacity for change, balance, and healing within the autonomic nervous system to be accessed (Dana, 2020).

Posttraumatic Growth (PTG)

For centuries, the uplifting belief that trauma can lead to positive changes has been prevalent across cultures worldwide (Henson et al., 2021). Tedeschi and Calhoun (2004), however, were the first to introduce the concept of PTG, which refers to the transformative positive psychological changes that can result from surviving a traumatic event.[28] Nonetheless, these authors argued that experiencing trauma alone does not lead to PTG. Rather, for PTG to develop, survivors need to make meaning (e.g., likewise referred to as sensemaking; Yuan, 2022) of the significant life changes they have experienced in the aftermath of trauma.[29]

Specifically, PTG has been observed to occur in five key domains. These include: (a) developing an enhanced appreciation for life, (b) strengthening relationships, (c) gaining confidence in the ability to overcome challenges, (d) identifying/establishing/pursuing new possibilities, and (e) deepening spiritual awareness (Tedeschi & Calhoun, 2004). PTG has also been reported in other areas, such as "an increased sense of the importance of the body and health" following an illness; Walsh et al., 2018, as cited in Berger, 2024, p. 29. Relevantly, Jayawickreme et al. (2021) provided recommendations for researchers from across a wide range of disciplines interested in rigorously examining the phenomenon of PTG.

Various factors have been shown to promote the development of PTG. Such factors include: (a) positive coping strategies (e.g., utilizing compassion-based practices), (b) altruistic behavior,[30] (c) optimism in nurturing and seeking social support, and (d) resilience (Jayawickreme et al., 2021). Regarding the latter term, whereas *resilience* has been defined as the ability to "bounce back" to pretrauma levels of functioning, PTG underscores the potential for surpassing pretrauma levels (e.g., Parry et al., 2023). Notably, within the workplace, a compassionate culture has likewise been referred to as a factor that can promote PTG (e.g., Maitlis, 2020).[31]

PTG Elements

The following elements for fostering PTG, adapted from Tedeschi (2020),[32] provide a framework through which helping professionals can not only enhance PTG in their clients but also navigate any unresolved personal traumatic experiences they may be facing. As such, these elements – *education, emotional regulation, disclosure, narrative development*, and *service* – offer proactive guiding principles to helping professionals in both their personal and professional capacities:

- *Education* – "To move through trauma to growth, one must first get educated about what the former is" (Tedeschi, 2020, para. 5). By engaging with resources that provide insights into trauma and related concepts, individuals can enhance their understanding of trauma and empower themselves in their journey toward PTG.
- *Emotional regulation* – By developing skills to manage their emotional responses, individuals can improve their emotional regulation capacities when navigating trauma.[33] This transformation necessitates, among other factors, a shift in perspective. For example, instead of focusing on worst-case scenarios, considering best-case possibilities (e.g., PTG).
- *Disclosure* – Disclosure holds significance as sharing traumatic experiences in a trauma-informed way with trusted and compassionate individuals (e.g., peers, family members, and therapists) can facilitate healing and growth. When individuals share their journeys, it can pave the way for both understanding and being understood.
- *Narrative development* – This involves constructing a coherent narrative that contextualizes the unresolved trauma within the broader framework of individuals' lives. By reframing their experiences as chapters of growth, narrative development can empower individuals to transform unresolved traumatic experiences into catalysts for PTG.
- *Service* – "People do better in the aftermath of trauma if they find work that benefits others" (Tedeschi, 2020, para. 18). By using their lived experiences as sources of insight, individuals can elevate their sense of purpose by helping others to overcome challenges similarly. In this way, trauma, transformed through PTG, becomes a conduit for compassion for others.

Section II

SECONDARY TRAUMATIC STRESS (STS)

STS and Related Terms – Definitions

The nomenclature in the field of indirect trauma exposure refers to several central terms: *secondary traumatic stress* (STS), *compassion fatigue, vicarious traumatization*, and the related term *burnout* (Gottfried & Bride, 2018; Sprang et al., 2021). These phenomena may negatively impact those who are in a helping relationship with survivors of trauma as well as those who respond and intervene in the aftermath of trauma (Ben-Porat et al., 2021; Craun et al., 2014; Duffy et al., 2015; Little, 2020; Pearlman & MacIan, 1995; Roberts et al., 2021).

Brief definitions of the aforementioned central terms are hereby provided, with *STS* recognized as the "most accurate and encompassing term" compared to the indirect trauma-related terms of *compassion fatigue* and *vicarious traumatization* according to Bride et al.'s (2023, p. 6) international expert consensus approach.[1]

In line with Figley (1999), a pioneering researcher in the field, the term *STS* is defined as the natural, consequent sensations, emotions, thoughts, and behaviors "resulting from knowing about a traumatizing event experienced by a significant other" (p. 7). It is the subsequent "stress resulting from helping or wanting to help a traumatized or suffering person" (p. 7). From a clinical perspective, STS can further be conceptualized as traumatic

DOI: 10.4324/9781003381747-3

stress originating from indirect exposure to trauma. It ranges from very mild/transient trauma symptoms without functional impairment to more frequent/more intense/longer-lasting trauma symptoms accompanied by functional impairment.[2] Once STS meets posttraumatic stress disorder (PTSD) diagnostic criteria, however, it can be referred to as PTSD without being qualified as STS-related. Nonetheless, from research or policy perspectives, STS-related PTSD may still be referred to as STS to accentuate the indirect trauma exposure qualifier (Bride et al., 2023; Sprang, Whitt-Woosley, et al., 2022; Sprang & Steckler, 2022).[3]

The term *compassion fatigue* has multiple meanings in the scholarly literature (Bride et al., 2023). Two such conceptualizations include compassion fatigue as: (a) a synonymous yet more user-friendly term than STS (e.g., Gottfried & Bride, 2018), and (b) a broader phenomenon comprising the combination of both STS and burnout (Adams et al., 2006; Cieslak et al., 2013; Stamm, 2010). The term *compassion fatigue* has also been cited as a misnomer, as social neuroscience research revealed that it is not compassion, but rather empathy, that leads to fatigue in caregivers. As a result, an example of a term that has been recommended in lieu of compassion fatigue is *empathic distress leading to empathic distress fatigue* (DeDecker, 2020; Dowling, 2018; Hofmeyer et al., 2020; Klimecki & Singer, 2011; Singer & Klimecki, 2014).

Comparably, the multifaceted term *vicarious traumatization* inclines primarily toward negative cognition shifts in beliefs, expectations, and assumptions about oneself, others, and/or the world as a result of trying to help survivors of trauma. Examples include adverse alterations in worldviews regarding key issues such as trust, safety, and/or control (Pearlman & MacIan, 1995; Pearlman & Saakvitne, 1995). The addition of the "negative alterations in mood and thinking" criterion to the DSM-5-TR PTSD diagnostic criteria (APA, 2022) strengthens the connection between vicarious traumatization and STS. Nonetheless, this addition may not comprehensively capture the phenomenon of vicarious traumatization within the definition of STS (Gusler et al., 2023).

Meanwhile, the term *burnout* signifies the state of feeling overwhelmed due to work-related stressors over a prolonged period of time. Examples include bureaucratic demands, time pressures, high workloads, and stressful interactions with colleagues. However, unlike the terms *STS, compassion fatigue,* and *vicarious traumatization,* those in careers outside the helping professions may also experience *burnout,* as this term is not necessarily associated with caring for individuals who have experienced trauma (Maslach et al., 2001).

STS Symptoms

The recognition of STS symptoms stands as a crucial initial step for helping professionals in addressing STS. A list of traumatic stress reactions associated with indirect exposure to trauma, divided into four categories, follows. Addressing these reactions can lead to improved personal and professional quality of life, with the latter including quality of services offered, job satisfaction, and job retention (see Appendix A for an associated self-assessment scale and scoresheet; e.g., Brend & Sprang, 2020; Gottfried & Bride, 2018).

Traumatic Stress Reactions

The following STS-related traumatic stress reactions are based on the DSM-5-TR PTSD core diagnostic criteria (APA, 2022):

Intrusive Reactions

Images, sensations, and/or memories associated with the indirectly experienced traumatic event that recur uncontrollably:

- Physiological reactions (e.g., rapid heart rate, hypertension, and/or elevated blood pressure)
- Disturbing thoughts/ruminations
- Flashbacks
- Nightmares

Avoidance Reactions

The process of distancing oneself from internal and/or external reminders of the indirectly experienced traumatic event:

- Internal reminders include physical sensations, thoughts, and/or emotions
- External reminders include people, places, objects, activities, situations, conversations, and/or certain times of the day/year

Hyperarousal and Reactivity Reactions

Intense psychological, emotional, and/or behavioral reactions associated with the indirectly experienced traumatic event:

- Hypervigilance
- Jumpiness or being quick to startle
- Difficulties with concentration
- Sleep disturbances
- Aggressive or irritable behavior
- Self-destructive, risky, and/or reckless behavior

Negative Alterations in Mood and Thinking Reactions

Adverse alterations in *mood* associated with the indirectly experienced traumatic event:

- Feeling detached/disconnected from others
- Persistent bad or sad mood (e.g., anger, sadness, and/or guilt)
- Difficulty experiencing positive emotions
- Extreme feelings of loneliness

Adverse alterations in *thinking* associated with the indirectly experienced traumatic event:

- Difficulty recalling parts of the traumatic event
- Decreased interest in previously meaningful matters
- Persistent exaggerated negative expectations about oneself, others, and/or the world
- Repeated distorted blame of oneself and/or others

Indirect Trauma Exposure Pathways

Although STS is not recognized in the DSM-5-TR as a formal disorder, revisions of the diagnostic criteria for PTSD stipulate that adverse reactions to trauma may also occur following indirect exposure. Specifically, indirect exposure includes learning about the trauma that was experienced by a significant other, and/or indirect exposure to aversive details of the trauma experienced by others. These inclusions demonstrate the ways in which helping professionals may be indirectly exposed to trauma during the course of their work (APA, 2022).

Helping professionals may thus develop STS as a result of listening to, reading, or otherwise learning about the traumatic events experienced by the individuals in their care. Similarly, they may develop STS due to exposure to the aftermath of the traumatic events experienced by their clients. Additionally, indirect exposure can occur when helping professionals (e.g., creative arts therapists) bear witness to artistically externalized trauma-related sensations, thoughts, emotions, and/or experiences expressed by those they assist (Lawson et al., 2019).

Alongside the dominant "recipient of care-to-caregiver" pathway, indirect trauma exposure can also occur when helping professionals render graphic details of their clients' traumatic experiences to colleagues (Sprang et al., 2014). Moreover, work-related media exposure to clients' traumatic events can also serve as an indirect trauma exposure pathway. Notably, helping professionals' indirect trauma exposure does not reflect any intentionality on the part of the individuals in their care or their colleagues (APA, 2022; Choi et al., 2021; Garfin et al., 2020; Silver et al., 2013).[4]

STS Prevalence – Overview

When considering the prevalence of STS among helping professionals, it is important to take into account possible variations across studies with regard to the way STS is defined and operationalized. These include differences in research methodologies (e.g., measurement instruments, response rates, sample sizes, and study limitations) as well as other methodological issues such as DSM PTSD diagnostic criteria revisions (e.g., Kilpatrick et al., 2013; North et al., 2016). This is relevant as the latter factors can make cross-sectional prevalence comparisons more challenging (Mordeno et al., 2017).

Furthermore, there may be a reluctance on the part of some helping professionals to disclose STS due to possible concerns regarding confidentiality and job security (Hensel et al., 2015). As such, Hensel et al. stated that in order to identify those at risk for STS within the workplace, it is advisable to ensure that helping professionals are guaranteed confidentiality as, otherwise, they may hesitate to disclose their STS experiences.

Due to the wide range of helping professionals that this resource guide seeks to address – it is beyond the scope of this literature review to present the prevalence of STS for all professional groups (e.g., health professionals, mental health professionals, first responders, and educators; e.g., Molnar et al., 2017).[5] It suffices to say that it is widely accepted that helping professionals who provide services to individuals who have experienced trauma are at high risk of developing STS and that STS is a prevalent occupational risk in the delivery of services to survivors of trauma (Bride et al., 2023). Indeed, the occupational risks in this field have emerged as a public health concern that jeopardizes workforce stability (Molnar et al., 2017).[6]

STS Risk Factors

A considerable number of STS-related risk factors relevant to helping professionals have been cited in the scholarly literature (e.g., Hensel et al., 2015). As these micro-level, mezzo-level, and macro-level risk factors largely overlap with respect to the terms *STS*, *compassion fatigue*, and *vicarious traumatization*, they are presented here together:[7]

At the *micro-individual level*, risk factors include heightened levels of trauma caseload volume, frequency, and ratio, as well as helping professionals' subjective interpretations of clients' traumatic narratives and helping professionals' own personal histories of trauma.[8] Additionally, helping professionals with an enhanced capacity for empathy may be similarly susceptible (e.g., Figley, 1995; Gottfried & Bride, 2018; Hensel et al., 2015; Rigas et al., 2023). Regarding the multifaceted term *empathy*, it is considered a double-edged sword as far as STS is concerned. Whereas *emotional empathy* may pose a risk factor for STS, *cognitive empathy* is viewed as serving a protective role (e.g., Dekel et al., 2018; Russell & Brickell, 2015).

This occurs because emotional empathy, which involves vicariously experiencing another person's emotional state as if it were "contagious," may lead to personal distress. Such distress, in turn, can contribute to the development of STS. By contrast, cognitive empathy, which signifies the ability to comprehend what another person may be feeling without sharing their actual emotion, involves perspective-taking, which implies a "caring distancing" (Inbar & Ganor, 2003, as cited in Cheng, 2014, p. 82; Reniers et al., 2011; Singer & Klimecki, 2014).[9] Of significance is that an enhanced capacity for empathy, as a risk factor for STS, validates the fact that helping professionals experiencing STS can be deeply empathic caregivers.

At a *mezzo-team level*, risk factors include listening to colleagues share graphic details of clients' traumatic events (Mathieu, 2012) as well as reduced or lack of work-related: (a) mentoring relationships, (b) opportunities for interdisciplinary team processing, and (c) coworker support (e.g., Gottfried & Bride, 2018; Isobel & Angus-Leppan, 2018).

At a *macro-organizational level*, risk factors encompass the allocation of excessive caseloads of clients who have experienced trauma, the provision of inadequate and irregular supervision, the lack of safe environments, and the lack of a supportive trauma-informed organizational culture (e.g., Gottfried & Bride, 2018; Hensel et al., 2015).

STS Recommendations

Micro-level, mezzo-level, and macro-level recommendations for addressing STS are hereby presented. As these recommendations may coincide with respect to the terms *STS, compassion fatigue*, and *vicarious traumatization*, they are presented here collectively. Significantly, implementing such strategies can assist helping professionals stay within and expand their STS-related window of tolerance:[10]

Micro-individual level recommendations include: (a) continued education for skill development and mastery of trauma-informed treatment methods, (b) regular and effective trauma-informed individual supervision within supportive supervisory relationships, (c) training in contemplative practices such as mindfulness-based stress reduction and compassion training, (d) anticipatory coping techniques (e.g., mental preparation), and (e) continuous self-assessment for indicators of STS warning signs (e.g., Delaney, 2018; Eastwood & Ecklund, 2008; Franco & Christie, 2021; Garcia et al., 2021; Gil & Weinberg, 2015; Gottfried & Bride, 2018; Kabat-Zinn, 2003; Knight, 2015; Owens-King, 2019; Siegel, 1999; Sprang & Craig, 2015).

Mezzo-team level recommendations involve: (a) socializing novice helping professionals and offering them mentorship, (b) enhancing team cooperation for optimizing problem-solving, (c) increasing team engagement in organizational change processes, (d) regular and effective trauma-informed group supervision within supportive supervisory relationships, (e) low-impact debriefing,[11] and (f) incorporating accountability partners, and peer-to-peer psychological first aid practices (see Appendix B for the "Compassion for STS" Partner Practice; e.g., Brach, 2019; Everly, 2020; Haans & Balke, 2018; Mathieu, 2012; Potocky & Guskovict, 2020; Pryce et al., 2007; Sprang et al., 2021).

Macro-organizational level recommendations encompass: (a) implementing trauma-informed approaches, (b) utilizing STS-related evidence-based policies and practices, (c) instituting STS-related critical incident management, (d) allocating resources for developing a system of ongoing mitigation and treatment of STS, (e) maintaining sustainable staff workloads, (f) establishing an STS champion within the organization,[12] (g) providing STS-related employment assistance programs, and (h) senior leadership who are engaged and well-informed about STS and model good self-care (e.g., Ben-Porat, 2015; Deaton et al., 2021; Isobel & Angus-Leppan, 2018; Potocky & Guskovict, 2020; Pryce et al., 2007; SAMHSA, 2014; Shea, 2021; Sprang et al., 2021; Zhang et al., 2021).

Key Organizational Foci for Addressing STS

Expanding on the aforementioned macro-organizational level recommendations, the following three key organizational foci for addressing STS, presented by O'Malley et al. (2019), are recommended. These foci are important to consider since work settings/conditions can inadvertently exacerbate STS rather than help alleviate it (Choi, 2011). This could result in reduced productivity, increased turnover (along with associated onboarding/training expenses), and even pose a risk to public safety if helping professionals find it difficult to carry out their duties effectively (e.g., Bloom, 2006; Handran, 2015; O'Malley et al., 2019).

Mitigation

To decrease the prevalence and severity of STS among their workforce, it is necessary for organizations to adopt an approach that centers on diminishing stigma/shame through promoting awareness and strengthening support structures. Particularly, concerning stigma/shame, professionals in the helping fields may hold the belief that their training should shield them from experiencing STS, and may be concerned that acknowledging the adverse effects of their work could be interpreted as an inability on their part to sustain their chosen careers. Likewise important to highlight is that such concerns may hinder effective problem-solving, including seeking compassion-based support (e.g., Lawson et al., 2019; Royle et al., 2009; Sprang & Steckler, 2022).

Additional examples of mitigating measures include displaying posters illustrating the signs and symptoms of STS, best practices to address the condition and information regarding relevant workplace resources in prominent areas throughout the organization. Pocket-sized cards outlining STS warning signs and symptoms, strategies for intervention, and available supports for employees to carry with them or place in their work areas have likewise been cited in this respect (e.g., O'Malley et al., 2019).

Encouraging professionals in the helping fields to self-assess for STS risk before symptoms hinder their work performance is advisable as well, along with promoting workers to commit to reducing negative coping strategies while enhancing positive ones (O'Malley et al., 2019). The latter can include mindful, compassion-based STS-related practices offered as part of ongoing professional development training programs.

Cultivation

Cultivating an STS-informed organizational culture requires leaders to exhibit an awareness of STS concerning their own wellbeing and to provide appropriate supports for the wellbeing of their employees. To this end, it is necessary that leaders take a proactive role in providing employees with appropriate STS-related workplace norms and associated resources (Molnar et al., 2017; Sprang, 2018a).

A negative organizational culture can perpetuate stigma/shame related to STS and hinder helping professionals from seeking support, which may lead to the exacerbation of their STS symptoms. Therefore, it is advisable to cultivate organizational norms that are informed by STS awareness, recognizing the challenging nature of caring for survivors of trauma as involving real and legitimate stressors (e.g., O'Malley et al., 2019; Sprang et al., 2021).

Organizations are further encouraged to align their practices with their STS-related norms to cultivate an STS-informed workplace culture. This can involve improving preservice orientation and training to include awareness of the signs and symptoms of STS, increasing opportunities for choice regarding work schedules, and enhancing helping professionals' access to confidential high-quality counseling supports aimed at addressing STS (Bloom, 2006; Sprang, 2018a).

Evaluation

Organizations are advised to evaluate the effectiveness of their STS-informed organizational policies and practices on a regular basis and involve employees in the evaluation process. Moreover, it is recommended that leaders be open to honest feedback regarding STS organizational policies and practices so that the workforce feels safe to voice such input without fear of retribution (Sprang et al., 2014).

Examples of organization-level evaluation tools for STS include the *Secondary Traumatic Stress-Informed Organizational Assessment* (STSI-OA) by Sprang et al. (2014). This 40-item measure includes six prevention and intervention strategy domains which are listed here for organizations to consider: (a) organizational promotion of resilience-building activities, (b) organizational promotion of physical and psychological safety, (c) the extent to which an organization has STS-informed policies, (d) the level of STS-informed practices for leaders, (e) the level of routine STS-informed organizational practices, and (f) the level at which an organization evaluates and monitors STS-informed policies and practices.

An additional recommended organization-level evaluation measure is the *Secondary Traumatic Stress Policy Analysis Tool* (STS-PAT). This 30-item tool can be utilized by internal teams and/or external consultants to guide a review of organizational STS policies and policy-making processes. As such, the STS-PAT can help organizations gain an understanding of STS-related policy-making, development, implementation, and evaluation processes (Sprang et al., 2022a).

Specifically, the STS-PAT is organized into four sections that focus on an analysis of: (a) existing STS policies, (b) the STS policy-making process, (c) how STS policies are being implemented/communicated/enforced, and (d) STS policy outcomes (Sprang et al., 2022a). The STS-PAT is also accompanied by an implementation guide that provides valuable guidance and supporting materials for organizations on how to effectively utilize the measure (Sprang et al., 2022b).

Furthermore, the *Secondary Traumatic Stress Core Competencies in Trauma-Informed Supervision Self-Rating Tool* can help guide supervisors using STS-related core competencies in trauma-informed supervision through each competency, step by step. It enables users to self-evaluate their proficiency levels in various competency areas, highlighting areas of confidence, those that require additional training, or those that are currently outside their skill sets. Parenthetically, there are two versions of the tool – one for mental health professionals and one for cross-disciplinary professionals (Sprang, 2018b, 2022).

STS Organizational Efforts

Over the years, strategies for addressing STS have focused primarily on individual self-care without taking into account the impact of workplace factors on the development, exacerbation, and persistence of STS-related symptoms (Sprang et al., 2019). Notwithstanding, research suggests that addressing STS requires a three-pronged approach that takes into account not only individual, but team and organizational-wide factors over time (e.g., Molnar et al., 2017; Sprang et al., 2021).

Sprang et al. (2021) conducted such a longitudinal study that revealed that organizational data-driven change efforts can improve outcomes related to STS. Results of this study further demonstrated that the improvements were sustained or enhanced postintervention, as evidenced by follow-up data. Moreover, since there is an interchangeable relation between individual, team, and organizational outcomes, it may be that positive changes at one level continue to bring about improvements at other levels over time (e.g., Nielsen et al., 2010).

Empowering helping professionals by demonstrating to them that they are seen and heard by their organizations, with respect to their STS-related needs, can lead to a chain reaction of favorable outcomes (Burris et al., 2013, 2017; Salanova et al., 2006). Further research is necessary, however, to determine the lasting impact of individual, team, and organization-wide gains and to identify the most effective approaches for maintaining such long-term improvements.

In line with Strand and Sprang (2018), human service organizations are, thereby, encouraged to establish a broad context in which STS can be acknowledged, openly discussed without stigma/shame, and addressed by all members of the organization. This necessitates a willingness to fully adopt a trauma-informed approach that is committed to addressing workers' secondary traumatic experiences and enhancing relevant cross-system collaborations.

STS Principles

Bride et al. (2023) put forth best-practice principles that organizational leaders and helping professionals are encouraged to implement in light of STS. These principles were formulated through a consensus-building process involving an international panel of experts, drawing from existing STS research in the field of behavioral health. As emerging research continues to provide new insights that shape best practices for mitigating STS, these principles can be further revised, updated, and expanded to encompass helping professionals from fields beyond behavioral health.

Organizational STS Principles

To create an STS-responsive work environment, organizations are encouraged to implement the following best-practice organizational principles (Bride et al., 2023):

- Organizations acknowledge the challenges of working in a trauma-exposed workplace and explicitly cultivate a psychologically safe culture that promotes team support and respects personal boundaries.
- Organizations demonstrate their commitment to workforce wellbeing via policies and practices that are responsive to trauma and STS.

- Organizational leaders model behaviors that are responsive to trauma and STS and actively cultivate a workplace that is supportive and resilient.
- Organizations provide advanced, ongoing, evidence-based, and culturally responsive STS training, which includes training to enable supervisors to support employees continuously.
- Organizations structure workloads to reduce the indirect trauma exposure of the work environment.
- Organizations dedicate resources (i.e., time and funding) to facilitate qualified supervision that is responsive to STS.
- Organizations prioritize workforce wellness via well-defined and continuously monitored metrics that are safeguarded for privacy and addressed with priority.

Individual STS Principles

On a personal level, helping professionals are encouraged to implement the following STS-related best-practice individual principles (Bride et al., 2023):

- Helping professionals are knowledgeable of STS-related risk factors and mitigating strategies.
- Helping professionals identify and monitor their personal profiles of vulnerabilities and strengths related to indirect exposure to trauma.
- Helping professionals actively monitor their own wellbeing and incorporate strategies for mitigating adverse indirect trauma exposure-related reactions.
- Helping professionals employ strategies to remain within their window of tolerance during exposure to indirect trauma and recovery from STS.
- Helping professionals cultivate and maintain beliefs that uphold their wellbeing in their roles as helpers.
- Helping professionals collaborate with a team of trauma-informed colleagues/peers with whom they can share indirect trauma exposure-related experiences.
- Helping professionals recognize when they can benefit from STS-related counseling or other external assistance, and seek out that assistance.

Vicarious Posttraumatic Growth (VPTG) – Definition, Domains, Predictors, and Interrelationships

Existing research on the impact of trauma work on helping professionals demonstrates that the outcome is not necessarily exclusively negative, as helping professionals may also report VPTG, likewise referred to as secondary posttraumatic growth and posttraumatic growth (PTG) by affiliation (e.g., Berger, 2024).[13] VPTG, in helping professionals working with individuals who have experienced trauma, is defined as "the experience of growth as a result of indirect trauma exposure" (Arnold et al., 2005, as cited in Deaton et al., 2023, p. 17).

VPTG is, therefore, a promising feature as it can signify experiencing positive psychological changes subsequent to or alongside the experience of STS (Bartoskova, 2017; Ben-Porat et al., 2021; Melinte et al., 2023). These positive changes are linked to the following five domains: (a) personal strength, (b) new possibilities, (c) appreciation of life, (d) spiritual growth, and (e) improved relationships. For example, research by Beck et al. (2017) demonstrated that VPTG can foster increased compassion toward others.

Nonetheless, VPTG does not imply that helping professionals are immune to experiencing negative impacts. Instead, the term suggests that, as helping professionals observe clients' PTG and navigate the challenging aspects of indirect exposure to trauma, they themselves may find opportunities for growth (Tedeschi & Calhoun, 2004). Manning-Jones et al. (2017) have argued, however, that in order to promote VPTG, posttraumatic stress needs to be challenging enough yet not so challenging as to hinder growth. A curvilinear relation may, thus, provide the most accurate explanation for the link between VPTG and STS. It suggests that VPTG may increase if STS symptom severity rises to a certain threshold but then plateaus or declines as STS symptom severity surpasses clinically significant levels (e.g., Morland et al., 2008).

Both personal and organizational factors have been identified as significant predictors of VPTG. The former involve internal factors such as actively pursuing self-care and social support to cope with STS. The latter involve external factors such as organizations encouraging and supporting helping professionals to take regular breaks for self-reflection and for processing STS-related traumagenic material (Tsirimokou et al., 2023). These authors further underscored the significance of organizations promoting healthy coping mechanisms, encouraging self-care practices at work, and advocating for work-life balance.

Furthermore, Tsirimokou et al. (2023) recommended that helping professionals providing specialized services to clients with trauma histories similar to their own, or those caring for large numbers of clients who have been exposed to trauma, should take special care to cultivate VPTG. This is important as these professionals have been found to be at an increased risk of experiencing lower levels of VPTG. Nonetheless, it is encouraging that Melinte et al. (2023) demonstrated a significant positive relation between STS and VPTG, supporting the idea that STS and VPTG can coexist.

Section III

COMPASSION FOR SELF
AND OTHERS

Compassion and Indirect Trauma Exposure –
A Buddhist Perspective

Introduction

Compassion is universally recognized as a central value that transcends cultural boundaries and resonates deeply across societies (Stevens & Benjamin, 2018; Strauss et al., 2016). Within Buddhism,[1] compassion plays a foundational role, representing an essential and integral feature of its teachings. For example, compassion has a historical connection to the earliest Buddhist meditations and aligns with the fundamental concept of *ahiṃsā* (i.e., nonharming in Sanskrit; a key principle in Buddhist ethics; Stevens & Benjamin, 2018; see Appendix C for Sanskrit pronunciation guidelines).[2]

Compassion is likewise associated with the Buddhist concept of *bodhicitta* (i.e., *bodhi* means "awakening" while *citta* means "heart-mind" and "consciousness") – encapsulating not only a wise and compassionate intention but also the manifestation of wise and compassionate actions aimed at alleviating the suffering of sentient beings (Śāntideva, n.d.). Pelden (2007) similarly referred to *bodhicitta* as encompassing both wisdom and compassion, as did Duckworth (2023), who stated that without the eyes of

DOI: 10.4324/9781003381747-4

wisdom and the legs of compassion, one cannot traverse the *bodhisattva-mārga* (i.e., *bodhisattva* means one who is cultivating *bodhicitta* and *mārga* means path).

Aligned with Buddhist thought, wisdom and compassion have likewise been likened to two wings of a bird working in tandem to steer the wise and compassionate resolution of suffering. This analogy underscores the significance of integrating both wisdom and compassion to skillfully navigate life's circumstances (Siegel & Germer, 2012). Notably, Buddhist traditions likewise refer to the twin wings of wisdom and skillful means (Skt. *upāya-kauśalya*; i.e., the variety of means that may be used to alleviate suffering in context-sensitive ways; e.g., Quaglia, 2023; Conze, 1973, as cited by Simmer-Brown, 2023).[3] That compassion is what motivates the skillful means is implicit, and the relation between the triad – wisdom, compassion, and skillful means – is assumed (Simmer-Brown, 2023).

The Wing of Wisdom

In English, the word *wisdom* derives from the Indo-European word "wede," meaning "to know" or "to see" (Holliday & Chandler, 1986, as cited in Siegel & Germer, 2012). In line with the Sanskrit term *yathābhūta-darśana* (i.e., seeing things as they are), wisdom (Skt. *prajñā*) involves recognizing the roots of suffering (Skt. *duḥkha*), impermanence (Skt. *anitya*), and no-self (Skt. *anātman*; e.g., Cheng, 2014; Olendzki, 2012). A brief outline of the latter three Sanskrit terms follows.

Duḥkha is commonly translated as suffering in English. However, it may be more precise to consider *duḥkha* as associated with the following three components (i.e., the threefold typology of suffering or unsatisfactoriness): (a) the existence of explicit painful/unpleasant experiences (Skt. *duḥkha-duḥkhatā;* i.e., the suffering of suffering), (b) the impermanence of pleasant experiences (Skt. *vipariṇāma-duḥkhatā;* i.e., the suffering of change), and (c) "the unsatisfactoriness belonging to any moment of experience in virtue of its dependence upon causal conditioning for its existence" (Skt. *saṃskāra-duḥkhatā*; i.e., the suffering of being conditioned; Harris, 2014, p. 4).[4]

Noteworthy is that Buddhist approaches provide valuable insights into understanding *duḥkha* and its management, guided by the *four noble truths* (Skt. *catvāry āryasatyāni*). These include recognizing the existence of *duḥkha*, understanding its causes, considering its prognosis, and exploring remedies to alleviate it (e.g., mindfulness is considered an essential element in this transformative process; Bodhi, 2005). Appropriately, Hanson (2020) suggested using the term *four ennobling truths*, as our innate nobility draws us toward these truths, and through them, we can mindfully cultivate noble qualities, such as wisdom and compassion, within ourselves.

Impermanence (Skt. *anitya*) encapsulates a profound insight into the ever-changing nature of existence. This concept emphasizes that all aspects of life, whether physical, mental, or emotional, are in a constant state of change. Gethin (1998) explained that if we try to hold on to things as if they were permanent, not realizing that they will inevitably change, we are bound to experience suffering. For instance, "A flower exemplifies both the beauty and impermanence of the world" (Harvey, 2013, p. 222). The following haiku conveys a similar sentiment:

> Impermanence…
> bare branches remember spring –
> snowflakes and sunsets

The notion of no-self (Skt. *anātman*) is linked to the multifaceted Buddhist concept of *emptiness* or *essencelessness* (Skt. *śūnyatā*), whereby each phenomenon is understood to be devoid of independent existence since it is intricately woven into an interdependent causal chain (e.g., Garfield, 2022; Tirado, 2008). Relatedly, the Buddhist term *pratītya-samutpāda* can be understood as expressing the notion of dependent co-arising (i.e., "the principle that all things arise in dependence upon multiple causes and conditions – nothing exists as a singular, independent entity;" Encyclopedia of Buddhism, 2024, para. 1).[5]

Of significance is that the transformative power of wisdom can only be fully cultivated/embodied through dedicated experiential practice. This is indicated by the following progressive pedagogical steps: (a) wisdom acquired through learning (Skt. *śruta-mayī prajñā*), (b) wisdom acquired through thinking (Skt. *cintā-mayī prajñā*), and (c) wisdom acquired through practice (Skt. *bhāvanā-mayī prajñā*), with *bhāvanā* commonly defined as mental development/cultivation (Keenan, 2000, as cited in Wu et al., 2019).

Sentimental vs. Untainted Compassion

Although Buddhist perspectives on compassion are prominent in the psychological literature, very little research has investigated the impact of indirect trauma exposure on helping professionals from a Buddhist perspective. One such study by Cheng (2014) utilized a hybrid research design that combined qualitative data from Buddhist participants who provided care services with references from the classic Sanskrit text *Vimalakīrti-Nirdeśa-Sūtra* (Study Group on Buddhist Sanskrit Literature, 2006).

This text includes a dialogue that stands as one of the most ancient references to the detrimental effects of indirect exposure to trauma. In this dialogue, a *bodhisattva* is questioned about the cause of their illness (Study Group on Buddhist Sanskrit Literature, 2006):[6]

- "Wherefore arose this sickness of yours? For how long will your sickness last and when will it cease?"
- *bodhisattva*: "When all living beings become free from sickness, then my sickness will cease. . . . For the *bodhisattva*, the world is the abode of living beings, and sickness is inherent in the world.[7] . . . Suppose that the only child of a merchant is sick. His mother and father would also become sick, and they would suffer for as long as the only child would not become free from sickness. Thus . . ., a *bodhisattva* loves all livings beings as if each of them were his only child. He becomes sick through the sickness of living beings, but he becomes healthy due to the health of living beings. Now, when you ask where my sickness comes from – the sickness of *bodhisattvas* arises from great compassion" (Chapter 4, para. 6–7).[8]

As also cited by Cheng (2014), the *Vimalakīrti-Nirdeśa-Sūtra* differentiates between two forms of compassion – sentimental vs. untainted compassion: (a) *sentimental compassion* is the type of compassion that led to the *bodhisattva's* sickness. This type of compassion signifies compassionate caregiving in which caregivers become emotionally overwhelmed by their reactions to the afflictions of the individuals in their care. On the other hand, (b) *untainted compassion* comprises the North Star of compassionate caregiving, as it is characterized by wisdom which entails emotional equanimity.[9]

Compassion – Evolution, Etymology, Definition, Phases, Flows, and Outcomes

From an evolutionary perspective, compassion is considered to have emerged as part of: (a) a benevolent caregiving response to offspring, (b) a preferred quality in mate-selection processes, and (c) a desirable characteristic in nonkin, cooperative relations (Gilbert, 2020a, 2020b; Goetz et al., 2010). Relatedly, Ash and colleagues (2021) differentiated between two forms of compassion: biological and extended. This distinction relates to the recipient of compassion. Biological compassion originates from the natural human inclination to show compassion toward kin. It serves as the building block for extended compassion, which transcends the boundaries of kinship. Nonetheless, without motivation and training, compassion may be restricted to one's immediate circle.

Furthermore, compassion, which originates from the Latin words *cum* and *pati*, signifying "with" and "to suffer" (i.e., to suffer with; Stevens & Taber, 2021), has been classified in various ways. These classifications of compassion include: an instinct (Keltner et al., 2010), an attitude, a trait, a state, a distinct emotion (Goetz et al., 2010), a blend of emotions (i.e., sadness and love; Shaver et al., 1987), a form of courage (Gilbert & Mascaro, 2017), a motivation, a temperament, an embodied virtue (Pessi et al., 2017, as cited in Horwitz et al., 2023), a mindset (Kim et al., 2020), a spiritual stance (Lee & Oh, 2019), and an absence (i.e., of harmfulness) – as depicted by the Sanskrit term *ahiṃsā* (i.e., nonharming; Kumar, 2023).

From a Buddhist perspective, compassion (Skt. *karuṇā*) is considered to be omnidirectional and inclusive of both oneself and others (Neff, 2023).[10] This is because offering compassion to others while excluding oneself, or vice versa, is seen as creating an artificial separation between the "interbeing" of all living beings (i.e., the term *interbeing* encapsulates the interdependence of all phenomena; Goleman et al., 2012; Hạnh, 1987; Quaglia, Cigrand, et al., 2021).[11] As such, compassion can be defined as comprising "a sensitivity to the suffering of self and others, with a deep commitment to try to relieve it" (i.e., the suffering; Dalai Lama, 1995, p. 16; Gilbert, 2014).[12]

Compassion for self and others has further been conceptualized as having several phases (Strauss et al., 2016). For illustration, by reviewing definitions from both Buddhist and Western perspectives, Strauss et al. identified the following five components of compassion as relevant for both self and others. These comprise the ability to: (a) recognize suffering, (b) understand the universality of suffering, (c) emotionally resonate with the suffering, (d) tolerate challenging emotions associated with the suffering, and (e) act, or be motivated to act, to alleviate the suffering. As the term *suffering* can mistakenly be viewed as a response solely to extreme crises, it is important to recognize that there are degrees of suffering and that compassion applies to them all (Dewar et al., 2011).

Building on the previously mentioned definition and conceptualization, compassion has the potential to "flow" both inward, from *self-to-self*, and outward, from *self-to-other* (Neff & Pommier, 2013; i.e., additional "flows" of compassion comprise *other-to-self* and *other-to-other*).[13] However, although the compassionate "flows" of *self-to-self* and *self-to-other* are interrelated (Quaglia, Soisson, et al., 2021), they can also be subjectively experienced as independent. This is demonstrated by helping professionals who may be good at directing compassion toward others yet struggle with including themselves within the circle of compassionate care (e.g., Jinpa, 2015; Kirby et al., 2019; López et al., 2018).[14]

Regarding outcomes associated with compassion for others, it has been shown to affect neurophysiological systems positively (Kim et al., 2020). For example, compassion has been found to activate brain regions linked to positive affect and social connection, making it a valuable coping strategy when dealing with distress in others (Klimecki et al., 2013). Moreover, helping professionals' other-oriented compassionate care has been shown to be positively correlated with improved patient outcomes, including patient satisfaction and patients' active involvement in their own healthcare (Sharp et al., 2016; Trzeciak et al., 2019).

Intriguingly, compassion for others has also been linked to possible negative outcomes. For example, researchers demonstrated that compassion can increase the allocation of resources for a suffering individual while unjustly exploiting the resources of the collective. This indicates that although the person for whom compassion is felt may benefit, compassion may also have possible negative consequences for others. It is important, therefore, to underscore the need for an all-encompassing understanding of compassion characterized by a balanced interplay between individual-focused compassion and broader communal needs (Batson, Batson, et al., 1995; Batson, Klein, et al., 1995).

Compassion for Others – Generous vs. Judgmental Interpretations

The interpretations that helping professionals utilize to understand the causes of suffering are crucial. Judgmental interpretations can impede compassion for others, in contrast to generous interpretations, which can promote and enhance this quality.[15] However, rather than judging themselves for judging others, helping professionals are advised to mindfully observe their judgments with self-compassionate curiosity, as this practice can enhance their self-awareness and help them develop a more nonjudgmental perspective (e.g., Maté, 2022).

The following three broad types of generous vs. judgmental interpretations, respectively, are associated with offering others compassion (Worline & Dutton, 2017):[16]

• Imbuing others with dignity/worth vs. jumping to the conclusion that others do not deserve compassion
• Withholding judgment/blame vs. jumping to the conclusion that others are blameworthy (i.e., responsible) and, therefore, undeserving of compassion
• Cultivating presence vs. jumping to the conclusion that one does not have the resources or capacity to respond to others compassionately

Regarding cultivating a sense of "presence," this involves the ability to "be" with others who are suffering without feeling that one immediately needs to "do" something to alleviate their suffering. As such, "being" with someone who is suffering may be considered a form of "doing" in and of itself. This notion is reinforced by Wiklund-Gustin and Wagner (2013), who stated that compassionate acts of presence do not necessarily center around intervening to alleviate symptoms or solve problems. Instead, they can involve such acts as voice-giving and compassionate listening.[17]

More generous interpretations offer others the benefit of the doubt and assume a no-fault assumption that others are worthy of compassion. Such a no-fault stance also implies that negative work events (e.g., colleagues' decline in performance, absences, and/or missed deadlines) may reflect suffering. This does not mean, however, accommodating irresponsible behavior or not holding colleagues accountable for consequences. It rather signifies suspending judgment and withholding blame (Worline & Dutton, 2017).

Nonadversarial Benevolence

From a Buddhist standpoint, compassion is offered to all in a nonadversarial benevolence, including to those who may have knowingly or unknowingly caused suffering (Cozart & Shields, 2018; Makransky, 2016). That is, rather than confining compassion solely to one's immediate circle (i.e., "biased compassion"), this entails extending compassion to perceived adversaries (i.e., "unbiased compassion").[18] Relatedly, the concept of *fierce compassion* can refer to the act of compassionately confronting individuals who act harmfully, not only for the benefit of those who are negatively impacted by their acts but for the sake of said individuals' own fuller humanity (Makransky, 2016).

With respect to helping professionals treating individuals who have committed an offense (e.g., restorative justice facilitators), Lamb (2002, p. 162) stated that "compassion . . . is crucial if we want to help them engage in self-reflection and make some difficult changes in character." Similarly, Witvliet et al. (2022) described compassionate reappraisal as viewing the offense as a signal that the person responsible for it is in need of learning and positive transformation.

Relevantly, compassion for others has been shown to predict subjective wellbeing through forgiveness of others (Roxas et al., 2019). Importantly, however, forgiveness does not imply (a) condoning unkindness, (b) denying or minimizing one's hurt, (c) forgetting that pain occurred, or (d) reconciling with the individual who caused the pain. Rather, it is a choice that individuals may wish to consider for enhanced wellbeing and health (Luskin, 2002). Compassion, as such, does not imply overlooking the deed – it rises above it, potentially leading to the release of heart-constricting feelings (Green, 2009).

Compulsory Compassion

The concept of *compulsory compassion* aims to foster compassion in individuals who have caused suffering toward those who have been harmed by their actions (Hargovan, 2007). In line with Acorn (2004), a key component of such restorative encounters is the practice of facilitating dialogues between survivors of trauma (who wish to participate in the process) and the individuals who perpetrated the trauma – creating a structured and safe environment for communication.

Ideally, survivor-centered encounters include the presence of all individuals who have been adversely impacted by the traumatic event, including those who were indirectly affected, thus enabling them to gain a sense of empowerment and closure. Moreover, it is often beneficial for this process to include disclosures from family members of the individuals who inflicted the trauma (Acorn, 2004; Wemmers et al., 2023).

In the latter mentioned disclosures, family members articulate their experiences of suffering as a result of the behavior of their kin. The underlying assumption is that the close relationships between the individuals who perpetrated the trauma and their family members may lead to a more compassionate response from the former. It is important to note, however, that a challenge in this field is the possibility that individuals who perpetrated trauma may offer a performance of compassion driven by self-serving motivations (Acorn, 2004).

Self-Compassion

Ongoing Challenge

There is an "ongoing challenge (and debate) regarding the nature of self-compassion" (Cha et al., 2023, p. 2665). Cha and colleagues further highlighted "the tensions between the definitions and conceptualizations of self-compassion in the scientific literature compared to Buddhist notions" (p. 2665). They noted that most contemporary self-compassion training and research has focused on evaluating outcomes related to the individualistic sense of "self" common in modern Western cultures. "Prima facie, however, this model is incompatible with the relational sense of self that is implied in Buddhist traditions" (p. 2665).

Although conceptualizations rooted in personal wellbeing have played a valuable role, there is a distinct need for further conceptualizations and measurements that encompass the interpersonal and social dimensions of self-compassion since these have received comparatively less attention (Cha et al., 2023). This recommendation aligns with Sahdra et al.'s (2023) focus on balancing self- and other-oriented compassion (i.e., "self-other harmony") for enhanced wellbeing as well as Condon and Makransky's (2023) emphasis on exploring mechanisms and outcomes that extend beyond self-centered perspectives, in order to enrich further the understanding of self-compassion.[19]

Conceptualizations and Interpersonal Outcomes

Thus far, self-compassion studies have primarily employed the *Self-Compassion Scale* (SCS) and its Short Form (SCS-SF; Neff, 2003a, 2003b;

Neff & Tóth-Király, 2022; Raes et al., 2011). In the SCS, Neff (2003b), a pioneering researcher in the field, conceptualized self-compassion as comprising three elements that contrast with three opposing mental states collectively referred to as self-coldness (Brenner et al., 2018).[20]

This seminal theory is hereby outlined specifically for helping professionals' experience of secondary traumatic stress (STS)-related self-compassion, which can range from tender to fierce (e.g., Neff, 2021). In line with Neff, *tender self-compassion* is characterized by inwardly comforting, soothing, and validating behavior. On the other hand, *fierce self-compassion* can refer to helping professionals outwardly taking action to protect, provide, and motivate themselves.[21] Ideally, as Neff and Germer (2018, p. 38) suggested, these two facets, representing the "Yin and Yang" of self-compassion, should be integrated and balanced to form a self-compassionate force:

- *Mindfulness* vs. overidentification – helping professionals' ability to hold their STS-related sensations, emotions, and thoughts in a mindfully balanced perspective rather than getting caught up and swept away by their negative reactivity
- *Common humanity* vs. isolation – helping professionals' ability to recognize that STS is a natural and often expected reaction to indirect trauma exposure – a shared challenge that other helping professionals may likewise encounter, rather than a phenomenon that they alone experience
- *Self-kindness* vs. self-judgment – helping professionals' ability to have a supportive attitude toward themselves, be self-accepting, and actively show themselves concern rather than being self-critical toward themselves concerning STS

Various queries have been raised regarding Neff's (2003a, 2003b) SCS conceptual framework. For example, scholars have highlighted essential elements not covered by the SCS, such as motivation, distress tolerance (i.e., the ability to endure adverse psychological situations), and the relational-self (Guyer, 2012, as cited in Cha et al., 2023; Muris & Petrocchi, 2017). In addition, Muris et al. (2016) recommended omitting the items that exhibit negative associations with self-compassion (i.e., overidentification, isolation, and self-judgment). This approach was endorsed by Muris and Petrocchi (2017), whose findings suggested that the inclusion of these items potentially yields an inflated relation with psychopathology symptoms.

Dodson and Heng (2022) proposed an alternative perspective, favoring the terms *noticing, feeling,* and *acting* over *mindfulness, common humanity,* and *self-kindness,* respectively. They conceptualized self-compassion as "a dynamic process that begins with mindful awareness of personal suffering (noticing), followed by appreciating and empathizing with one's own pain (feeling) which culminates in a response to alleviate it (acting)" (p. 184). These three steps which can be recursive and/or iterative rather than linear, are hereby presented as pertaining to STS:

- *Noticing* – helping professionals' ability to notice their STS-related reactions and the triggers that elicit said reactions. This is necessary, as, without this initial step, self-compassion is unlikely to commence/flow. In essence, noticing their symptoms related to STS is a needed catalyst for the process of self-compassion to unfold.
- *Feeling* – helping professionals' ability to self-empathize with their STS-related reactions. This step also emphasizes the importance of helping professionals feeling worthy of compassion and validating their own feelings as a fundamental aspect of addressing STS (e.g., Donald et al., 2018; Porges, 2017).
- *Acting* – helping professionals' ability to take self-compassionate actions to reduce their personal suffering. These actions can encompass various measures to alleviate STS, which are not only intrapsychic (e.g., self-kindness) but include behavioral forms of self-care. This aligns with the perspective of researchers such as Gilbert et al. (2017), who broadly defined enacted self-compassion as "I take the actions and do the things that will be helpful to me" (p. 13).

Importantly, Dodson and Heng (2022), as well as Neff and Pommier (2013), referred to interpersonal outcomes associated with self-compassion, aligning with the notion that "actions should result in wellbeing for both the self and for others – neither being sufficient on its own" (Mitra & Greenberg, 2016, p. 420). For example, Dodson and Heng stated that self-compassion has been linked to improved interpersonal outcomes among workers and their clients as well as between colleagues and their supervisors. Neff and Pommier likewise reported that self-compassion is associated with potential benefits for others, such as increased empathetic concern, altruism, and self-reported compassion for humanity (particularly among individuals who practice meditation). That being said, self-compassion alone may not be enough to foster compassion for others (Marshall et al., 2020).

Relevant Interrelations

Regarding interrelations, self-compassion has been shown to be negatively correlated with posttraumatic stress disorder (PTSD) symptom severity in a systematic review conducted by Winders et al. (2020). This review suggested that interventions focusing, either partially or entirely, on self-compassion have the potential to alleviate PTSD symptoms. A systematic review and meta-analysis by Luo et al. (2021) similarly demonstrated that self-compassion-focused interventions, particularly those of longer duration, provide a protective effect against PTSD.

The integration of self-compassion into existing psychological treatments for PTSD has indeed shown promising results (Braehler & Neff, 2020). These authors reported that elevated levels of self-compassion alleviated the shame of PTSD. Moreover, self-compassion has been linked to increased resilience to stress, providing potential benefits for helping professionals in coping not only with PTSD but with challenging conditions such as burnout and STS (Eriksson et al., 2018; Lefebvre et al., 2020).

With respect to STS, Xie et al. (2021) recommended the inclusion of self-compassion training within comprehensive interventions designed to address STS. Correspondingly, results by Rushforth et al. (2023) provided preliminary evidence that self-compassion training could reduce STS among healthcare professionals. Relatedly, Rushforth and colleagues also called for enhanced methodological rigor in this field and for future investigations that prioritize diversifying geographical locations to encompass nonwestern countries.

Lastly, Tsirimokou et al. (2023) recommended that organizations offer specialist trainings not only to mitigate adverse reactions following indirect trauma exposure but also to enhance helping professionals' awareness regarding their potential for personal growth through their work (i.e., vicarious posttraumatic growth; VPTG). This aligns with Ogińska-Bulik and Juczyński (2024), who highlighted that self-compassion and self-care can contribute to VPTG in the face of trauma. Significantly, Poli et al. (2022) recommended self-compassion interventions as a beneficial noninvasive strategy for a wide range of clinical and nonclinical populations, offering advantages for physiological and psychological wellbeing.

Self-Compassion From a Buddhist Perspective

Background

As a backdrop for this exploration, Anālayo (2017) presented a distinction in Buddhist teachings between caring for oneself and caring for others.[22] This distinction assesses four types of individuals based on whether they prioritize their own and/or others' wellbeing, ranging from least to most favorable (p. 85): (a) "those who benefit neither themselves nor others," (b) "those who benefit others," (c) "those who benefit themselves," and (d) "those who benefit both themselves and others."

In this ranking, it might seem surprising that those who benefit themselves are more favorably viewed than those who benefit others (Anālayo, 2017). Schmithausen (2004, as cited in Anālayo, 2017) elucidates this by explaining that those who are solely focused on others may merely offer advice on virtuous conduct but fail to practice it themselves. By contrast, those who practice virtuous behavior themselves, even if they do not actively encourage others, embody the values they advocate.

Self-Compassion as Skillful Means

The concept of *self-compassion*, considered separately from the cultivation of compassion toward others, has gained prominence as a distinct field of contemporary Western compassion training and research (e.g., Neff & Germer, 2018).[23] However, its purported Buddhist roots have received relatively little attention in academic discourse. To this end, the following are two examples of Buddhist precedents, or lack thereof, of self-compassion as a stand-alone notion (Anālayo & Dhammadinnā, 2021; Dunne & Manheim, 2023).

In early Buddhist teachings, the meditative practice of compassion involved visualizing compassion radiating outward in all directions (Anālayo, 2019; Anālayo & Dhammadinnā, 2021). As cited by these authors, this approach is exemplified in the *Kālāma-Sutta* found in the Pāli Canon (*Tipiṭaka*; i.e., the primary scriptural collection of Theravāda Buddhism). This meditative practice emphasizes boundless compassion extended to the entire world without specific mention of a personified object of compassion (Anālayo, 2019; Anālayo & Dhammadinnā, 2021).[24]

This altruistic nature of compassion assumed a central role in Mahāyāna Buddhist literature, philosophy, and practical teachings (Gethin, 1998). Within the Mahāyāna theoretical texts, compassion is directed to others, and the very concept of *self-compassion,* as a stand-alone concept, "is tantamount to speaking of a square circle" (Dunne & Manheim, 2023, p. 2376).[25] Anālayo and Dhammadinnā (2021, p. 1355) likewise observed that "self-compassion is conspicuous by its absence in any of the constructs of compassion inherited or developed by the Mahāyāna traditions." This absence is not only a theoretical observation but is also evident in contemplative Mahāyāna practices (Dunne & Manheim, 2023).[26]

Dunne and Manheim (2023) emphasized the disparities between self-compassion and traditional Buddhist theory and practice. Their intention, however, was not to undermine self-compassion but rather to highlight its potential effectiveness as a "skillful means" (Skt. *upāya-kauśalya*), particularly for individuals entangled in self-destructive narratives (e.g., self-hatred). The Buddhist concept of *skillful means* – broadly described as the variety of means that may be used to alleviate suffering in context-sensitive ways (e.g., Quaglia, 2023) – recognizes that customized approaches, motivated by both wisdom and compassion, can be creatively tailored to individuals' needs within diverse contexts (e.g., Condon & Makransky, 2023; Quaglia & Simmer-Brown, 2023).[27]

In line with Simmer-Brown (2023),[28] to classify self-compassion as a skillful means within contemporary compassion trainings, practitioners would need to engage in the practice of self-compassion with several key considerations. These include: (a) approaching self-compassion with an altruistic orientation, (b) discerning what others may need, even if only provisionally, (c) evaluating potential actions and anticipating their outcomes, (d) maintaining humility regarding the ability to foster change, and (e) ensuring that the actions that stem from self-compassion are offered with a strategically precise, and gentle approach that aligns with all the aforementioned considerations.

Thus, considering self-compassion as a skillful means involves recognizing interdependence and looking beyond oneself (Condon & Makransky, 2023).[29] It necessitates broadening the scope of self-compassion-related outcomes to encompass others, thereby cultivating a perspective that integrates both wisdom and compassion. Such an altruistic orientation contributes to a more comprehensive understanding of self-compassion and more accurately reflects (self-)compassion from a Buddhist perspective (e.g., Cha et al., 2023; Garfield, 2022).[30]

The Phenomenon of Exchange

The term *exchange* highlights the subtle ways in which we are interconnected with others. As *exchange* is a bidirectional term, when helping professionals emanate compassion, their compassion can be "contagious" (i.e., similarly to the traumatic stress reactions of the individuals in their care; Isobel & Angus-Leppan, 2018). This implies that cultivating compassion not only provides helping professionals with resources to address STS but can also have a positive impact on their clients through the activation of their clients' mirror neurons (i.e., neurons that enable individuals to perceive what other people are experiencing, as if the individuals themselves are sharing the same experience; e.g., Rizzolatti et al., 2023).

Relevantly, Hatfield and colleagues (2014) defined *emotional contagion* (i.e., the likelihood of "catching" the emotions of others) as "the tendency to automatically mimic and synchronize facial expressions, vocalizations, postures, and movements with those of another person's and consequently to converge emotionally" (p. 161). In line with this definition, and taking clients' own empathic responses into account, helping professionals' expressions of compassion through such processes as mimicry of vocal, facial, and postural feedback can produce similar expressions in their clients (Hatfield et al., 2014; Horwitz et al., 2023; Louchakova-Schwartz, 2020). Consequently, the expression of compassion can support helping professionals' own wellbeing and contribute to bringing out this potential in their clients (Makransky, 2012).

The preceding can also be conceptualized by the term *mirror flourishing* – defined as the flourishing/growing together that can occur naturally and reciprocally when a care recipient is in the presence of a compassionate caregiver (e.g., Cooperrider & Fry, 2012). *Mirror flourishing*, as such, can be described as "an intimacy of relations between entities to the point where we can posit that there is no outside and inside, only the creative unfolding of an entire field of relations or connections" (Cooperrider & Fry, 2012, p. 8).

Notably, the concept of *mirror flourishing* can also refer to an organizational phenomenon whereby when organizations help the world "out there" flourish, helping professionals cannot help but benefit "in here" as well (i.e., within their organizations). In other words, working for an organization that compassionately helps others can increase helping professionals' perception of their organizations as compassionate workplaces (Cooperrider & Fry, 2012).

Section IV

COMPASSION WITHIN AND BEYOND ORGANIZATIONS

Compassion at Work

Helping professionals may spend around 100,000 hours of their lives at work, with some dedicating even more time (e.g., Worline & Dutton, 2017). It is, therefore, safe to say that their work can have a profound impact on their quality of life. Likewise, it follows that suffering – a fundamental component of human existence – may be present within such a considerable investment of time and effort (e.g., Worline & Dutton, 2017).

Suffering can be pervasive within workplaces, with common sources including suffering that originates from outside work boundaries, such as when employees suffer from financial pressures, addictions, or other hardships. Forms of suffering can also arise from within the workplace itself through heavy workloads, performance pressures, exposure to work-related indirect trauma, secondary traumatic stress (STS), and burnout (e.g., Driver, 2007; Dutton et al., 2014).

Without compassion, workplaces can unintentionally amplify suffering. Unfortunately, however, compassion, both in general and in the context of STS, can be diminished due to workplace demands such as time constraints, overload, and other organizational pressures. Fostering a compassionate workplace culture, therefore, is crucial to counteract such challenges and to promote wellbeing among employees (Worline & Dutton, 2017).

DOI: 10.4324/9781003381747-5

Compassion can radically improve employees' day-to-day work lives (Salzberg, 2013). Specifically, cultivating compassion within the workplace can have strategic organizational advantages such as improved service quality, employee and customer engagement, retention of talented staff, collaboration, and relational wealth (i.e., the latter concept highlights the economic advantages of cultivating interpersonal connections within the workplace; Jinpa, 2015; Leana & Rousseau, 2000; Worline & Dutton, 2017).[1] Furthermore, compassionate work environments create the potential for a spillover effect, whereby employees carry compassion home with them, thereby extending the positive impact beyond the workplace (Simpson et al., 2020).

Dutton et al. (2014) conceptualized compassion as having several attributes/phases within organizational settings. Accordingly, workplace compassion involves helping professionals' ability to: (a) notice others' suffering, (b) interpret suffering in a way that leads to their desire to alleviate it, (c) feel *empathic concern* for the individuals who are suffering, and (d) act to alleviate the suffering in some way. Notably, Wong (2015) highlighted another pivotal aspect – that compassion initiates through a visceral bodily response, entailing a reflexive movement toward those who are suffering.

Specifically, regarding *empathic concern,* this signifies an other-focused emotional response of concern rooted in the understanding of another person's adverse emotional state without actually experiencing the same emotions (Stevens & Taber, 2021). This implies not succumbing to personal distress, which is a self-focused response to another person's suffering. Compassion training can help guide helping professionals to cope with empathic distress and cultivate empathic concern (e.g., Chierchia & Singer, 2017; Stevens & Taber, 2021).[2]

Compassion Competence

Workplaces wherein individuals collectively notice, interpret, feel, and subsequently act to alleviate suffering in a coordinated, emergent, effective, and customized way exhibit *compassion competence* (Worline & Dutton, 2017). In line with Worline and Dutton, this form of competence includes the dimensions of *speed, scope, magnitude*, and *customization of resources.* These, as well as the added dimension of *quality*, are described here as pertaining to STS and refer to such compassionate organizational resources as: (a) compassion-informed STS trainings, (b) compassion-informed supervision and peer-support opportunities for addressing STS, and (c) a compassionate STS champion within the organization (e.g., Shea, 2021).

Regarding champions, they have been shown to play a key role in the successful formalization and implementation of new practices (e.g., Miech et al., 2018; Nair, 2022). Compassionate STS champions' qualities can encompass: (a) awareness of how compassion relates to STS, (b) agreement that compassion-based practices can help improve STS outcomes, (c) enthusiasm to actively involve and inspire additional employees, through peer engagement, to join the cause of compassionately addressing STS, and (d) initiative in compassion-based problem-solving strategies for addressing challenges associated with STS (e.g., Sprang et al., 2023).

Dimensions of Compassion Competence

The following five *compassion competence* dimensions are described specifically for STS (e.g., Eisler, 2017):

- *Customization*: *The degree to which compassionate actions for addressing STS are individualized to the workforce* – This dimension includes an organization's ability to take action to ensure that staff members encountering STS are provided assistance, taking their individual needs, preferences, and circumstances into account.
- *Magnitude*: *The number of compassionate actions generated by an organization for addressing STS* – This dimension includes an organization's ability to evaluate the magnitude of resources needed to address STS and to provide such resources even if many resources are required.
- *Scope*: *The breadth of compassionate actions generated by an organization for addressing STS* – This dimension includes an organization's ability to evaluate the full spectrum of requirements for addressing STS and to provide the requisite resources accordingly.
- *Speed*: *The timing of compassionate actions generated by an organization for addressing STS* – This dimension includes an organization's ability to respond promptly to STS and to quickly initiate and adjust appropriate actions.
- *Quality*: *The quality of STS-related compassionate actions generated by an organization* – This dimension highlights the organization's proficiency in delivering high-quality resources that are supported by evidence-based approaches.

Self- and Other-Oriented Compassionate Leadership

Leader Role Self-Compassion

Due to the key role that leaders play in organizations, the field of management has focused much-deserved attention on effective leadership. Recognizing the demanding nature of their role, leaders need to find ways to navigate it skillfully (e.g., Badura et al., 2020; van Knippenberg, 2020). To this end, Lanaj et al. (2022) demonstrated that adopting a self-compassionate outlook toward their leadership responsibilities can be an effective tool for leaders, fostering a stronger connection to their leadership role and resulting in leaders being more inclined to assist coworkers with both task-related and personal matters. As a result, these authors introduced the term *leader role self-compassion,* which entails adopting a compassionate stance toward oneself in the face of the challenges inherent in leadership.[3]

Operationalizing Compassionate Leader Behavior

As part of their responsibilities, leaders also play a significant role in establishing other-oriented compassion within the work environment. By modeling compassionate behaviors toward others, leaders shape the organizational culture that their employees perceive, react to, and replicate (Lilius et al., 2008, 2011).[4] Shuck et al. (2019) operationalized compassionate leader behavior to comprise the following six distinctive themes: *authenticity, integrity, presence, empathy, dignity,* and *accountability.* These provide a pathway for considering "*how*" work is getting done, not just "*how much*" work is getting done (Frost, 2003, as cited in Shuck et al., 2019, p. 558):[5]

- *Authenticity* is evident in how compassionate leaders strive to maintain their genuineness. As one leader aptly expressed, "Compassion is authentic, it's genuine, it's real, it's caring for those you have the privilege to either lead or work with" (Shuck et al., 2019, p. 547). This is also exemplified by compassionate leaders displaying vulnerability and openness when sharing their experiences (i.e., both successes and challenges) with others.
- *Integrity* is rooted in the concept of *professional transparency* and the alignment of compassionate leaders' personal and professional actions with their words, idiomatically referred to as "walking the talk." Specifically, integrity is understood as the practice of sharing information in a timely, accurate, and transparent manner, openly communicating motivations and goals rather than concealing agendas, and addressing conflicts or disagreements in a straightforward manner (e.g., versus exhibiting passive-aggressive behavior).
- *Presence* is exemplified in compassionate leaders' ability to remain attentive to their employees in the present moment. This characteristic signifies leaders' proficiency in actively listening to employees, perceiving not only what employees convey verbally but also through their non-verbal cues. Presence requires leaders to master their emotional and cognitive capacities, enabling them to prioritize employees' needs even amidst other pressing organizational matters. This signals to employees that they are both valuable and valued.
- *Empathy* is illustrated by compassionate leaders' ability to empathize with their employees. This includes a balance of both understanding their employees' thoughts and emotions and vicariously experiencing what their employees might be feeling by symbolically putting themselves in their

employees' shoes. Importantly, compassionate leaders also demonstrate in their actions that they empathize with their employees. Consequently, compassion can be seen as the practical application of empathy.[6]

- *Dignity* is reflected in how compassionate leaders uphold the inherent worth and humanity of every employee. Such leaders stress the importance of openly embracing an attitude of acceptance and tolerance toward differences, including skills, opinions, and lifestyle choices. They also emphasize a consistent sensitivity to employees' wellbeing. This involves flexibly seeking and creating options for employees to maintain self-worth as well as celebrating employees' successes.

- *Accountability* centers around the principles of action-oriented responsibility. It includes compassionate leaders establishing high-performance standards, clearly communicating expectations, providing feedback on work quality, and instituting recognition for high performance. Significantly, compassionate leaders also hold employees accountable for their work, address challenging performance issues, and enforce consequences for underperformance.

Compassionate Leaders' Relational Practices

The following four relational practices of *attuning, wondering, following*, and *holding* can be learned, practiced, and mastered by compassionate leaders. These relational practices are described here specifically for leaders' interactions with helping professionals dealing with STS (e.g., Koloroutis & Pole, 2021; Koloroutis & Trout, 2012). Meaningfully, as described further by Long and Smith (2017), these relational practices can likewise be practiced by leaders as self-care:

- *Attuning* plays a crucial role in establishing compassionate human connections. It necessitates compassionate leaders consciously setting aside distractions and fully focusing on the present interaction or situation. By tuning in to both verbal and nonverbal cues – as also referred to in the aforementioned theme of "presence" (Shuck et al., 2019) – leaders can gain valuable insights into helping professionals' STS-related needs. Moreover, attuning encompasses leaders mindfully tuning in to themselves, as this introspective practice can allow them to better recognize any preconceived notions, assumptions, and biases that may be impacting their interactions.

- *Wondering* involves compassionate leaders cultivating curiosity and showing a genuine interest in understanding helping professionals' STS experiences. This entails leaders avoiding making hasty assumptions, judgments, and conclusions and asking open-ended questions such as "What worries you?" and "What do you need?". When leaders wonder, they suspend their own agendas and become open to new information, allowing them to compassionately embrace curiosity and engage in a process of continuous learning.

• *Following* involves compassionate leaders actively listening and remaining attentive to what is being communicated by helping professionals without interruption. This approach also involves leaders saying such things as "Tell me more about that" and "Did I understand this correctly?" Encouraging helping professionals to express their STS-related thoughts and feelings creates a space for them to feel heard and validated, fostering a sense of trust and psychological safety within the interaction. This open and nonjudgmental atmosphere allows helping professionals to explore their STS-related experiences more deeply, facilitating meaningful dialogue and promoting a collaborative approach to addressing their needs related to STS.

• *Holding* involves compassionate leaders creating a safe and supportive environment that enables helping professionals to feel seen and acknowledged further. It likewise encompasses leaders actively doing their best to resolve issues and concerns and to follow through on their commitments (e.g., "I will see this through and ensure that . . ."). By holding space for helping professionals' STS-related needs, compassionate leaders cultivate a culture in which those caring for others also feel cared for. This reciprocal support enhances helping professionals' ability to provide compassionate care while maintaining their own wellbeing.

The STS-Related Organizational COMPASSION Compass

Creating a compassionate infrastructure for addressing STS within the workplace is imperative. Identifying and articulating such a compassionate infrastructure includes the following recommendations presented via the acronym COMPASSION – which can serve as an STS-related organizational compass for leaders (see Table 1).

Table 1. STS-Related COMPASSION Recommendations for Leaders

Letter of Acronym	Recommendations
C	Cultivate an organizational culture characterized by compassion for STS.
O	Open channels for employees to voice their experiences and suggestions regarding compassionate support for STS.
M	Make compassion for STS a core organizational value, ensuring that it is provided in a trauma-informed, inclusive, and culturally sensitive manner.

(Continued)

Table 1. (Continued)

Letter of Acronym	Recommendations
P	Provide financial and instrumental support for customized, individualized, team-oriented, and organization-wide STS-informed compassionate resources.
A	Acknowledge that compassionate responsiveness to STS is an essential leadership skill.
S	Support and model the practice of self-compassion in relation to STS as *altruistic self-care.*
S	Share evidence-based and culturally responsive knowledge on the benefits of approaching STS with compassion within the organization.
I	Interpret suffering due to STS generously, letting it evoke a compassionate response.
O	Oversee the implementation of compassionate organizational policies and practices related to STS as well as their ongoing assessment.
N	Navigate barriers that may hinder the ability to engage in compassionate responses within the organization in the context of STS.

Note. These recommendations are not necessarily exhaustive or mutually exclusive, nor are they listed by significance or recommended order. It is also worth mentioning that the term *altruistic self-care* goes beyond the conventional understanding of personal wellbeing, emphasizing the connection between self-care and the wellbeing of others (Bhalla & DiCuirci, 2023).

Compassion for Indirect Trauma – A Public Health Perspective

Throughout history, societies have focused primarily on the immediate survivors of traumatic events, generally overlooking those who indirectly experienced the aftermath. However, over time, societies began to acknowledge the impact of trauma on those indirectly exposed, recognizing that the repercussions of trauma extend beyond immediate survivors. This evolving understanding underscores the importance of addressing the far-reaching consequences of traumatic events on a broader scale (e.g., Blanch, 2012; Hinton & Good, 2016).

Exposure to trauma is widespread in societies worldwide, making it a global public health concern (Magruder et al., 2017; Watson, 2019), with this exposure recognized as encompassing both direct and indirect forms.

Significantly, "Indirect trauma has become equally important as direct trauma" (Choi et al., 2021, p. 1) and "is a problem of huge proportions in the world" (Horesh, 2016, p. 348). The term *indirect trauma*, as referred to in this context, is broader, however, than helping professionals' indirect exposure to the traumas experienced by the individuals in their care.

Indeed, indirect exposure to trauma extends beyond helping professionals caring for survivors of trauma. It encompasses indirect exposure via the media (Silver et al., 2013) and the indirect exposure of family members, friends, and community members to the traumatic events experienced by those they are empathically trying to support (e.g., Casas & Benuto, 2022; Landers et al., 2020; Zerach et al., 2022). The latter also extends to support offered to individuals responsible for perpetrating trauma (Munger et al., 2015).[7]

"The implications of a society being trauma-literate could be immense. Since trauma is the core dynamic undergirding so much ill health, we need to develop the eyes and ears to spot it to begin with" (Maté, 2022, p. 486). This capacity extends not only to direct but also to indirect exposure to trauma (e.g., Lawson et al., 2019). Fostering a culture of trauma literacy encompassing indirect trauma can equip us with the knowledge and sensitivity to address what still often goes unnoticed, thereby paving the way for more compassionate communities.

Public health relies heavily on the notion that our perception of health is contingent on robust and sustainable social foundations that include compassionate community engagement, partnerships, and social support systems. Compassion, as such, can be viewed as the foundational pathway by which trauma is addressed within social structures and subsequently transformed into opportunities for positive growth. This includes trauma experienced indirectly in personal, professional, community, and larger-scaled social contexts (e.g., Centers for Disease Control and Prevention Foundation [CDC], 2023; Kellehear, 2004).

Terms such as *compassionate activism*, *radical compassion*, and *compassion spheres* are relevant in this context (Brach, 2019; Garavan, 2012; Harris, 2023; Makransky, 2016; Quaglia, 2023).[8] Embedded within these terms are the requisite levels of commitment and courage to compassionately confront large-scale systemic suffering with unwavering care. This holds significance because, much like direct trauma, addressing indirect trauma may necessitate the compassionate confrontation of systemic suffering on a broader scale – underscoring the importance of an interconnected compassionate perspective (e.g., Bronfenbrenner, 1989; Garavan, 2012; Harris, 2023; Jackson-Preston et al., 2023; Kornfeld, 2009; Lampert, 2005; Strolin-Goltzman et al., 2020).

Compassion compels each of us to take action that promotes the collective wellbeing in the context of trauma, whether experienced directly or indirectly. As King (2023, p. 2516) emphasized, "compassion can be . . . and should be manifested in concrete action on all levels, from an individual's personal life all the way to society-wide social action." This aligns with the profound perspective that "compassion is what impels you to act for the sake of the larger whole – or put more accurately, it is the whole acting through you" (Macy, 2022, para. 2).

Summary of the Literature Review

This literature review highlights selected topics organized in four sections. Section I provides a comprehensive exploration of trauma-related concepts, responses, and care principles. Building on that foundation, Section II delves into the realm of secondary traumatic stress (STS), shedding light on the associated challenges encountered by helping professionals caring for survivors of trauma. Next, Section III highlights the interplay between wisdom and compassion, as well as between self- and other-oriented compassion, along with an examination of related constructs. Finally, Section IV considers the transformative potential of compassion within and beyond organizational settings, as pertaining to STS and exposure to indirect trauma more generally.

Upcoming is a comprehensive collection of transformative individual and group practices as well as associated self-reflection prompts. In line with Bronfenbrenner's (1989) ecological systems theory, these extend beyond the self-care of individual helping professionals working with survivors of trauma. They encompass the wellbeing of their colleagues and the cultivation of a trauma-informed and compassionate culture within their respective organizations. It is hoped that these practices and self-reflection prompts provide meaningful benefits, enabling helping professionals to continue their invaluable work with dedicated compassion.

Part II

SECONDARY TRAUMATIC STRESS-RELATED COMPASSION-BASED PRACTICES

Reestablishing Pure-Hearted Motivation[1]

May compassion become your compass and passion:
A guiding light for you and yours and all creation.[2]

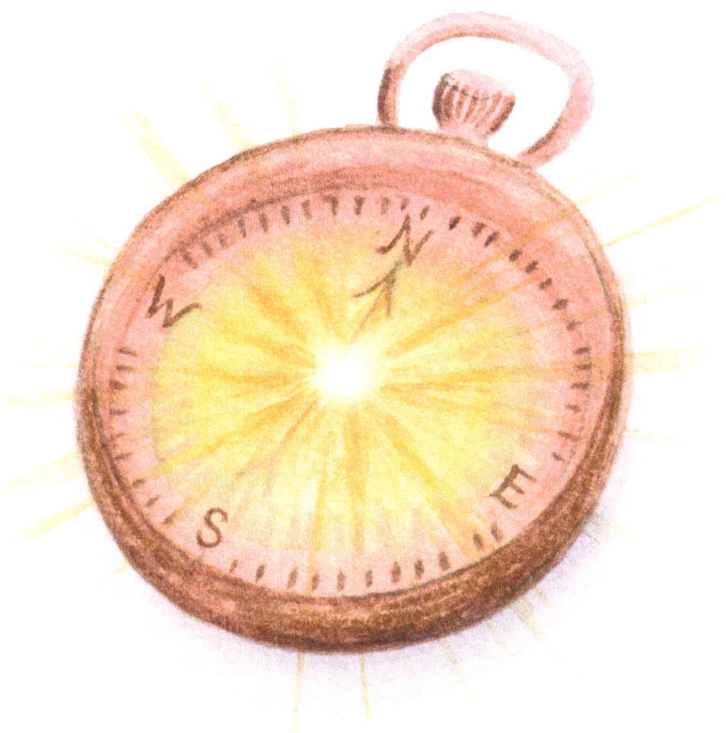

Inner Compass

A compassion compass

Opening Words

A comprehensive collection of personal and group practices, as well as associated self-reflection prompts are hereby presented, preceded by introductory segments that feature: (a) mental preparation recommendations prior to engaging with the practices and reflection prompts, (b) a reference to the Buddhist metaphor of the two arrows, (c) a recommended reading and practice approach, and (d) a quote by Śāntideva (n.d.; late 7th to mid-8th century CE) – a Buddhist monk, philosopher, and Sanskrit poet (Goodman, 2016). Following these introductory segments, three categories of practices are presented, with each category serving a specific purpose (see Appendices D and E for the practices' orientation and type, respectively).

These categories include: (a) "Foundational Practices" – designed to establish the foundation for engaging with the secondary traumatic stress (STS)-related practices, (b) "Practices for Addressing STS" – tailored to support helping professionals navigating STS-related challenges, and (c) "Practices for Promoting Vicarious Posttraumatic Growth (VPTG)" – created to enhance helping professionals' wellbeing in line with the VPTG framework. These practices incorporate a wide range of creative approaches, predominantly contemplative in nature, including contemporary Buddhist-inspired compassion-based practices relevant for helping professionals from diverse backgrounds.

Closing segments, including a summary of the practices, a call to compassionate action, and guidance for group facilitation, are then presented. While primarily intended for group leaders, the latter guidance contains insights that helping professionals practicing within group contexts will likewise find valuable. These insights shed light on (a) the benefits of practicing within a group setting (see Appendix F for specifics of practicing online), and (b) considerations associated with promoting compassion while incorporating principles of East Asian philosophy within interreligious, intercultural, and intersectional group contexts. These considerations are relevant as helping professionals from different backgrounds, working in diverse settings, may require customized adaptations (Dodson-Lavelle, 2015).

Correspondingly, the Dalai Lama was once invited to lead a guided group meditation at Harvard University. Surprisingly, he declined, explaining that as every person in the audience was dealing with different challenges and had different strengths, it would not make sense to guide them all through the same meditation (2009, as cited in Pollak et al., 2014). Similarly, Thích Nhất Hạnh (1998) – a Buddhist monk, peace activist, author, and poet – emphasized that the true measure of a practice's relevance is its capacity to alleviate suffering and enhance the wellbeing of those who engage in it. This underscores the importance of tailoring practices to meet individual needs and recognizing the diversity of experiences and perspectives within group settings.

Mental Preparation Recommendations

Mental preparation is a dynamic process that involves readying yourself to cope with various challenging situations. Whether it is an athlete preparing for a competition, an individual getting ready to navigate a challenging life event, or a helping professional readying to address secondary traumatic stress (STS) – mental preparation can play a pivotal role. The following five Cs of mental preparation, adapted from Strycharczyk et al. (2021),[3] are applicable for helping professionals and serve as recommended guidelines prior to engaging with the practices that follow:

• *Control* – Cultivate an inner belief that you have sufficient control over your behavior to achieve your goals. For example, if you have decided to engage with the STS-related practices provided in this resource, have faith in your resolve to follow through. Believing in your ability to steer your actions can serve as a valuable anchor.
• *Commitment* – Dedicate yourself to a committed practice of STS-related compassionate care, ensuring that wellbeing remains a priority. Sometimes described as "stick-to-itiveness," commitment, in this context, refers to your ability to continue caring for yourself and others despite obstacles that may arise. Maintaining a steadfast commitment to compassionate care can lead to favorable changes.
• *Confidence* – Develop a sense of confidence in your ability to offer yourself and others compassionate care in the context of STS. Should you encounter moments of uncertainty, embrace this confidence by reaching out for assistance (e.g., supervision, peer support, and continuous learning). Your self-confidence can empower you to navigate the complexities of STS with compassion and seek the necessary resources to sustain your efforts.
• *Challenge* – View challenges associated with STS as opportunities for self-development (as well as team and organizational enhancement). By reframing your outlook in this way, you can harness the challenges posed by STS to deepen your understanding of compassionate coping strategies. This perspective is grounded in the notion that labeling something as a challenge inherently opens up the prospects for positive transformation (Goldberg et al., 2019).[4]
• *Connection* – Connect with an altruistic aim by grounding your practice in the understanding that addressing STS with compassion not only benefits you but can also positively impact others. This includes your clients, colleagues, organization, and community. Recognizing compassion's ripple effects amplifies the significance of your endeavors.

Notably, the Buddhist metaphor of the two arrows that follows these recommendations is likewise beneficial to contemplate as mental preparation before reading this resource guide.

The Metaphor of Two Arrows

In Buddhist teachings, the metaphor of being struck by two arrows, discussed in the *Salla-Sutta* (e.g., Feldman & Kuyken, 2011), serves as a well-known metaphor differentiating between the physical sensation of pain, which may be unavoidable, and the mental reaction to it, which can be controlled. From this perspective, pain and suffering are delineated as distinct entities. Pain is acknowledged as inherent in human existence. By contrast, suffering is considered a secondary response, comprising the adverse mental, emotional, and behavioral reactions that may potentially follow (Gethin, 2015).

This metaphor holds significance for helping professionals indirectly exposed to their clients' traumatic experiences. This is so, as the first arrow resonates with the inherent challenges faced by helping professionals caring for clients who have experienced trauma. Conversely, the notion of the second arrow encourages helping professionals to recognize that while indirect exposure to trauma may be an inherent aspect of their work, they have the capacity to mitigate potential related suffering by choosing skillful responses, such as the forthcoming STS-related mindful compassion-based practices.

> storm clouds grow, rain falls –
> mountains watch the raindrops flow –
> rivers choose their course

This haiku subtly mirrors the aforementioned Buddhist metaphor, depicting life's inevitable challenges through the imagery of storm clouds and stormy weather, reminiscent of the physical pain represented by the first arrow. The mountains, observing the raindrops, may be seen as symbolizing the practice of mindfulness – akin to observing one's own experiences from a higher, metacognitive perspective. Similarly, rivers, in proactively choosing their course, embody the mindful selection of compassionate responses to life's inevitable storms, reinforcing the teaching that while pain may be inevitable, suffering is optional and shaped by the responses chosen.

Recommended Reading and Practice Approach

The following recommendations are designed to help you effectively engage with the upcoming practices:

- Commencing with the "Foundational Practices" is recommended. It is suggested, however, that you view these practices as more than initial steps and instead consider them as enduring practices. While they lay a strong foundation, their value does not diminish as you progress through subsequent practices, as they are transformative in and of themselves.
- Since secondary traumatic stress (STS) and vicarious posttraumatic growth (VPTG) can co-occur – even though you do not necessarily need to wait until STS completely subsides to commence the VPTG-related practices, it is, nonetheless, advisable to begin by addressing STS. By doing so, you pave the way for the subsequent cultivation of VPTG (Wheeler & McElvaney, 2018).
- Within each of the three main practice sections – "Foundational Practices," "Practices for Addressing STS," and "Practices for Promoting VPTG" – you have the flexibility to practice sequentially or selectively, depending on your preferences. The order of the practices within each section can be tailored to your individual needs, preferences, and circumstances, allowing you to create a customized practice order.
- Certain precursory conditions being in place can facilitate the realization of the desired outcomes. These include practicing in a setting characterized by physical attributes that are calming and soothing. Throughout history and in different cultures, contemplative practices have been performed in tranquil and safe surroundings. Such environments have a neurophysiological effect that soothes defensive physiological reactivity, potentially also serving as a neural catalyst for cultivating compassion (Porges, 2017).[5]
- The practices incorporate a wide range of approaches, the majority of which can be classified as contemplative (e.g., guided meditations, reflection prompts, and journaling prompts) as well as practices that are arts-based. Appropriately, you are encouraged to select the practices that resonate with you the most while considering the value of exploring them all.

- It is advisable to practice in a setting that supports the expressive nature of the creative arts activities. This involves ensuring that the space you practice in accommodates movement and is appropriately equipped with the following: a yoga mat, a candle, the option of listening to music, visual arts materials, one or more cushions and/or blankets, and ideally, a natural setting nearby.
- Regarding the visual arts, feel encouraged to integrate culturally relevant visual arts materials. This suggestion aligns with Wang's (2022) perspective on the significance of self-exploration through culturally meaningful creative activities as a means of promoting wellness following indirect exposure to trauma. Wang illustrated this by incorporating the use of a Chinese calligraphy brush and ink on rice paper for artistic expression.
- For practices involving movement, you can choose to visualize yourself moving instead of physically performing the movements. The concept of *motor imagery* provides a means for engaging in movement even when physical limitations present challenges. Incorporating imagined movement, either as a substitute for or in concert with physical movement, is thereby a possibility you may wish to consider (e.g., Dana, 2020).
- Consider keeping a notebook handy as you practice. Jotting down reflections, highlighting key points, and noting personal insights may enhance your engagement and heighten your comprehension and retentive capacity.
- As many practices invite you to close your eyes, familiarize yourself with the instructions by reading them thoroughly beforehand prior to transitioning into the practices themselves. Thereby, you may more fully engage with the practices, drawing from your memory while immersing yourself in the experience. Notably, trauma-sensitive recommendations suggest that practicing with open eyes may be advised, including looking at an external object that evokes positivity while practicing (Treleaven, 2018).[6]
- Prioritize wellbeing. If a certain practice does not feel right, you can revisit it later, skip it altogether, or practice it with the support of a trusted individual. Also, take breaks between practices to digest their benefits fully. Furthermore, as a way of gradually building up your compassionate resources in practices that invite you to recall clients or colleagues who have experienced primary or secondary trauma, it is advisable to first concentrate on trauma-related recollections of mild to moderate severity.

• Lastly, for further exploration and enrichment, associated endnotes offer explanations and reading recommendations relevant to the practices. While endnotes are sometimes overlooked, please think of these as hidden gems, filled with extra insights and bonus content aimed at enhancing your practice (see the "Hidden Gems" section).

"Just as a blind person might uncover a gem in heaps of dust,
so too, this *bodhicitta* of mine has somehow arisen."[7]
Śāntideva[8]

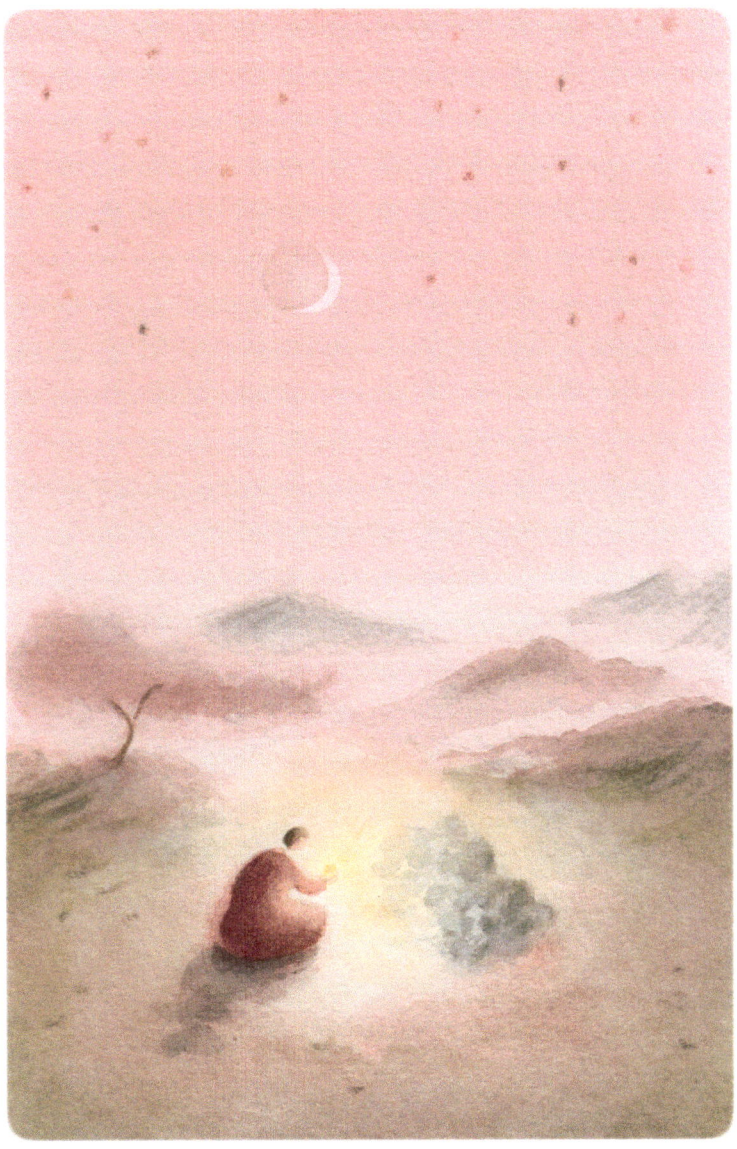

Precious Gem

Figure uncovering an illuminated gem symbolizing compassion

FOUNDATIONAL PRACTICES

DOI: 10.4324/9781003381747-7

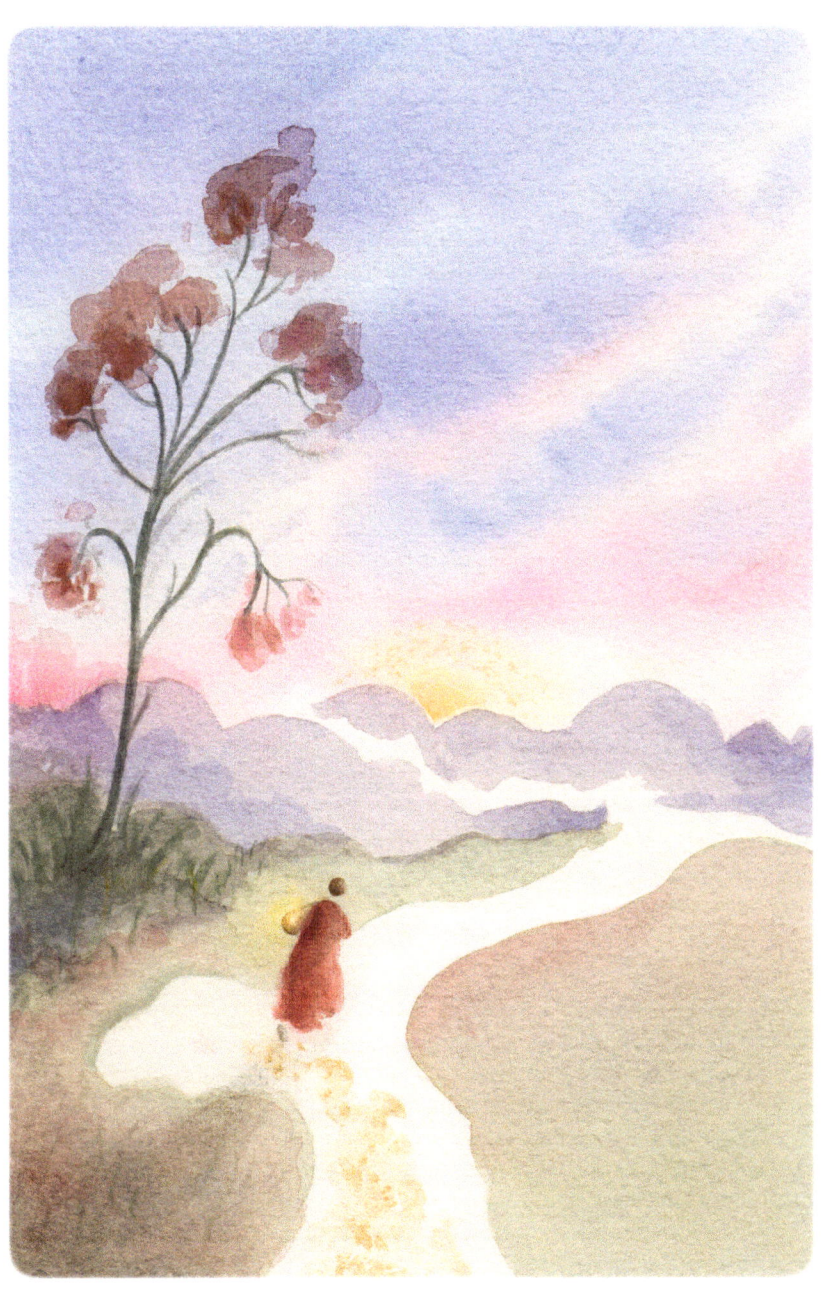

Embarking on the Path

Figure setting out on a path

Seeking REFUGE

Practice Orientation and Type:
Other- to Self-Orientation – Reflection Prompts

Personal Practice

In Buddhist traditions, taking refuge entails finding a sanctuary within the wellspring of compassionate wisdom passed down by a lineage of teachers, exemplified by Buddhist teachings, and nurtured within a community of fellow practitioners. Essentially, practitioners become an extension of the caring environment that envelops them. Hence, taking refuge serves as a secure base from which one can engage in extending compassionate care to others (Condon & Makransky, 2020a).

Inspired by this tradition and by scientific knowledge in the field of attachment priming,[1] the following six-step opening practice adapted from Condon and Makransky (2020a, 2020b; see Table 2) serves as a touchstone for helping professionals from diverse backgrounds.[2] The emphasis is on positive moments of compassionate connection that can take various forms, and which helping professionals can revisit as they engage with the subsequent practices.

Find a sitting posture that is kind to you, with your back, neck, and head aligned, and take a few deep and relaxing breaths. With your eyes preferably closed or your gaze lowered to reduce distractions,[3] allow your awareness to gently sweep through your body while relaxing areas of tension, tightness, or pressure. You might also consider placing one or both hands on your heart to enhance your connection with this practice.

Like a ship finding refuge in a secure harbor, allow this practice to function as an anchor, reconnecting you with the compassion you have received. Even if such compassionate moments feel distant and/or small, they hold significance as the building blocks of your ability to care for and nurture both yourself and those you serve.

Table 2. Seeking REFUGE Reflection Prompts

Letter of Acronym	Reflections
R	*Recall a compassionate moment* – Begin by recalling a time in your life when you received compassion. It may be from a beloved relative, mentor, teacher, friend, caring stranger, cherished pet, or even nature itself.
E	*Embrace the compassionate memory* – Immerse yourself in the memory as if it were happening now. Allow the recollection of receiving compassionate care to envelop you fully.
F	*Focus inward* – Let go of external distractions that may arise, and focus on thoughts and emotions linked to your experience of receiving compassionate care.
U	*Uncover your felt-sense* – Shift your focus toward bodily sensations, including subtle ones, linked to your experience of receiving compassionate care. Allow the sensations that arise to be recognized and acknowledged.
G	*Gateway to refuge* – Let your memory become as nuanced as possible. This can help it evolve into an inner refuge, offering a sense of connection, care, and inspiration to be revisited in times of need.
E	*Extend self-affirmations* – Inwardly repeat to yourself relevant self-affirmations. For example, you might repeat the following or similar words of your preference: "Compassion flows through me," and "I share the gift of compassion with others."

Note. As you return to this practice time and again, consider creating a "relational map" that captures memorable moments of receiving compassion. This map can take various textual or visual forms (e.g., a diagram, a flowchart, or a series of sketches/drawings that symbolize these compassionate moments).

Self-Reflections

• Dupasquier et al. (2018) suggested that the more helping professionals fear receiving compassion, the less likely they are to disclose secondary traumatic stress (STS). Does this resonate with me in any way?[4]
• Reflecting on a time when I was the recipient of compassion, how might that memory guide my approach to extending compassion toward others?

Group Context

Within a group setting, *Seeking Refuge* can transition into the following expressive movement activity:

The facilitator can invite participants to form a circle and extend their arms outward to their sides, creating a symbolic shared space within the circle. Participants can then be encouraged to make eye contact with each other and, one by one, after lowering their arms back down to their sides, translate their memories into brief movement sequences or gestures that capture the essence of their compassionate experiences.

After each participant shares their movement sequence or gesture, group members mirror the shared expression, physically reflecting the movement/ gesture as closely as possible. This process of mirroring can foster secure and trusting relationships within the group, allowing each member to feel seen and acknowledged (e.g., Levine & Land, 2015, as cited in Mintarsih & Azizah, 2020). Sharing sessions in pairs, small groups, and/or the whole group can complete this activity.

Surfing the Waves

Practice Orientation and Type:
Self- to Self-Orientation – Guided Meditation[5]

Personal Practice

This practice draws inspiration from two classic Buddhist meditations originally introduced in the *Satipaṭṭhāna-Sutta* (e.g., Freese, 2023). These meditations are referred to as *ānāpāna-smṛti,* which signifies "mindfulness of breathing," and *vipaśyanā,* which signifies "insight" and "clear seeing."[6] With this practice, helping professionals are encouraged to observe their breath and accompanying bodily sensations in an equanimous and nonreactive way (Bhikkhu, 1980; Jeebodh-Desai et al., 2022; Kusala, 2020).[7]

Bodily sensations can be likened to ever-changing waves that you can symbolically learn to surf. Similar to waves, sensations arise, appear to stay the same for a while, and eventually fade away. Directly experiencing the transient nature of your shifting sensations opens a gateway to recognizing *anitya,* which translates to "impermanence" in Sanskrit. This understanding can, in turn, empower you to respond to your sensations in a composed and mindful manner (e.g., Harvey, 2013; Papies, 2016).[8]

Find a sitting posture that allows for both comfort and wakefulness. To minimize distractions, you are welcome to either softly close your eyes or, if you prefer, lower and relax your gaze. Gradually, bring your attention to the sensations of your breath naturally flowing in and out of your nostrils without trying to control your breath in any way.[9] As you settle into this practice, welcome a sense of grounding and presence as you anchor yourself in the here and now (De Tord & Bräuninger, 2015).

At some point, you may notice your attention drifting. If you do, bring your attention back, nonjudgmentally, to the naturally unfolding sensations of breathing while keeping in mind that when you fall out of presence with your breath, it is actually mindfulness that is bringing you back. Your intention, as such, is to become increasingly skilled at returning your focus to the sensations of breathing whenever you notice that you have become distracted.

With your breath as an anchoring point, start to cultivate an even deeper awareness of the natural ebb and flow of the sensations accompanying your breath, including subtle ones, within and around the area of your nostrils. This includes paying attention to such sensations as the temperature and the touch of each incoming and outgoing breath. Observe how these sensations naturally emerge and then gently subside as part of a continuously shifting, dynamic flow.

While observing your sensations, try to refrain from reacting to them by wishing them away or wishing that they stay. Simply observe, objectively and equanimously, whatever sensations are manifesting in the present moment in and around the area of your nostrils as these sensations arise and fade away like waves in the sea.

By developing experiential insight into the impermanence of your sensations, from the time they arise to the time they "merge back into the sea," you can cultivate greater composure. This, in turn, allows you to develop the ability (and privilege) to respond mindfully rather than automatically react to your sensations. Regardless of how high the waves are or how forceful they may be, they are inherently a part of the ocean – compassionately guiding each wave until it reaches the shore.

Self-Reflections

- As I transition out of this practice, can I maintain mindfulness of my sensations and their impermanent nature in an equanimous way?
- What is it like to be with and clearly feel a moment of discomfort without automatically reacting to it?
- "The repeated practice of mindfulness is a path that leads one to transcend self-focused needs and to increase one's prosocial disposition" (Mitra & Greenberg, 2016, p. 418) – How does this understanding resonate with my own experience?[10]

Group Context

Within a group setting, *Surfing the Waves* can be carried out as follows to further facilitate a shift in focus to encompass others:

The facilitator can invite participants to engage in the personal practice together, setting aside a few minutes at the beginning of group sessions for this shared experience. Practicing at the start of each session can serve as a settling-in exercise – a mindful transition that allows participants to arrive fully in the present moment. Moreover, this practice can set the tone for a cohesive and centered group experience, creating a safe container for authentic participation.

Significantly, even though each group member is directing their focus inward, this practice is inherently other-centered as well. By engaging in this practice alongside others, group members are collectively contributing to a mindful environment. This is because, as they deepen their own capacity to be mindful, they become better equipped to relate to others in a mindful way. Sharing sessions in pairs, small groups, and/or the whole group can complete this activity.

Finding Equilibrium

Practice Orientation and Type:
Self- to Self-Orientation – Visualization and Breath Awareness

Personal Practice

This practice, adapted from Halifax (2018),[11] draws inspiration from the Buddhist concept *strong back, soft front,* which relates to the relationship between equanimity and compassion, respectively. The strong back of equanimity is linked to the capacity to maintain patience and composure in the face of challenging experiences. Importantly, however, equanimity does not equate to passive acceptance of the status quo when change is necessary. Instead, it entails responding to challenges in a balanced way, which can ultimately enable more effective action.

Conversely, the soft front of compassion involves being receptive to things as they are, including vulnerability. It emphasizes accepting and being present with life's inherent challenges rather than turning away from them and wishing for a challenge-free existence. It is within this dynamic interplay between a receptive, compassionate attitude (a soft front) and equanimous resolve (a strong back) that the potential for meaningful, positive change can emerge.

The following visualization and breath awareness exercises aim to cultivate a harmonious balance between a *strong back* and a *soft front*:

Embodying centeredness – To connect with your strong back, practicing a variation of spinal breathing is recommended. This visualization and breath awareness technique, drawn from traditional yogic practices, invites you to envision the breath's ascent from the base of the spine to the crown of the head with each inhalation and its descent down the spine with each exhalation. Each natural breath cycle symbolizes the quality of centeredness in the face of life's ups and downs, fostering a connection with the metaphor of a strong back representing equanimity through life's challenges.

Embodying receptivity – As a reflection of your soft front, gently rest one or both hands on the front side of your body (i.e., your belly and/or chest).

This tactile connection serves as an embodiment of receptivity, with your breath flowing in and out like the ocean's tide and your hand(s) like the shoreline – compassionately receiving the ebb and flow.

Self-Reflection

• In what ways does equanimity enhance my capacity for compassion both toward vulnerability within myself and others?

Group Context

Within a group setting, *Finding Equilibrium* can be carried out as follows to further facilitate a shift in focus to encompass others:

The facilitator can encourage participants to engage in this practice together, allocating dedicated time for this shared experience. This practice can serve as a valuable exercise, accessible to participants not only during designated shared moments but consistently as a personal practice throughout the group sessions. It underscores the ongoing importance of cultivating equanimity and compassion both in active caregiving and within the group dynamics. Sharing sessions in pairs, small groups, and/or the whole group can complete this activity.

Grounding Connections

Practice Orientation and Type:
Self- and Other-Orientation – Guided Meditation and
Expressive Movement

Personal Practice

The concept of *grounding* originates from the word *ground*, referring to the earth's surface (Merriam Webster, 2024b). Within the framework of trauma-informed care, grounding signifies being physically, mentally, and emotionally well-balanced and engaged in the here and now (e.g., Clark & Sonsiadek, 2023; De Tord & Bräuninger, 2015; Meekums, 2002). This state of presence can be enhanced by consciously focusing on immediate sensory experiences and the process of breathing (De Tord & Bräuninger, 2015).

Accordingly, the following practice, which comprises two sequential steps, invites you to first focus on the connection between your feet and the ground while observing your breath and associated sensations. This preliminary grounding step then serves as a gateway to the second, where you will embark on a related symbolic visualization practice rooted in the act of grounding.

In a standing position, with your feet slightly apart and your arms resting by your sides, bring your attention to the connection between your feet and the ground. Take a few moments here, allowing your eyes to gently close, or alternatively, soften and lower your gaze. While standing in this grounded position, attend to the sensations in your feet, the nuances of weight distribution, and the gentle cadence of your breath. These elements provide an opportunity for you to center yourself, anchoring your awareness in the support of the ground beneath you, the sensations of your body, and the rhythm of your breath.

When you feel ready, you are invited to imagine roots extending out from the soles of your feet, like redwood tree roots. Redwoods are among the tallest trees in the world, yet, surprisingly, their roots are not very deep. What gives redwoods their strength is that their roots are intertwined with each other so that every redwood is interconnected with every other red-wood nearby. That is, their ability to stand tall and be resilient, even against the strongest storm, is due to their united interdependence.

Visualize your roots interlinked in this way and yourself, not apart, but a part of a community of redwoods. Then, gradually, begin to gently shift your weight back and forth and right and left, varying the direction and speed of your movements, much like a tree swaying in the wind. This intentional movement serves as a symbol of resilience and is a metaphor for achieving balance amid challenging or "stormy" circumstances.

Continue with this embodied visualization practice while raising your arms above your head. This gesture can serve as a symbol of how red-woods, connected to the ground and interconnected with each other, extend their branches, much like outstretched arms, toward the raindrops – as if to support and hold space for tears of trauma. Finally, as you lower your arms back down to your sides and return to center, allow the sense of grounding and connection to linger within you as you slowly open or raise your eyes again.

Self-Reflections

• Do I give myself mindful moments (even micro-moments) throughout the day to ground and reground by focusing on my body's "touch points" (e.g., sitting and feeling the support of my chair and/or noticing the connection of my feet with the floor; Salzberg, 2013, p. 63)?[12]
• Can I recall an instance when my ability to stay grounded in a challenging circumstance had a ripple effect, benefitting others as well?

Group Context

Within a group setting, *Grounding Connections* can be accompanied by the following yoga, *mudrā*, and visual arts activities:

The facilitator can invite participants to practice the yoga "tree posture" together (Skt. *vṛkṣāsana*; with *vṛkṣa* meaning "tree" and *āsana* meaning "posture"; e.g., Spence, 2021) while reflecting on their interconnectedness, much like a community of redwoods.[13] To practice, group members (a) begin by taking a few moments to feel their feet connected to the ground, (b) shift their weight onto their right foot while lifting their left foot, (c) bend their left leg and bring the sole of their left foot onto their inner right thigh (or lower according to each participant's comfort level), (d) raise both hands to their heart center in a prayer gesture (Skt. *añjali-mudrā*; Le Page &

Le Page, 2013),[14] (e) hold the posture for a few moments, while releasing any unnecessary tension, (f) come out of the posture by lowering their left foot back to the ground, and relaxing their arms by their sides, and finally (g) practice the posture on the other side while balancing on their left leg.[15] Notably, this yoga posture can likewise be practiced in pairs (Skt. *dvi vṛkṣāsana*; i.e., two tree posture).[16]

Akin to "peace poles" (*May Peace Prevail on Earth International*, 2020), another possible activity is for the facilitator to invite participants to create "compassion poles" by decorating wooden poles with creative elements and then "planting" (i.e., securely placing) them outside in a garden.[17] The act of symbolically "planting" the poles can serve as a reminder to remain grounded while also reinforcing the notion that the seed of compassion, like a perennial seed, takes time to establish and fully grow. However, when it is nourished and properly taken care of, it can grow into a flourishing ecosystem of support. Inviting participants to choose inspiring quotes to inscribe on their "compassion poles" is likewise recommended. This is similar to how the inspiring quote, "May peace prevail on earth," is inscribed on "peace poles" (*May Peace Prevail on Earth International*, 2020). A sharing session with the whole group can complete these activities.

redwood *dharma*...[18]
when challenges cloud your path,
remember your roots

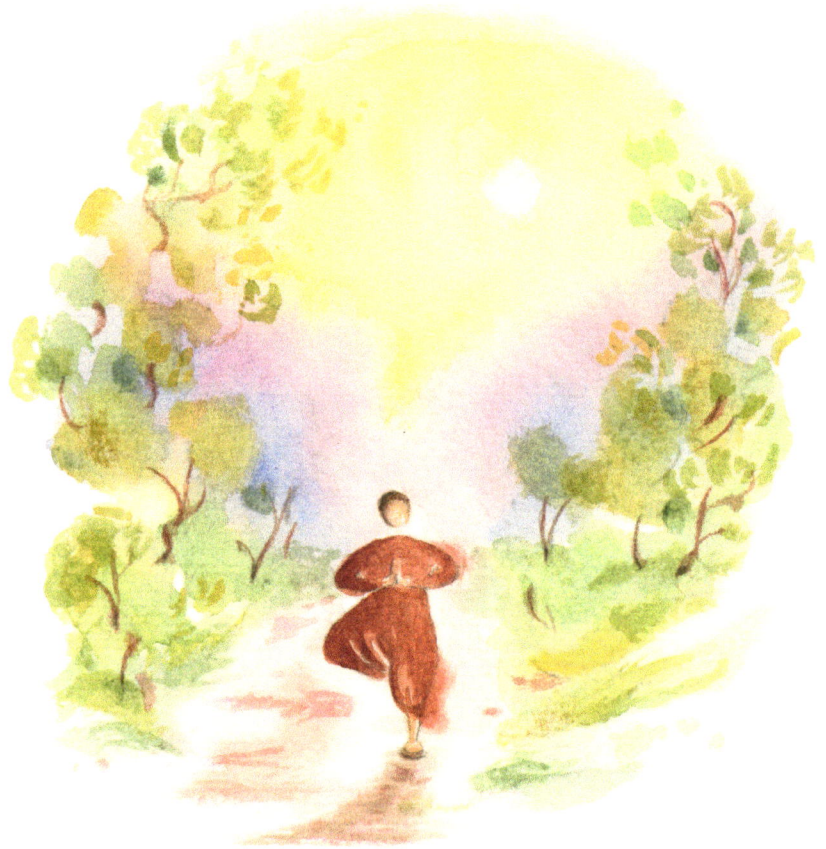

Inner Grounding

Figure practicing the tree posture in yoga

Recollecting Positivity

Practice Orientation and Type:
Self- and Other-Orientation – Reflection Prompts

Personal Practice

Working as a helping professional can be a profoundly rewarding experience in spite of the many challenges it may entail. In the midst of stressful work-related circumstances – and as a touchstone to return to even on the best of days – it helps to reconnect to your work-related resources. Such resources encompass everyone and everything that nurtures and supports your wellbeing at work.

Settle into a comfortable seated position that offers you optimal support. As you relax into stillness and presence with yourself, you are likewise invited to tune in to your bodily sensations. This is relevant as mindfully connecting to your *felt-sense* can enhance your experience of this practice (see Table 3). The term *felt-sense* refers to the bodily-felt awareness of a particular thought, emotion, or experience. It goes beyond intellectual understanding and involves tuning in to the sensations that arise in your body in response to different stimuli, resulting in a more holistic experience (Gendlin, 1988).

Table 3. Recollecting Positivity Reflection Prompts

	Breathing in Positivity	**Breathing out Positivity**
1.	What are you most grateful for with respect to your work?	In what way(s) do you contribute to a work environment for which others can be grateful?
2.	Describe work-related positive feedback that you have received.	Describe work-related positive feedback that you have offered others.
3.	What internal and/or external source(s) of strength do you draw upon at work?	In what way(s) are you a source of strength for others at work?

(Continued)

Table 3. (Continued)

	Breathing in Positivity	**Breathing out Positivity**
4.	Which of your talents and areas of expertise enhance the quality of your work?	Which of your talents and areas of expertise enhance the quality of your work environment?
5.	Highlight the qualities of someone who inspires you at work.	In what ways do you strive to be an inspiration for others at work?
6.	Describe how your work offers you opportunities for learning and growth.	In what ways do you contribute to a work environment of learning and growth?
7.	Recount one or more enjoyable moments that you experienced at work.	How do you contribute to an enjoyable work environment?
8.	Describe one or more rewarding experiences that you have encountered at work.	In what way(s) do you help facilitate rewarding workplace experiences for others?
9.	Describe how you have benefited from open lines of communication and effective collaboration at work?	In what way(s) do you contribute to open lines of communication and effective collaboration at work?
10.	What does your workplace already do well in addressing secondary traumatic stress (STS)?	How do you contribute to cultivating a work environment that addresses STS?

Note. The headings "Breathing in Positivity" and "Breathing out Positivity" refer to more inward- vs. outward-oriented reflections, respectively.

Self-Reflections

• Amid the daily challenges of caring for individuals who have experienced trauma – can I make it a practice to savor what went well today at work (i.e., savoring involves cultivating awareness of positive experiences as they occur; Neff & Germer, 2018)?[19]
• Have I taken time today to consider how my colleagues' workday is unfolding? Is there anything I can do to support or enhance their day in some way?

Group Context

Within a group setting, *Recollecting Positivity* can be carried out as follows:

The facilitator can invite participants to form two circles – one inward and one outward circle – with participants in the inner circle facing outward and participants in the outer circle facing inward. In this way, pairs are formed, with each pair comprising one member from the inner circle and one member from the outer circle facing each other.

Next, the facilitator can initiate the group activity by inviting partners to share their reflections regarding the first set of prompts (i.e., "What are you most grateful for with respect to your work?" and "In what way(s) do you contribute to a work environment for which others can be grateful?"). After a set duration, the facilitator can ask participants in the outer circle to move one step to their right, forming new pairs. This rotation process continues until participants have addressed all the prompts needed to complete a full circle. A sharing session with the whole group can complete this activity.

PRACTICES FOR ADDRESSING SECONDARY TRAUMATIC STRESS

DOI: 10.4324/9781003381747-8

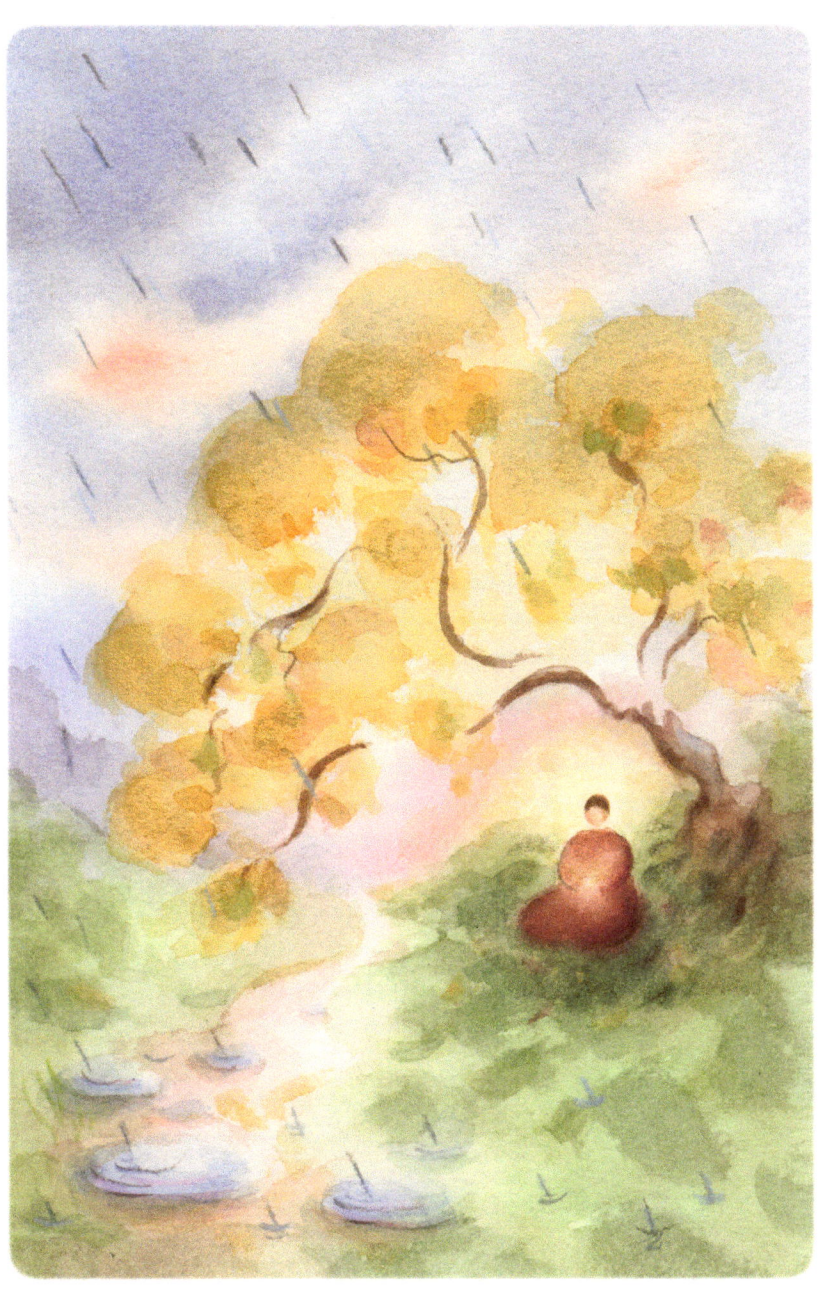

Sanctuary From the Storm

Figure sheltering under a tree

compassion takes flight,
guided by wisdom's insight:
two wings of a bird

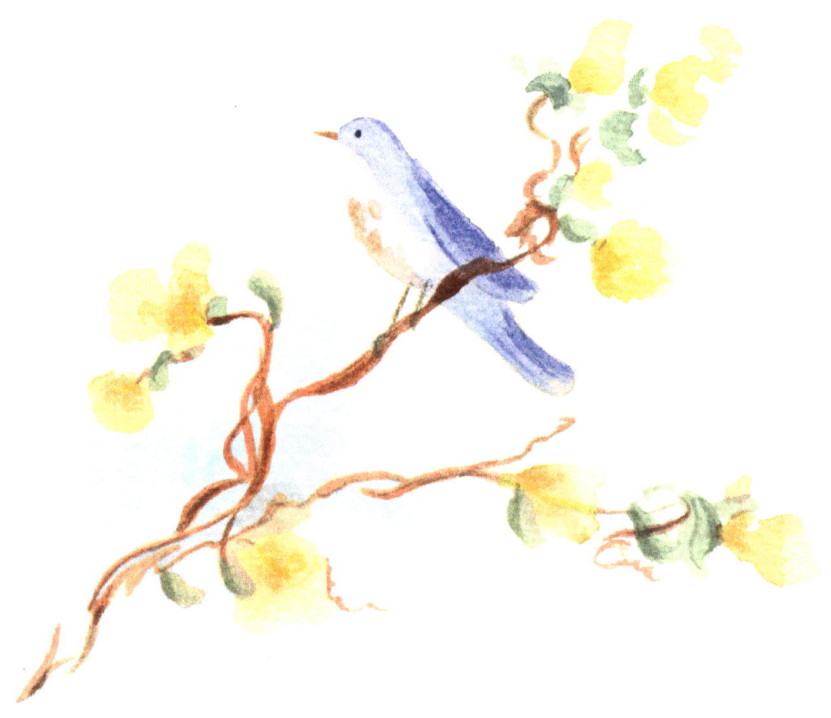

Wisdom and Compassion[1]

A bird resting on a branch with flowers

Lighting the Candle of Compassion

Practice Orientation and Type:
Other-to-Self and Self- and Other-Orientations – Guided Meditation

Personal Practice

The practice of *trāṭaka*, also referred to as concentrated gazing, is considered a cleansing technique in yoga that can assist helping professionals in achieving a state of one-pointed concentration by focusing on a single visual point.[2] In addition to improving concentration, *trāṭaka* has also been shown to enhance equanimity and mental calmness (Husain & Hasan, 2021; Senthil & Britto, 2022).

The object selected for the purpose of concentration should be small and can either be a virtual or real external object or an object that one visualizes internally. The Sanskrit terms for *trāṭaka* incorporating an external or internal object, respectively, are *bahir-aṅga* ("external") and *antar-aṅga* ("internal;" Patra, 2017). For illustration, an external *trāṭaka* candlelight gazing practice is described with a symbolic reference to compassion and secondary traumatic stress (STS).[3]

Candlelight can be likened to the light of compassion. Prior to lighting your candle, bring to mind one or more individuals who have offered you compassion and inspired your own desire to be compassionate. This offers you the opportunity to start this practice with a focus on receiving compassionate care. Then, as you light your candle, you can light it in honor of that lineage and as a tribute to your intention to address STS compassionately.

Subsequently, in a quiet and dimly lit space, sit in front of your lighted candle at a comfortable distance, with the flame preferably at eye level. Make sure your sitting posture is as comfortable as possible, with your head, neck, and back in alignment. Next, begin to gaze at the flame, and after a while, close your eyes and focus your attention on the flame's negative afterimage. With your eyes still closed, try consciously to bring the negative afterimage to the placement between your eyebrows, also referred to as the third eye.[4]

A negative afterimage is a visual illusion that is opposite in hue or brightness to the original stimulus (Merriam-Webster, 2024a). When you no longer see the flame's negative afterimage, you can continue this practice by starting another round. After completing several rounds, rub your hands briskly together in order to generate warmth. Then, gently cup the palms of your hands over your closed eyes, allowing your eyes to relax. When you feel ready, take a few deep breaths and gradually open your eyes again.

Throughout this process, you are invited to reflect on how the bright light of the candle's flame and the negative afterimage may be likened to compassion and STS, respectively. Namely, consider how the flame's negative afterimage, representing STS, gradually fades away, whereas the actual flame, representing compassion, continues to shine bright throughout this practice. You may likewise wish to consider how the colors within the flame come together to create the candle's bright light. Similarly, with respect to compassionately addressing STS, the collective benefits of compassion converge to create a transformative impact – benefiting both your personal wellbeing and your ongoing support for others.

Self-Reflection

• In line with the saying, "A candle loses none of its light by lighting another candle" (Renzenbrink, 2011, p. viii) – what steps can I take to embody this principle in the context of supporting others dealing with STS?

Group Context

Within a group setting, *Lighting the Candle of Compassion* can be carried out as follows:

The facilitator can invite participants to practice while sitting in a circle,[5] with a candle placed at eye level in the center of the circle. Alternatively, each participant can practice with their own candle within the group setting. This group practice can be complemented by inviting participants to tune in not only to their individual intentions but also to their shared intention, as a group, of compassionately addressing STS. Notably, this practice calls for a dim setting, which can potentially be triggering. Therefore, before dimming the lights, the facilitator should inform the group and seek their permission to proceed. Sharing sessions in pairs, small groups, and/or the whole group can complete this activity.

generosity –
candles shine just as brightly
when they share their light

Light of Compassion

Candlelights

Extending a Helping Hand

Practice Orientation and Type:
Self- to Self-Orientation – Guided Meditation and
Expressive Movement

Personal Practice

This practice, adapted from Brach (2019),[6] can support helping professionals in compassionately addressing secondary traumatic stress (STS). The five steps of this practice, all beginning with the letter "**I**," offer a memorable and practical framework: Identify, Include, Investigate, Imbue, and Implement. These steps serve as a reminder for helping professionals to remain mindful of their own wellbeing, ensuring that they can continue to extend a helping hand to those in their care.

Significantly, the visual metaphor of extending a helping hand can reinforce the idea that, just as your five fingers work together, these five steps are interconnected and essential for nurturing your wellbeing in light of STS. In this metaphor, each finger symbolizes one of the letter "I" recommendations, highlighting their collective role in supporting your inclusion within the circle of compassionate care you extend to others.

Find a comfortable sitting posture with your back, neck, and head aligned, and take a few deep and relaxing breaths. If you wish to close your eyes, you are welcome to do so to minimize distractions. When you feel ready, consider one or more clients who have experienced trauma and any STS-related thoughts, emotions, and underlying somatic sensations that you may be experiencing.

To differentiate between thoughts, emotions, and sensations – which is relevant as reactions to thoughts and emotions originate from reactions to sensations (Levine, 2010) – follow these steps: (a) become mindful of the narratives associated with your thoughts/emotions, (b) facilitate the release of these narratives, (c) redirect your attention to the realm of bodily sensations tied to these narratives, and (d) experience your sensations in a direct, physical manner.

Step 1: Identify

To help yourself identify STS-related sensations, you can ask yourself "what-" and "where-" rather than "why-" type questions. For example, "What sensations am I most aware of related to STS?" and "Where do I experience them in my body?" It may also be helpful to label each sensation (e.g., heaviness, numbness, pressure, tenseness, or tightness).

As you label your sensations in this way, pay attention to the language you choose to use. For example, to effectively label sensations, it is recommended that you use the phrase "I observe" rather than "I am." This approach avoids labeling yourself as the sensation and instead acknowledges this as an observation (e.g., "I observe tension" vs. "I am tense;" McHale, 2022). "A part of me is feeling . . ." or "'Something' inside is feeling . . .," are additional recommended phrasing possibilities, as they disentangle your wholeness from the experience (e.g., Dearly, 2019, p. 13).

Step 2: Include

If you identify STS-related sensations, include them in your awareness without ignoring, judging, or trying to control them in any way. Let your sensations be as they are. They may get stronger, stay the same, or change in additional ways. This step is important as self-compassion cannot come to full maturity if you reject or resist the reality of your own suffering (Super, 2015).

Step 3: Investigate

Gently bring your attention to your felt experience with kindness and curiosity, framing your felt experience as valuable data. Ask yourself related questions such as: "What is the most challenging sensation I am experiencing related to STS?" "If this sensation could communicate, what would it say/express?" and "What area of my body needs my attention so I can offer it attention and make choices from there?" See also if you can tell the difference between the objective sensations in your body and your subjective reactions to them.

Additionally, you can enter into an inner dialogue with your STS sensations. For example, by talking with the most challenging sensation as if it were a character. You could ask questions such as: "What are you trying to tell me?" "What do you need?" "How do you want me to be with you?" and "How can I help?" Finally, allow the sensation to respond, permitting yourself to be surprised by any insights that may emerge through this introspective dialogue.

Step 4: Imbue

As you become attuned to what your sensations related to STS are expressing, consider gently placing your hand on the area of your body where these sensations manifest, symbolically imbuing them with compassion. Take your time, allowing yourself to rest in the soothing comfort of your own compassionate presence. An example of a compassionate phrase that you may also wish to contemplate during this step is: "Compassion is guiding me through."

Step 5: Implement

Following the first four contemplative steps, if you feel inspired to do so, express your inner experience with an associated gesture or with authentic, expressive movement. The latter involves moving compassionately "from the inside out," focusing your attention on the present moment, and acting out your inner experience through improvised movement. Allow yourself to embody the STS-related compassionate care and let the gesture/movement soothe you like a breath of fresh air.

Self-Reflections

• As self-compassion can be practiced anywhere and at any time, can I practice a shortened version of this practice with my eyes open, even when I am actively caregiving (e.g., during the fourth and fifth steps of this practice, I might incorporate a simple gesture, such as giving myself a gentle hug)?[7]
• To what extent does self-compassion extend outward to create a more compassionate environment for those in my presence?

Group Context

Within a group setting, *Extending a Helping Hand* can be accompanied by the following visual arts activity to further facilitate a shift in focus to encompass others:

Participants can be encouraged to enhance their engagement with this practice by crafting an associated *maṇḍala,* meaning "circle" in Sanskrit. This artistic endeavor involves providing participants with visual arts supplies and having them draw a circle on a sheet of paper. Next, participants can be invited to partition their circle into six sections (not necessarily of equal size). Within each section, they can then artistically convey their experiences related to each of the five steps of this practice, including their reflections pertaining to expanding their compassion toward others as a sixth step. Following this creative expression, the facilitator can invite participants to share their *maṇḍalas* and associated reflections in pairs, small groups, and/or with the whole group.

Strengthening Inner Resolve

Practice Orientation and Type:
Self- and Other-Orientation – Guided Meditation

Personal Practice

This practice is inspired by the time-honored yogic tradition of *yoga-nidrā*. *Yoga-nidrā* – from the Sanskrit words yoga, meaning "union," and *nidrā,* meaning "sleep" – is recognized for its profound rejuvenating and self-transforming effects (e.g., Saraswati, 2009). This eight-step variation of the practice is tailored for compassionately addressing secondary traumatic stress (STS). Notably, the second step of this practice, which involves welcoming opposites, invites you to recall your STS experience.

The eight steps of this variation of *yoga-nidrā* include: (a) preparation, (b) welcoming opposites, (c) personal intention or resolution (i.e., *saṅkalpa*), (d) rotation of awareness, (e) breath awareness, (f) repetition of the personal intention or resolution (i.e., *saṅkalpa*), (g) completion, and (h) dedicating merits.

Prepare yourself for the practice of *yoga-nidrā*.

Step 1: Preparation

Find a quiet, uninterrupted space, and dim the lights to support drawing your attention inward. Set up the space so that you can relax comfortably on your back by placing a yoga mat beneath you. You may also choose to cover yourself with a blanket for warmth and place another folded blanket or cushion under your knees for support. If you wish, you can place a cushion under your head for comfort and an eye cushion over your eyes to enhance relaxation. With your feet slightly apart and your palms facing upward by your sides, scan your body for areas of tension or discomfort.

Step 2: Welcoming Opposites

Gradually shift your focus toward recalling the experience of STS. To facilitate this process, the progressive muscle relaxation technique can be utilized, as it has been recommended for addressing STS (Sprang et al., 2019). In line with this technique, you are invited to tense each of the following muscle groups deliberately and hold the tension, simulating the experience of STS, for a period of several seconds.

These muscle groups include: (a) the right foot and leg, (b) the left foot and leg, (c) the chest, belly, and back, (d) the right hand and arm, (e) the left hand and arm, (f) the shoulders, and finally (g) the face (McCallie et al., 2006). After tensing each muscle group, release the tension, focusing your attention on each muscle group as it relaxes, and gradually allow the sense of relaxation to envelop you. Feel the relaxation spreading throughout your body while maintaining wakefulness and focus. If necessary, adjust your posture accordingly so you are as comfortable as possible.

Step 3: Personal Intention or Resolution

Create your *saṅkalpa* – that is, a few positively phrased words in the present tense associated with self-compassionately addressing STS, such as "Compassion is guiding me through." Inwardly repeat your *saṅkalpa* three times to yourself.

Step 4: Rotation of Awareness

Allow your awareness to rotate throughout your body, and feel each part of your body as you rest on your back.

Begin with the right side of your body:

Feel your right-hand thumb, first finger, second finger, third finger, fourth finger, four fingers and thumb together, palm, back of hand, right wrist, lower arm, elbow, upper arm, right shoulder, right armpit, right chest, right side waist, right hip, right upper leg, knee, lower leg, ankle, heel, top of foot, sole of foot, right big toe, second toe, third toe, fourth toe, fifth toe, five toes together – whole right side of the body.

Repeat with the left side of your body:

Feel your left-hand thumb, first finger, second finger, third finger, fourth finger, four fingers and thumb together, palm, back of hand, left wrist, lower arm, elbow, upper arm, left shoulder, left armpit, left side chest, left side waist, left hip, left upper leg, knee, lower leg, ankle, heel, top of foot, sole of foot, left big toe, second toe, third toe, fourth toe, fifth toe, five toes together – whole left side of the body.

Now, bring your awareness to the back of your body:

Feel your right lower back, left lower back, right middle back, left middle back, right upper back, left upper back, right shoulder blade, left shoulder blade, spinal cord, back of the neck, back of the head – whole back side of the body.

Next, bring your awareness to the front of your body:

Feel the top of the head, forehead, right temple, left temple, right ear, left ear, right eyebrow, left eyebrow, space between the eyebrows, right eye, left eye, bridge of the nose, right nostril, left nostril, tip of the nose, right cheek, left cheek, upper lip, lower lip, chin, jaw, neck, right collarbone, left collarbone, right side of chest, left side of chest, center of chest, navel, abdomen – whole front side of the body.

Finally, widen your awareness to your whole body:

Feel the whole right leg, whole left leg, whole right arm, whole left arm, whole head, whole face, whole torso – whole body.

Step 5: Breath Awareness

Become aware of your breath as it flows in and out of your nostrils and as it moves naturally through your body. There is no need to alter the rhythm or depth of your breath. Allow yourself simply to feel its natural flow and observe it as it is without any effort to change or control it.

Step 6: Repetition of the Personal Intention or Resolution

Come back to the *sankalpa* that you created in the third step of this practice (e.g., "Compassion is guiding me through"). Inwardly repeat your *sankalpa* three more times to yourself.

Step 7: Completion

Reconnect with the sensation of your breath flowing in and out of your nostrils. As you maintain awareness of your breath, notice your bodily sensations as well. Notice the weight of your body as it rests on the mat and focus your awareness on all the points that are in contact with the mat (e.g., the back of your heels, thighs, upper back, arms, hands, and head).

Before opening your eyes, visualize your surroundings. Imagine where you are and the objects that are around you. Rest quietly until you feel ready to move. Then, start by wiggling your fingers and toes, taking your time and stretching slowly. Finally, gently roll to one side and sit up. Sit silently for a few more moments with your eyes still closed and with the palms of your hands resting on your lap.

Step 8: Dedicating Merits

If you recognize any positive effects from this practice, consider symboli-cally sharing these benefits with someone who might find them beneficial. In your mind's eye, picture this person receiving and experiencing the posi-tive benefits of your compassionate offering. When you feel ready, gradu-ally open your eyes again.

The practice of *yoga-nidrā* is now complete.

Self-Reflections

- If I were to wake up tomorrow morning and realize that STS has sub-sided, how would I know? What would be different?
- What was my experience of dedicating the merits of my practice to others?

Group Context

Within a group setting, *Strengthening Inner Resolve* can be carried out as follows:

The facilitator can incorporate the *yoga-nidrā* practice into the group context by first creating a supportive and safe environment for partici-pants. Beginning with an introduction to the practice's purpose and emphasizing the voluntary nature of participation, participants can be encouraged to find a comfortable posture while being mindful of indi-vidual preferences. Additional recommendations include making modifi-cations for participants who wish to practice with their eyes open or in a seated position (e.g., Treleaven, 2018). Through these preliminary steps, which include seeking participants' permission before dimming the lights, the facilitator can set the stage for a meaningful *yoga-nidrā* experience. Sharing sessions in pairs, small groups, and/or the whole group can com-plete this activity.

Reciting a Mantra

Practice Orientation and Type:
Self- and Other-Orientation – Reflection Prompts

Personal Practice

In this practice, adapted from Neff and Germer (2018) to compassionately address secondary traumatic stress (STS),[8] helping professionals are guided to create their own personalized STS-related self-compassion mantra. The term *mantra*, rooted in Sanskrit and denoting an "instrument of thought," refers to one or more phrases that can be committed to memory and inwardly recited as needed. Utilizing a self-compassion mantra can prove beneficial when facing distressing sensations, thoughts, emotions, and/or behaviors triggered by STS.

An example of a four-line STS-related mantra follows. This mantra aligns with the three elements of self-compassion described by Neff and Germer (2018), namely mindfulness, common humanity, and self-kindness, while also embracing an altruistic orientation:

This is a challenging situation.
(mindfulness)
Other caregivers experiencing STS may feel similarly challenged.
(common humanity)
May I offer myself the compassion I need —
(self-kindness)
And extend it forward to others.
(altruistic orientation)

Self-Reflections

• What are the consequences of engaging in negative STS-related self-talk?
• How might reciting an STS-related self-compassionate mantra better serve me and those with whom I interact?
• What is my experience of integrating self-compassion into a broader understanding of compassion for others?

Group Context

Within a group setting, *Reciting a Mantra* can be carried out as follows:

After participants have created their own STS-related mantras, they can be invited to anonymously write down their mantras on separate pieces of paper and place them into a designated container. Once all the mantras are collected, each participant can take a turn choosing a mantra from the container and reading it aloud to the group. As participants listen to and share each other's mantras, they can gain a sense of common humanity, recognizing that their fellow group members are facing similar challenges related to STS. This group-sharing session can provide a platform for validation, inspiration, and collective growth within the group.

Transforming Technique

Practice Orientation and Type:
Self- to Self-Orientation – Guided Meditation

Personal Practice

This practice, adapted from the Applied Compassion Training (ACT, 2021) at Stanford University's Center for Compassion and Altruism Research and Education (CCARE),[9] fosters acknowledging, expressing, and verbally releasing challenging secondary traumatic stress (STS)-related sensations, thoughts, feelings, and experiences. Verbally expressing in this way may reduce activity in the amygdala and increase activity in the prefrontal region of the brain, thereby diminishing emotional reactivity and producing a calming effect (e.g., Lieberman et al., 2007).[10]

Moreover, this practice can help train your mind to overcome its innate negativity bias by shifting your focus to positive intentions and qualities. Negativity bias refers to our tendency as humans to place more significance on negative events compared to positive or neutral ones. This is due to evolutionary and neurological factors, as our brains are naturally inclined to be more acutely attuned to negative events for the sake of survival (Norris, 2021).

The following four steps describe this transformative practice:

Step 1: Express Challenging STS Reactions

In a comfortable sitting position, take a few deep breaths to begin this practice. When you feel ready, place both hands on your lap, with your right hand facing upward in a loose fist. With your eyes preferably closed, verbally express, in the first person, one or more challenging STS reactions you may be experiencing. Speak out loud, even though you are practicing this technique on your own while imagining that your right hand is symbolically holding your STS-related challenges.

While speaking, try to remain aware of your bodily sensations. If distressing emotions arise, pause and allow yourself to mindfully experience the bodily sensations associated with these distressing emotions until the sensations become less intense or subside.[11] Likewise recommended is to name distressing emotions (i.e., affect labeling; e.g., "Fear is arising," or "This is sadness") while taking into account that the idea is not necessarily to feel better but to become better at feeling. To conclude this step, take a few deep, cleansing breaths.

Step 2: Connect to Intention and Positive Qualities

Form a loose fist with the palm of your left hand facing upward. Then, verbally articulate a future scenario where you have already compassionately addressed STS (i.e., express this scenario audibly in the present tense). Moreover, from this vantage point, describe the positive qualities you are now able to access within yourself. In essence, you are encouraged to speak as if your intention and positive attributes have already manifested. To conclude this step, take a few deep, relaxing breaths.

Step 3: Integrate with Compassion

Open your right hand and place your right palm, symbolically holding your STS reactions, at heart center, allowing your compassionate heart to hold them metaphorically. Then, open your left hand and gently place your left palm, over your right hand, at heart center. With this gesture, you symbolically and compassionately welcome your positive intentions and qualities into your heart as well. Continue holding both hands in this way at heart center, and take a few deep, calming breaths.

Step 4: Compassionate Response and Acceptance

Lower both hands to your lap, with your palms facing upward, and take a few more deep breaths. Consider what compassionate responses you might choose to move your present situation forward in alignment with your intentions, taking your positive qualities into account. While keeping in mind that some circumstances may be beyond your control, consider also saying words such as, "These are my STS reactions, these are my positive intentions and qualities, and these are my compassionate responses." After speaking such phrases out loud, rest with your palms on your lap facing upward, inviting acceptance. Conclude this practice by taking a few deep, rejuvenating breaths, and then gently open your eyes again.

Self-Reflections

• What step(s), no matter how small, can I take today to help turn my intended compassionate responses into a reality?
• Is there a colleague I can compassionately share this technique with who might benefit from its application?

Group Context

Within a group setting, the *Transforming Technique* can be carried out as follows to further facilitate a shift in focus to encompass others:

After explaining and demonstrating the technique, the facilitator can invite participants to form pairs and together practice two rounds of this technique. This allows each participant the opportunity to both practice and serve as a facilitator. As facilitators, participants are instructed to lead the practice while refraining from unnecessary conversation and remaining mindfully aware of their own as well as their partner's experiences.

Having group members facilitate a practice themselves offers several additional benefits. For example, it can (a) empower participants by giving them the opportunity to take an active role in guiding others, (b) encourage a sense of shared responsibility within the group, (c) foster an inclusive environment where everyone has a chance to contribute, (d) deepen participants' understanding and mastery of the practice, and (e) inspire creativity and innovation as participants bring diversity and fresh insights into the practice. Lastly, after each round, pairs can be invited to debrief, and once participants have completed the rounds, a group sharing session can complete this activity.

Inspiring Rituals

Practice Orientation and Type:
Self- and Other-Orientation – Reflection Prompts

Personal Practice

Making compassion a daily practice is an important key to nurturing compassion for secondary traumatic stress (STS). Cultivating compassion for STS requires time and dedication, just as a skill becomes refined through repeated practice. This is so, as each repetition strengthens relevant key neural circuits – like strengthening your compassion muscle at the gym. It is also valuable to emphasize that rather than being a fixed attribute that one either has or does not have, compassion is a quality that can be cultivated through practice (e.g., Hanson, 2009).[12]

The following morning and evening rituals can help make STS-related compassion practices an integral part of your day:

Morning intention practice – Morning sets the tone for the rest of the day. After you wake up, take a moment to set an intention that will inspire and guide your actions throughout the day.[13] Consider the words you might speak and the actions you might take to treat both yourself and others experiencing STS with compassion in the face of STS challenges.

Evening dedication practice – Take a few moments each evening before you go to sleep to reconnect with your morning intention and reflect on your day. Did you have the opportunity to act with compassion toward yourself and others dealing with STS? How much alignment was there between your morning intention and the way your day actually unfolded? Rejoice in whatever you achieved, keeping in mind that every day offers a chance to reaffirm your intentions.

Self-Reflections

• What will help me incorporate this morning intention and evening dedication practice into my schedule?

• Considering my existing commitments and obligations, what can help me maintain this practice over time for the ultimate benefit of survivors of trauma?

Group Context

Within a group setting, *Inspiring Rituals* can be accompanied by the following reflection prompt and guided meditation:

As some participants may find it challenging to include STS-related compassionate practices into their daily routine, the facilitator can encourage them to first reflect on the following sentence stem: "I give myself permission to . . ." Participants can then complete this sentence stem by reflecting on the self- and other-oriented compassionate actions that they wish to undertake, but for some reason are resisting (e.g., Brown, 2017).[14]

Next, the facilitator can invite participants to assume comfortable seated positions, preferably with their eyes closed, and guide them as follows:

Envision a gentle, calmly flowing river, symbolizing your STS-related self- and other-oriented compassionate intentions. Now, imagine the riverbanks that frame this river. These riverbanks represent your morning intention and evening dedication practice, which serve to support your intentions "flowing" on course throughout the day. Take a deep breath, inhaling the tranquility of this imagery, and release any unnecessary tension as you exhale. With your intentions at the forefront of your mind, visualize how you move through your day, compassionately responding to both your own and your colleagues' STS challenges. Picture yourself embodying compassion in this way, and trust that the river, supported by its riverbanks, flows steadily within you . . .

riverbanks embrace
morning's promise, evening's grace –
compassionate flow

Sharing sessions in pairs, small groups, and/or the whole group can complete this activity.

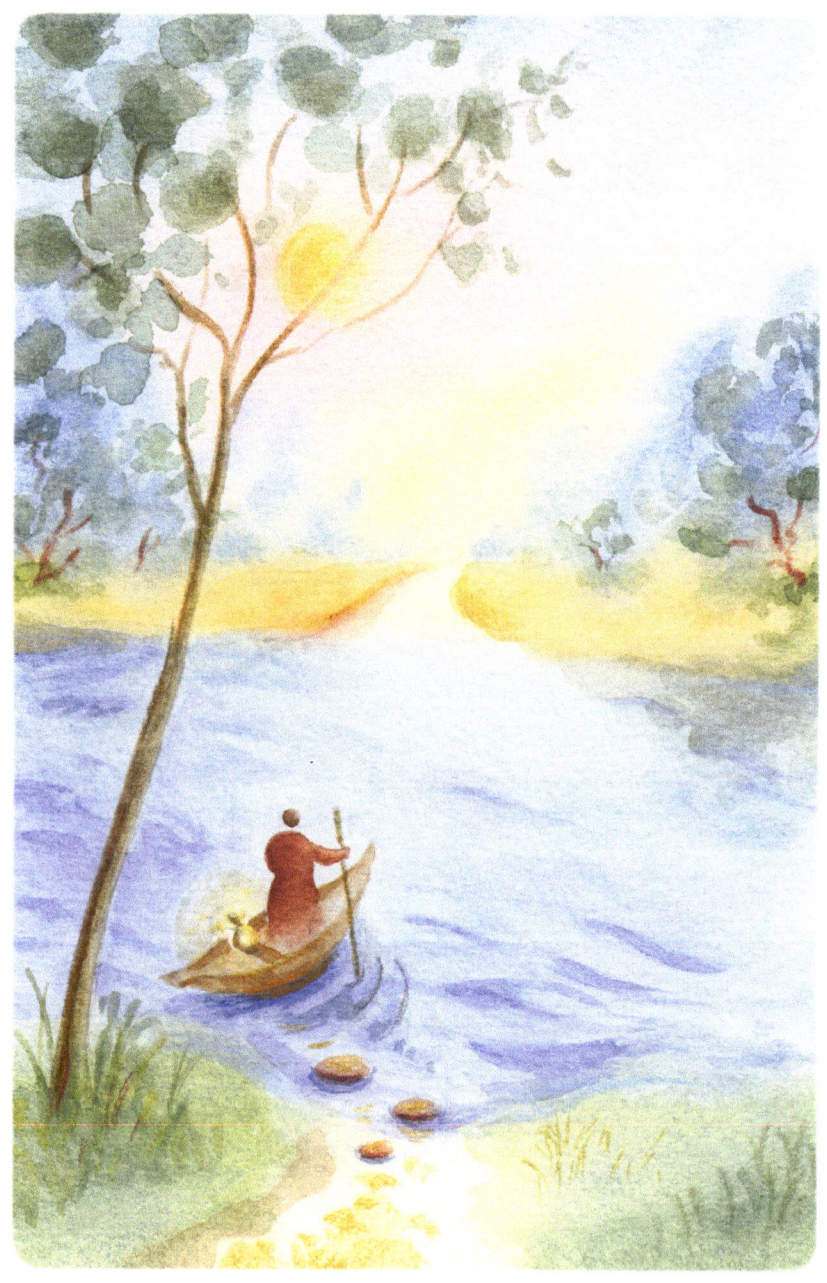

River Crossing

Figure crossing a river in a small boat

Turning Toward vs. Away

Practice Orientation and Type:
Self- to Self-Orientation – Journaling Prompts

Personal Practice

In this practice, the concept of "turning away" signifies a tendency to avoid or ignore secondary traumatic stress (STS)-related vulnerability, whereas "turning toward" represents embracing STS-related vulnerability with self-compassion. "Turning away" may manifest through maladaptive stress responses (e.g., denial and/or social withdrawal), while "turning toward" involves self-compassionately acknowledging vulnerability and actively engaging in compassion-based practices as an empowering coping strategy (e.g., Atkins et al., 2019; Hayes, 2020; Polk et al., 2016).

The notions of "turning toward" vs. "turning away" are closely related to the concepts of *approach coping* vs. *avoidant coping*, respectively. The former involves proactively engaging with the somatic, cognitive, emotional, and behavioral aspects of stressful experiences in order to promote trauma processing.

By contrast, the latter involves defensive tendencies, such as trying to ignore or distort aspects of one's experience in an attempt to divert attention from stressors and minimize immediate distress. Although avoidant strategies may provide temporary relief, they are often maladaptive in the long run as they fail to address the underlying stressors, which may persist or even worsen over time (Moos, 2002, as cited in Maddock, 2023; Rauch & Foa, 2006).

Notably, "turning toward" can likewise signify welcoming challenging sensations, thoughts, and emotions via a gentle "Yes-And" approach.[15] Here, the "Yes" serves to validate STS-related reactions, while the "And" serves to reorient you toward a beneficial, compassionate response (Polk et al., 2016, p. 13). Ultimately, this approach can enhance your ability to navigate STS with increased equanimity and resourcefulness (e.g., "Yes, I am experiencing STS, and I will respond with compassion").

Settle into a sitting position that allows you to maintain an upright posture comfortably. Place your attention on your breath to help anchor yourself within the present moment. As thoughts and feelings come into your mind, become aware of these phenomena and gently return your focus to each cycle of breath. This process of returning to the breath cultivates a foundation of calmness and concentration. Gradually, when you feel ready, transition into the following six-step practice presented via the acronym TOWARD (see Table 4).

Table 4. Turning Toward vs. Away Journaling Prompts

Letter of Acronym	Journaling Prompts
T	*Turn within* – Begin by recalling times in your life when you encountered vulnerability (not related to STS) and reflect on whether your tendency was to turn away or toward it.
O	*Observe Reactions* – Notice your sensations, thoughts, and emotions as you reflect on the first step of this practice.
W	*Write Compassionately* – Express your observations with self-compassion, capturing the nuances of your experience in a written format.
A	*Assess Orientation* – Within the context of STS, evaluate whether you tend to lean toward avoiding or accepting vulnerability.
R	*Revisit Reactions* – Observe your inner landscape, connecting with STS-related sensations, thoughts, and emotions.
D	*Detail Insights* – Conclude by articulating your insights regarding STS in writing in a self-compassionate manner.

Self-Reflections

- Do I experience any warning signs leading to "turning away" behavior associated with STS (e.g., anxiety, fatigue, and/or overwhelm)?
- Do I experience "turning away" behavior associated with STS (e.g., using distractions to avoid STS sensations, thoughts, and/or emotions)?
- What can best help me minimize STS-related "turning away" tendencies, ultimately enabling me to be more fully present?
- If I tend to "turn away" from acknowledging STS-related vulnerability in others, how can I cultivate "turning toward" them with compassion instead?

Group Context

Within a group setting, *Turning Toward vs. Away* can be accompanied by the following activity to further facilitate a shift in focus to encompass others:

The facilitator can invite participants to use their journaling as storytelling prompts in pairs or small groups. Before starting, participants should be guided to incorporate low-impact debriefing recommendations in order to reduce listeners' exposure to traumatic information. As described by Mathieu (2012), low-impact debriefing involves four sequential steps that pertain to the individual who is sharing: (a) increased self-awareness, (b) giving others fair warning, (c) waiting for their consent, and (d) limiting disclosure.

Participants, thereby, have the opportunity to "story themselves" in a mindful, regulated, and trauma-informed way. This can help facilitate a gradual transition from "turning away" tendencies to "turning toward" STS-related vulnerability. The practice of self-narration serves as a catalyst for this transition, allowing participants to potentially uncover deeper insights, challenge unhelpful patterns, and cultivate compassion in response to STS.

Interestingly, the facilitator can also promote taking a "step outside the story line," aligning with the concept of *dereification* (Dunne & Manheim, 2023, p. 2381). This concept is defined as "the degree to which thoughts, feelings, and perceptions are phenomenally interpreted as mental processes rather than as accurate depictions of reality" (Lutz et al., 2015, p. 21). In other words, dereification involves the ability to engage flexibly with various lines of thought without presuming that any particular line of thought is the exclusive truth (Lutz et al., 2015).[16]

Meanwhile, listeners can be encouraged to remain mindful of their own inner reactions; and respond by listening compassionately, not interrupting the shared narratives, and reflecting back a compassionate gesture and/or appreciative verbal feedback.[17] Regarding compassionate listening, Hạnh (2001, p. 98) offered the following guidance:

"Deep listening, compassionate listening is not listening with the purpose of analyzing or even uncovering what has happened in the past. You listen first of all in order to give the other person relief, a chance to speak out, to feel that someone finally understands . . . During this time, you have in mind only one idea, one desire: to listen in order to give the other person the chance to speak out and suffer less . . . First of all, listen with compassion."

A sharing session with the whole group can complete this activity.

Healing Hands

Practice Orientation and Type:
Self- and Other-Orientation – Guided Meditation

Personal Practice

The first part of this practice guides helping professionals to self-compassionately address secondary traumatic stress (STS) by incorporating self-holding gestures that provide a sense of security and calm (e.g., Dana, 2020; Davis, 2017; Dreisoerner et al., 2021; Huseinagić & Hodzić, 2008; Seoane, 2016; Tal, 2006).[18] The practice then transitions to focus on *karuṇā-mudrā,* encompassing both self- and other-oriented compassion (i.e., in Sanskrit, *karuṇā* means compassion, and *mudrā* denotes specific hand positions or gestures; Le Page & Le Page, 2013). Notably, in the context of this practice, self-compassion is offered in light of STS, and compassion for others is directed toward clients with a history of exposure to trauma and/or colleagues experiencing STS.

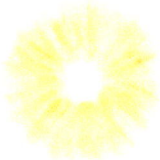

To begin this practice, find a comfortable sitting position, and, if you wish, gently close your eyes while directing your attention toward your breath. After taking a few deep and intentional breaths, take a moment to recall individuals in your care who have a history of exposure to trauma and/or colleagues experiencing STS. Recall aspects of their trauma-related narratives, paying attention to any associated somatic sensations that you may perceive as uncomfortable while observing your sensations as they are.

Gradually, begin to rub your hands together to generate warmth. Then, explore which self-holding gestures might feel genuinely comforting and supportive. Some possibilities of offering yourself compassion in this way include holding the area of your body that is experiencing discomfort, placing one hand on your heart and the other on your abdomen as a self-holding gesture, or giving yourself a gentle hug. Interestingly, even when you only imagine these gestures, they can offer stress-buffering effects (Jakubiak & Feeney, 2016).

Next, consider holding your hands together in *karuṇā-mudrā* as follows:

With both hands gently cupped, place your left fingertips at the base of your right fingers. Then, rest your left thumb's outer boarder alongside the outer boarder of the lower part of your right thumb (the left thumb's upper digit should be resting on the right thumb's lower digit). Hold your hands in front of your chest, near your heart center, and slowly rotate the gesture so that the left palm is oriented more toward your heart center (as a symbol of self-compassion) and the right palm is facing slightly outward (symbolizing compassion for others).

Hold this *mudrā* for several slow, deep breaths, reflecting on the interconnectedness of self-and other-oriented compassion. You may also wish to consider the symbolic significance conveyed through the positioning of your hands. In this *mudrā,* self-compassion serves as the foundation upon which compassion for others rests, with compassion for others held higher up and altruistically poised to reach out and uplift those in need.[19]

Self-Reflections

• As I engage in this practice, do any attachment-related challenges emerge, and if so, how can I compassionately address them?[20]
• What is my experience of self-compassion as the foundation for extending compassion to others?

Group Context

Within a group setting, *Healing Hands* can be accompanied by the following expressive movement activity:

Participants can be invited to create various symbolic hand formations as a group while standing in a circle, reinforcing their collective efforts in cultivating self- and other-oriented compassion. Some hand formation possibilities include: (a) joining hands to create a unified/interconnected circle, (b) extending palms toward the center of the circle to symbolize unity, and (c) elevating hands upward to embody a sense of aspiration and growth. Given that this activity involves physical contact, participants' consent is necessary. Notably, if participants agree, the facilitator can photograph the hand formations they create as a group. These photographs, capturing moments of collaboration and shared intention, allow for visual documentation of their collective commitment to address STS compassionately. A sharing session with the whole group can complete this activity.

Embodying a Path to Compassion

Practice Orientation and Type:
Self- to Self-Orientation – Expressive Movement and
Journaling Prompts

Personal Practice

This practice offers helping professionals a kinesthetic perspective for self-compassionately addressing secondary traumatic stress (STS). It involves exploring how the following manifest expressively through movement: (a) STS, (b) the path leading from STS to self-compassion, and (c) self-compassion itself. Feel free to use the provided journaling prompts (see Table 5) to gain deeper insights into your experience. Also, feel free to incorporate music to complement your movement. No prior background in dance/movement is necessary.

During the first three steps of this practice, you are encouraged to engage in authentic and spontaneous movement expressions rather than relying on preplanned choreography. Then, in the fourth step, you are invited to create a choreographed movement sequence that incorporates the previous steps. In this context, a movement sequence refers to a connected series of movements that embody and communicate inner experiences through the language of movement.

Choose whether to begin this practice standing, sitting, or lying down. As an initial grounding practice, take a few deep breaths, allowing your body to relax. Focus your attention on the connecting points between your body and the ground. Notice the bodily sensations that accompany the feeling of support beneath you and recognize that your connection to the ground is a source of stability and safety. Inwardly saying to yourself, "I am" with each inhalation and "here" with each exhalation, as an anchor, is likewise encouraged (e.g., De Tord & Bräuninger, 2015; Spence, 2021). Gradually, when you feel ready, proceed with the following four-step practice:

Step 1: STS Movement Exploration

Reflect on your experience of STS, and create a movement sequence that symbolizes and embodies it. Allow your body to guide you in an authentic and improvised manner, using gestures, postures, and movements to express your experience.

Step 2: Path from STS to Self-compassion Movement Exploration

Imagine that you are embarking on a journey from STS to self-compassion, and create a movement sequence that represents this transition. Significantly, if you experience natural somatic release responses such as sighing, crying, or shaking during this step, embrace them and let them occur. By welcoming and honoring such natural bodily expressions, you create space for the release of pent-up STS-related reactions (e.g., Levine, 2010).

Step 3: Self-compassion Movement Exploration

Focus on cultivating a self-compassionate response to STS and create a movement sequence that embodies this compassionate response. Allow your body to express gestures, postures, and movements that align with self-compassion. Importantly, let yourself explore movements that symbolize comforting, soothing, and validating yourself (i.e., tender self-compassion) or alternatively, protecting, providing for, and motivating yourself (i.e., fierce self-compassion; Neff, 2021).

Step 4: Integrated Movement Sequence

Combine the previous three movement sequences into a cohesive sequence. The goal is to create a seamless flow that represents the process of acknowledging STS, finding a path from STS to self-compassion, and embodying a self-compassionate response to STS. You can practice refining this integrated sequence, allowing it to become a more fluid movement narrative.

The following journaling prompts can help you further explore and integrate your experience in relation to this expressive movement practice:

Table 5. Journaling Prompts for Embodying a Path to Self-Compassion

Step	Journaling Prompts
1.	Describe the movement sequence you created to simulate your STS-related experience.
	Did any specific movements resonate strongly with your experience of STS? If so, please describe them.
2.	Describe the movement sequence you developed to symbolize the path from STS to self-compassion.
	What is the symbolic meaning behind the movement sequence marking the transition from STS to self-compassion?

(Continued)

Table 5. (Continued)

Step	Journaling Prompts
3.	Describe the movement sequence you created to embody a self-compassionate response to STS.
	Were there specific movements that stood out as particularly reflective of self-compassion? If so, please describe them.
4.	What added value did expressing your entire journey from STS to self-compassion through movement have for you?
	When reflecting on the four steps of this embodied movement practice, what insights have emerged for you?

Self-Reflections

• What expectations, if any, did I have before I began this expressive movement practice, and how do I feel after completing it?
• What gestures, postures, and movements would I choose to illustrate the path from self-compassion to compassion for others?

Group Context

Within a group setting, *Embodying a Path to Compassion* can be complemented by the following movement and visual arts activities to further facilitate a shift in focus to encompass others:

The facilitator can invite participants to share their integrated final movement sequences with each other in pairs while further extending their sequences to incorporate gestures, postures, and movements that symbolize compassion for others. Partners can be encouraged to illustrate what they observe through a variation of *blind contour line drawing*. This can be carried out by partners abstractly illustrating the movement with single pencil strokes without lifting their pencils from the paper or diverting their gaze from the movement (e.g., Dobkin, 2022; Murphy, 2021).

After each presentation, while still in their respective pairs, "movers" can engage in a reflective sharing process. In response, "observers" can be encouraged to share their drawings and articulate their kinesthetic empathy experience, which involves experiencing empathy solely by observing the movement of another individual (Lauffenburger, 2020). "Observers" can also add a compassionate gesture and/or appreciative verbal feedback.[21] For example, they may reflect back on one aspect of the movement that they genuinely found inspiring and/or meaningful. A sharing session with the whole group can complete this activity.[22]

Breathing Compassion

Practice Orientation and Type:
Self- and Other-Orientation – Guided Meditation and
Visualization and Breath Awareness

Personal Practice

Adapted from Neff and Germer (2018) to compassionately address secondary traumatic stress (STS),[23] this practice can help ensure that helping professionals remember to include themselves within the circle of compassion they offer others. As this practice involves deep breathing, it is also valuable to mention that research demonstrates that deepening your breath can potentially help you shift from a stress to a relaxation response (Perciavalle et al., 2017).

Find a comfortable sitting posture with your back, neck, and head aligned and your hands gently resting on your lap. Close your eyes or lower and soften your gaze, and consider synchronizing your breath with a gentle inward count of four for each inhalation and each exhalation for several cycles of breath. As you do so, mindfully release any lingering tension and allow your breath to flow with simplicity and ease.

Gradually, with each incoming breath, imagine that you are breathing in compassion for yourself for any STS-related reactions you may be experiencing, feeling the quality of compassion with each inhalation. It may also be helpful to imagine a compassionate image flowing in on your incoming breath.

Next, consider your outgoing breath and call to mind either a client who has experienced trauma or a colleague experiencing STS. Visualize your client or colleague clearly in your mind's eye and begin directing your out-breath toward this individual, offering them compassion with each exhalation. It may also be helpful to imagine a compassionate image flowing out on your outgoing breath.

Now, shift your focus to the sensations of breathing both in and out. Inhaling STS-related compassion for yourself and exhaling compassion for your client or colleague, for the trauma or STS-related reactions they may be experiencing, respectively.

Feel your breath flowing in and out like an ocean tide, and yourself, a part of, rather than apart from, this limitless flow. Drawing from this well-spring of compassion, if additional clients and/or colleagues come to mind, you are invited to share compassion with them, too, with each exhalation. Slowly, when this practice feels complete, take a few deep and refreshing breaths and gently open or raise your eyes again.

Self-Reflections

- "There is the in-breath and there is the out-breath, and it's easy to believe that we must exhale all the time, without ever inhaling. But the inhale is absolutely essential if you want to continue to exhale" (Brown, 2017, p. 147). What are my perspectives regarding this metaphor?
- The in-breath and out-breath are distinct yet interconnected. What insights emerge when I reflect on self-compassion and compassion for others as similarly intertwined?

Group Context

Within a group setting, *Breathing Compassion* can be carried out as follows:

The facilitator can invite participants to practice one or both of the following practice variations: (a) *practicing individually* – with each participant practicing independently within the group context, and/or (b) *practicing together* – with participants sitting in a circle and practicing breathing in compassion for themselves and out for the entire group. Expanding this practice to compassionately encompass a wider circle of helping professionals, even those who may be unfamiliar to participants, is likewise encouraged. A sharing session with the whole group can complete this activity.

Flowing RIVER

Practice Orientation and Type:
Self- and Other-Orientation – Reflection Prompts

Personal Practice

This practice is based on the premise that just as a river nourishes the land-scape through which it flows, helping professionals are naturally imbued with compassion by nurturing compassion for others. Reilly and Stuyvenberg (2023) similarly suggested that practices focusing on other-oriented compassion may also increase self-compassion. In other words, "it is in the giving that we receive,"[24] or to paraphrase Saraswati (2021, p. 290) – as we embrace the world with loving compassion, we are included within that very embrace.

The five steps of this practice, presented via the acronym RIVER (see Table 6), offer a memorable and inspiring framework for reexamining the interdependence between self- and other-oriented compassion and how this may be relevant for compassionately addressing secondary traumatic stress (STS). As an initial step, dedicate time to the simple yet profound act of "just sitting." As you sit in stillness, cultivate an open awareness, allow-ing your thoughts to flow like a gentle river without clinging to any specific thought/mental narrative.[25] Gradually, following your own pace, transition into the subsequent steps of this practice:

Table 6. RIVER Reflection Prompts

Letter of Acronym	Reflections
R	Recall one or more clients who have a history of exposure to trauma.
I	Inwardly cultivate compassion for your client(s).
V	Visualize how compassion flows through you toward your client(s).

(Continued)

Table 6. (Continued)

Letter of Acronym	Reflections
E	Embrace the idea that just as a river nourishes the landscape through which it flows, you are being nourished by the compassion that flows through you.
R	Reflect on how you might incorporate this insight into your understanding of STS-related self-compassion.

Self-Reflections

- Are there additional metaphors that come to mind to describe how the flow of compassion toward others not only nurtures them but also has the potential to nourish my own inner landscape, including my experience of STS?
- In line with the following haiku, what is it like for me to practice integrating self-compassion and compassion for others without drawing a clear line between them?

> compassionately,
> self and other harmony:
> rivers merge as one

Group Context

Within a group setting, *Flowing RIVER* can be carried out by incorporating the following visual arts activity:

After the five steps of this practice, the facilitator can invite participants to gather around a large sheet of paper. Participants can then be encouraged to collectively sketch the outline of a winding river, symbolizing the flow of compassion that they extend to those in their care.

Next, each participant can select a section of the river to focus on and express their creativity by drawing their section of the river and its surrounding landscape. This landscape serves as a visual representation of the inherent benefits of being a conduit through which compassion flows.

The facilitator can further prompt participants to consider how well their drawings interconnect. This focus on interconnectedness can nurture a shared sense of purpose among participants, reinforcing their mutual commitment to providing compassionate care. Sharing sessions in pairs, small groups, and/or the whole group can complete this activity.

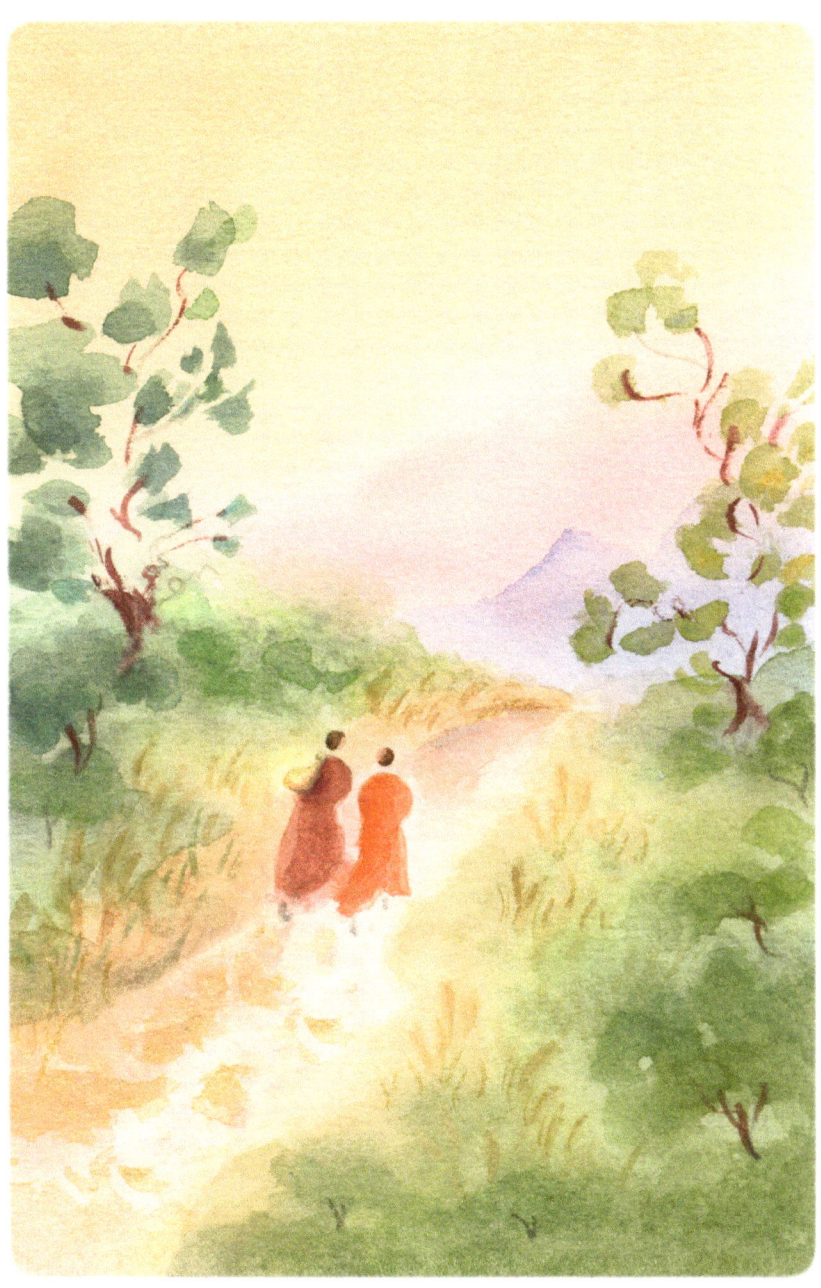

Together on the Path

Two figures walking on a path

Identifying Compassionate Words

Practice Orientation and Type:
Self- to Self-Orientation – Reflection Prompts and
Various Creative Expressions

Personal Practice

Helping professionals may struggle with negative self-talk when confronted with secondary traumatic stress (STS)-related challenges. In such cases, this internal dialogue can perpetuate a negative self-fulfilling prophecy. Compassionate self-talk can counterbalance this inclination. As you consistently embrace such positive self-expression, it can gradually become your default approach when navigating challenges associated with STS (e.g., Latinjak et al., 2023).

Find a comfortable sitting position, letting your hands rest comfortably on your lap. With your eyes preferably closed, take a few deep breaths, inhaling through your nostrils and exhaling through your mouth. While breathing out, let a soothing sigh accompany your breath, allowing this moment to bring a sense of calm and presence to your practice.

When you feel ready, consider what compassionate words you would like to hear from a trusted other with respect to the STS-related challenges you are facing. For example, you may wish that someone would show solidarity with your compassionate STS-related intentions, endorsing self-compassion as an altruistic self-care approach that can sustain the compassionate care you offer survivors of trauma.[26] As Graff (2020) eloquently expressed, "For helping professionals, restoring compassion requires seeing ourselves as recipients, not just dispensers of compassion. We are like a conduit through which compassion flows" (p. 145).

Give yourself the opportunity to receive such self-compassionate words in the context of STS. This can manifest in diverse ways, such as reading an associated poem, listening to meaningful song lyrics, or reflecting on inspiring quotations that include the compassionate messages you wish to hear. While considering that this self-compassion practice is rooted in the altruistic intention of ultimately sharing compassion with others, explore different avenues to find what resonates most deeply with you, what nurtures you, and what uplifts your spirit.

Self-Reflections

• What STS-related compassionate words do I wish to receive from a trusted other, and can I compassionately extend such words to myself?
• What compassionate words can I offer others experiencing STS?

Group Context

Within a group setting, *Identifying Compassionate Words* can be accompanied by the following role-playing activity to further facilitate a shift in focus to encompass others:

The facilitator can utilize the psychodrama technique known as *doubling,* as it is applicable for addressing trauma and STS (e.g., Chesner, 2020; Kraybill, 2015). In line with this modified version of the technique, participants form groups of three wherein each participant is designated one of the following roles (i.e., to foster a well-rounded experience, participants are encouraged to switch between these roles):

• *The protagonist* – The participant in this role describes one or more STS-related symptoms in a trauma-informed manner and articulates their desired response(s) from a trusted source.
• *The double* – The participant in this role metaphorically "steps into the protagonist's shoes" whenever the double senses it would be beneficial, assisting the protagonist in articulating their STS-related desired response(s) from a trusted source.
• *The witness* – After the protagonist and the double have completed their interaction, the participant in this role offers appreciative feedback, emphasizing what they perceive the protagonist most wishes to hear from a trusted source.[27]

Importantly, before sharing, the protagonist is encouraged to identify a personal quality (e.g., courage) to support them throughout this process. This initial step holds significance as it enables the protagonist to tap into their personal resources. By acknowledging and embodying their chosen quality, the protagonist creates a self-affirming environment for effective communication.

Regarding the double, the participant in this role should seek the protagonist's consent before speaking. This step ensures that the protagonist maintains agency and control throughout the process. The double then compassionately speaks on behalf of the protagonist, using the first-person perspective. The double's role, as such, is to serve as a compassionate mirror, reflecting the protagonist's needs, with the ultimate goal of deepening the protagonist's awareness with respect to the compassionate words they wish to hear.

The protagonist can then choose to incorporate the double's words, either by echoing the central message or by adapting the message to better resonate with their own feelings. The protagonist may alternatively be inspired to voice their inner wishes independently. Throughout this process, the double can stand alongside the protagonist, offering a reassuring presence.

Following the protagonist and the double's interaction, the participant in the role of the witness provides positive feedback. This feedback can focus on what the witness believes the protagonist most wishes to hear from a trusted source. In this way, the protagonist has the opportunity to listen to their own compassionate words reflected back to them compassionately. Sharing sessions in groups of three and/or the whole group can complete this activity.

Letting the Words Sink in

Practice Orientation and Type:
Self- to Self-Orientation – Journaling Prompts

Personal Practice

This practice, adapted from Neff and Germer (2018),[28] invites helping professionals to compose a compassionate message in response to their secondary traumatic stress (STS)-related challenges. Moreover, in line with Howe's insight (as cited in Joyce, 2010, p. 16) that "letters are sounds we see," helping professionals are encouraged to reflect not only on the literal meaning of their compassionate message but also on how the words might be conveyed. This includes considering subtle aspects such as intonation and the emphasis placed on certain words or phrases. This perspective is expected to facilitate a deeper internalization of the essence of the compassionate message.

Envision yourself receiving a compassionate message from an actual or imaginary colleague – someone who understands the challenges you have faced or are currently facing concerning STS. As you write to yourself from this perspective, try to write with a sense of your colleague's care and best wishes for your wellness and health. Also, considering how your colleague might help you, describe the compassionate suggestions they may offer.

After you finish writing, read and reread the message several times, allowing the compassionate words to resonate fully.[29] As you do so, tune into subtle nuances such as the tone of voice in which you imagine the message would be communicated, allowing the full resonance of the compassionate expression to sink in. To effectively address STS, actively putting into practice compassionate suggestions that are mentioned in the message would likewise be advised.

Self-Reflections

• How can I deepen my sense of interconnectedness during this practice to avoid self-objectification? In this context, self-objectification signifies treating myself as a separate "other" to whom compassion is directed, which contradicts the interconnected and nondualistic perspective found in Buddhist teachings.

• As the compassionate message related to STS sinks in, what new possibilities arise?

• Do I know a colleague dealing with STS to whom I could respond in such a compassionate way?

Group Context

Within a group setting, *Letting the Words Sink in* can be accompanied by the following activity to further facilitate a shift in focus to encompass others:

Participants can be prompted to form pairs and share all or parts of their compassionate messages with each other. This sharing process allows participants to cultivate a more profound understanding that their fellow group members are navigating similar challenges related to STS and may be equally open to receiving support. As participants realize that others share similar needs, it can nurture an atmosphere of mutual support and compassion within the group. This, in turn, can stimulate the exchange of valuable insights and strategies to address these shared challenges collectively.

While listening to each other, participants can engage in *embodied listening*. This comprises a whole-bodied approach to listening that involves being fully attuned to one's own bodily sensations as well as to the nonverbal communication cues of the individual who is speaking. Additional listening recommendations include: (a) aligning eye level with the speaker, (b) making and maintaining eye contact, and (c) remaining still while listening (i.e., avoiding unnecessary movements or distractions to fully engage with the speaker; Mundle & Smith, 2013). After listening in this way, listeners can be encouraged to respond with a compassionate gesture and/or appreciative verbal feedback.[30] Sharing sessions in small groups and/or the whole group can complete this activity.

Journaling Journey

Practice Orientation and Type:
Self- to Self-Orientation – Journaling Prompts

Personal Practice

A secondary traumatic stress (STS)-related self-compassion journal is dedicated to compassionately enhancing helping professionals' wellbeing in light of STS. When beginning your journaling, it can be beneficial to utilize journal prompts, as prompts can provide you with ideas and inspiration for writing, help you stay focused on a specific topic, and encourage you to explore new perspectives. In time, feel free to expand your journaling experience by incorporating different types of journaling prompts, such as sentence starters, thought-provoking quotes, and picture-prompts.[31] These supplementary prompts can serve as creative catalysts for your journaling practice (e.g., Cutler et al., 2014; Shannon et al., 2014).

Find a quiet place to sit and let your attention turn inward, becoming aware of your body's breathing. In this state of relaxed attentiveness, choose one or more of the following journaling prompts to reflect on and write about:

• Looking back, what STS-related self-compassionate guidance would you have given yourself when you began your career as a helping professional?
• List one obstacle that hinders your ability to approach STS with self-compassion, and consider two potential solutions to initiate the process of overcoming this obstacle.
• Imagine a memoir about your life. What title would you give the chapter that encompasses your experience with STS? Does self-compassion play a role in this chapter?
• List sources of stress in your life (excluding STS) and propose specific self-compassionate actions to address them, recognizing that lightening these stressors may indirectly ease STS.

Self-Reflection

- We are all stars in the same sky, lighting our way together. Given the interdependence of my wellbeing with others, in what ways does this journaling practice help me sustain my compassionate care of others?

Group Context

Within a group setting, *Journaling Journey* can be carried out as follows to further facilitate a shift in focus to encompass others:

Participants can be invited to "write alone together," which signifies that each participant journals independently within the supportive group environment (Cutler et al., 2014, p. 18). The following three-step group activity can provide a practice ground/safe harbor for journaling, with the journaling prompts providing added structure and containment:

Step 1: Time for Writing

The facilitator can begin by suggesting a timed writing session centered around one or more of the journaling prompts. Timed writing involves setting a time limit, which can encourage free-flowing expression, reduce self-editing/self-censorship, and help group members place an emphasis on the writing process rather than on the final product.

Step 2: Time for Sharing

After journaling, participants can reflect on their writing experience and then share their journaling entries, a portion of their writing, or even just a few words in pairs or small groups. This process can enable insights to surface in those who choose to share. It can likewise serve as a learning opportunity for listeners who may resonate with and gain clarity from the shared reflections.

Step 3: Time for Feedback

Journaling can be a catalyst not only for personal growth but also for meaningful conversations and mutual support. In this stage of the practice, participants can be invited to offer each other appreciative verbal feedback, fostering a sense of connection and compassionate reinforcement. This way of interacting with fellow group members honors who they are and what they have shared.[32] Notably, feedback need not focus on grammar, spelling, and/or punctuation. A sharing session with the whole group can complete this activity.

Externalizing STS

Practice Orientation and Type:
Self- to Self-Orientation – Reflection Prompts

Personal Practice

The following is a self-compassion-based visualization and externalization practice for addressing secondary traumatic stress (STS). Regarding visualization, evidence suggests that "vividly imagining a situation simulates that experience in the brain as if it were, to a degree, actually happening" (Wilson-Mendenhall et al., 2023, p. 2532). The concept of externalization is beneficial as well, as it can help you perceive the externalized issue with enhanced objectivity and assist you in distinguishing your identity from the challenges at hand (e.g., White & Epston, 1990). This perspective is valuable as it can help you perceive STS-related challenges as distinct rather than intrinsic and unalterable aspects of yourself.

The following five steps, all starting with the letter "**C**," provide a coherent framework and help in easy memorization of the steps:

Step 1: Commencing the Practice

Find a quiet and comfortable space, settle into a relaxed seated position, and come into stillness. In this relaxed posture, simply observe your breath without attempting to alter it in any way, paying close attention to the subtle sensations associated with each inhalation and exhalation. Mindfully fostering a connection with your breath and bodily sensations allows you to immerse yourself in the here and now.

Step 2: Concentrating on Your Felt Experience

Bring to mind a client who has experienced trauma, along with one or more aspects of their traumatic narrative. Pay attention to any ensuing physical sensations related to STS that may be causing you discomfort, and notice where these sensations are most noticeably located.

Step 3: Considering STS as External to Yourself

Contemplate the attributes that most accurately symbolize your physical experience of STS, such as shape, size, weight, color, and/or movement, and then visualize these attributes as a tangible image. For instance, if you identify "heaviness" and "darkness" as key attributes, you might imagine STS as a dense, grey cloud. Then, gradually visualize this symbolic form, representing STS, externalized in front of you, and compassionately ask it questions such as: "What do you need?" and "How can I help you?"

Step 4: Changing Places

Imagine yourself answering the questions you previously posed from the perspective of the externalized form representing STS: "What I need is . . .," and "It would be helpful if you could . . ." Try to answer in as much detail as possible, and notice if your initial STS-related physical sensations are transformed by this process in any way.

Step 5: Coming out of the Practice

Take a moment to reconnect with your surroundings by visualizing the space you are in. When you feel ready, gradually open your eyes and allow your gaze to seek out something with which you resonate positively. Let this visual focal point inspire optimism, reinforcing your commitment to compassionately address STS in line with any insights you may have gained from this practice.

Self-Reflections

• The concept of *decentering* refers to the metacognitive awareness that thoughts and emotions are essentially no more than mental events transpiring within your mind. Consequently, decentering involves adapting a more objective or impartial stance toward these mental processes, potentially allowing for a more objective and balanced perspective (Papies, 2016). Decentering, as such, can be viewed as a form of externalization as it can enable you to metacognitively observe thoughts and emotions without necessarily automatically identifying with them.

Reflecting on the metacognitive concept of *decentering*, to what extent can its practice potentially help me manage STS-related distressing reactions?

• In what ways can subtle changes in the language I use to refer to STS help me recognize that STS is not an inherent reflection of my character or capabilities (e.g., "STS is causing me to feel hypervigilant" vs. "I am hypervigilant")?

• What will help me keep in mind that STS-related challenging behaviors in colleagues are not necessarily reflective of their inherent character or capabilities?

Group Context

Within a group setting, *Externalizing STS* can be accompanied by the following visual arts activity to further facilitate a shift in focus to encompass others:

After participants have had a chance to practice individually within the group setting, the facilitator can introduce the following activity, providing a creative outlet for externalizing STS. This activity calls for participants to depict, via the use of visual arts, the attributes and/or associated images that most accurately symbolize their experience of STS. This can be done figuratively or abstractly.

When participants complete their artwork, the facilitator can invite them to sit in a relatively large circle, with a group member volunteering to position their artwork at the center of the circle. This artwork then serves as the starting point for a meaningful connection-building group activity intended to leverage the common humanity element in self-compassion – reinforcing the idea that "we are all in this together."

As the circle of participants views the artwork in the center of the circle, each member of the group can be encouraged to consider their own artwork and whether it resonates in some way with the central piece. If a participant feels that their artwork shares a connection with the central one, they are invited to place their own artwork next to it. This process continues as each participant takes their artwork and, guided by their own sense of connection, places it alongside any artwork already within the circle.

As this process draws to a close, time for silent observation can provide participants with the opportunity to absorb the intricate tapestry of interconnected experiences more fully. During this pause, participants can also be invited to reflect on how this activity ultimately fosters greater compassion for others, creating ripples of care that extend beyond the self. Sharing sessions in pairs, small groups, and/or the whole group can complete this activity.

Composing a Haiku

Practice Orientation and Type:
Self- to Self-Orientation – Poetic Expression

Personal Practice

In this practice, you are invited to create a haiku – a traditional Japanese poetry form – as a means of self-compassionately addressing secondary traumatic stress (STS). This approach is consistent with the idea that poetry can be a valuable resource for helping professionals seeking to process and heal from STS. As Sax (2019) explained, "Poetry holds, for many, the power of processing and healing from trauma" (para. 4).

An English-language haiku is typically an unrhymed short poem consisting of 17 or fewer syllables, usually arranged in three lines, following a five-seven-five syllable count, respectively. While this definition provides a starting point, it is oversimplified, as there are facets to haiku that may be more significant than syllable count (Haiku Society of America, 2004).

Writing a haiku provides a path for you to highlight a now-moment of insight, in which mother nature and human nature intertwine (Kelsey, 2020). Moreover, haiku has been defined as comprising two elements: "an experience and an expression of that experience in words, after it has passed through the poet's heart" (Gurga, 2003, as cited in Kelsey, 2020, para. 13).

To find inspiration for your haiku, immerse yourself in a natural setting, recognizing that noticing nature, intentionally and preferably every day, can help you foster a deeper connection with the world around you. The natural world offers countless opportunities for observation and reflection and can serve as a profound source of inspiration for the creation of haikus (Antonelli et al., 2022).

For a meaningful haiku-writing experience that delves into the world of STS while drawing inspiration from the natural world, consider the following example. This haiku captures the essence of compassionately addressing trauma (including STS):

> transforming trauma
> through tears, compassion blossoms:
> the lotus flower

In this haiku, the lotus flower is used as a symbol of compassionately trans-forming trauma (e.g., Hạnh, 2014). Mirroring the lotus's emergence, tears born from trauma carry their own symbolic significance. They serve as a natural release of pain and thereby embody the capacity for healing and growth (Levine, 2010).

Self-Reflections

- Are there additional forms of poetry or creative writing that I would like to try as a way of self-compassionately addressing STS?
- Can I reach out to a colleague who is navigating STS and share my haiku with them as a gesture of extending compassion?

Group Context

Within a group setting, *Composing a Haiku* can be carried out as follows to further facilitate a shift in focus to encompass others:

The facilitator can suggest that participants compose their haikus as part of the group session and, if the circumstances allow, offer participants the opportunity to compose their haikus in a natural setting nearby. The latter option allows for a potentially deeper immersion into the creative process, encouraging participants to engage in mindful observation, deep contem-plation, and poetic expression in nature.

Once the haikus are written, participants can create a "Poet-tree" by carefully hanging their haikus on a designated tree outdoors or on a cre-atively crafted tree indoors. This group activity not only decorates the "Poet-tree" with poetic beauty but also serves as a shared reflection. As more haikus find their place on the "Poet-tree," it becomes an evolving tes-tament to the common humanity within the group (e.g., De Britos, 2016).

When group members recognize that they are not alone in their STS-related struggles, this activity can enhance their compassion toward them-selves and also create a natural bridge for the flow of compassion toward others. In this way, self-compassion becomes a catalyst for the development of compassion for others, nurturing a sense of interconnectedness within the group. Sharing sessions in pairs, small groups, and/or the whole group can complete this activity.

stillness…
bluebird resting on a branch:
nature's poetry

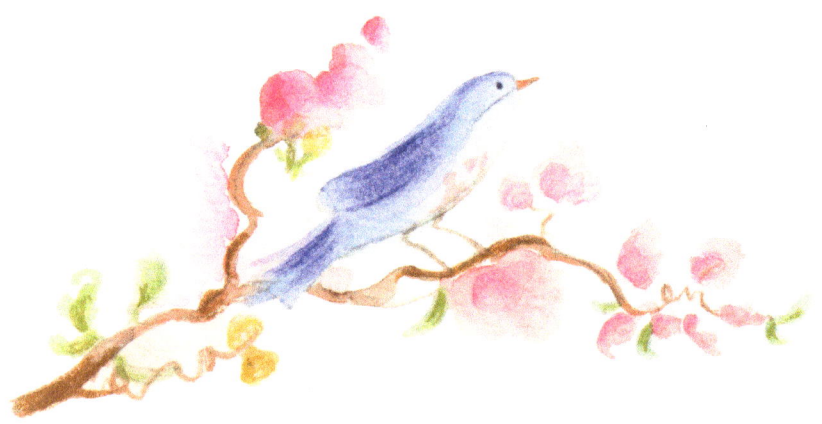

Time to Pause

A bird perched on a branch with flowers

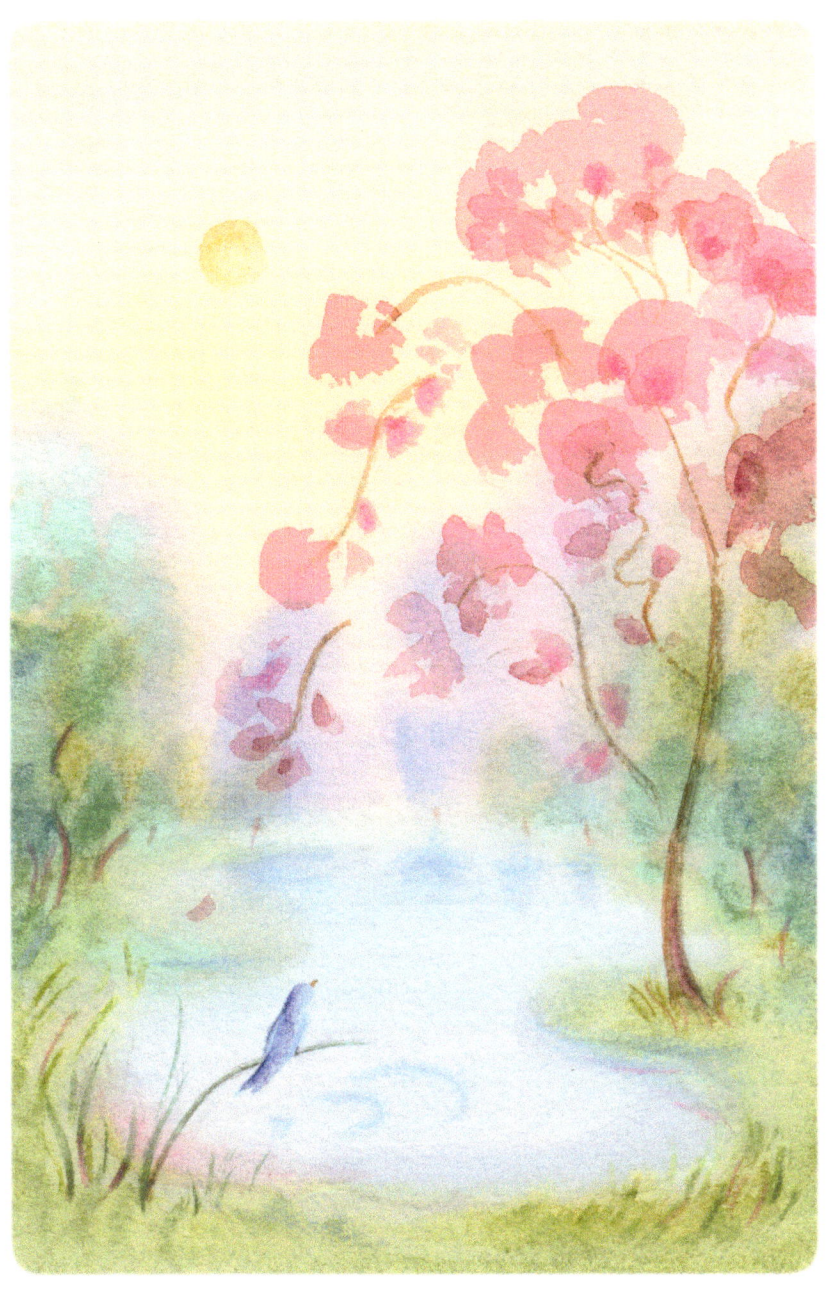

Mother Nature

A nature scene overlooking a lake

Preparing a Playlist

Practice Orientation and Type:
Self- to Self-Orientation – Musical Expression

Personal Practice

In this practice, adapted from Rook (2016),[33] helping professionals are invited to create a personalized playlist as a way of self-compassionately addressing secondary traumatic stress (STS). Listening to music has been shown to have a positive impact on reducing physiological arousal and regulating the autonomic nervous system after experiencing stressful events (Dana, 2020; Yehuda, 2011). Studies have likewise demonstrated that individuals who have experienced trauma can benefit from music-based therapy (Landis-Shack et al., 2017; Yehuda, 2011). Encouraging helping professionals to develop a playlist may enable them to realize some of these therapeutic benefits (Landis-Shack et al., 2017).

When selecting music for your playlist, begin by bringing a gentle awareness to your current sensations, thoughts, and emotions. Are you experiencing STS symptoms? In what ways would you like to feel better? Select music that will gradually bring you to your goal, whereby the music first resonates with how you currently feel, and then transitions to how you wish to feel. In other words, before attempting to improve your mood with music, try to mindfully and empathically match it.

Consider the following musical elements, as they can help you prepare your playlist:

• *Harmony* is a musical element that represents unity, cohesion, and consonance, embodying a sense of agreement and coherence within a composition. When creating your playlist, consider the role of harmony in the music you select. For example, if STS leads you to feel detached or disconnected from others, your playlist could start with music that creates a sense of discord or dissonance, gradually shifting toward more harmonious melodies.

- *Texture* in music refers to the manner in which various musical elements are combined and layered together within a composition. When creating your playlist, consider the role of texture in the music you select. For example, if you are feeling overwhelmed by intrusive thoughts due to STS, you might start your playlist with music that has a complex texture that resonates with that experience. Then, gradually shift toward music with a simpler texture, which can act as a form of relief and release from that experience.
- *Tempo* is a musical element that indicates the speed or rhythmical pace of a given musical composition. When creating your playlist, consider the role of tempo in the music you select. For example, if you are experiencing physiological reactions such as a rapid heart rate or hypertension due to STS, you might first resonate with music that has a faster tempo and gradually shift to slower-paced music.
- *Dynamics* is a musical element that denotes the intensity of a musical composition. When creating your playlist, consider the role of dynamics in the music you select. The music you select can be suddenly shifting or gradually changing and can help to create a sense of tension or release. For example, if you are feeling jumpy and quick to startle due to STS, and your goal is to induce a feeling of relaxation – you might consider choosing music that gradually diminishes in intensity, resulting in a more refined dynamic range.
- *Volume* is a musical element that relates to the loudness or softness of a musical composition. When creating your playlist, consider the role of volume in the music you select. For example, if you are having difficulty experiencing positive emotions due to STS, you might choose to start your playlist with a lower volume level and end your playlist with a higher volume to help boost your energy and mood. Alternatively, you might feel that beginning with louder music better reflects the challenges you are presently facing and that a lower volume offers you relief.

Furthermore, incorporating music without lyrics can help you avoid "hermeneutic contamination." This signifies that word-free music can expand your experience, as your rational mind is not constrained to following the content of the words (Theodore, 2020).[34] Additionally, consider that although sad music could be expected to induce parallel feelings of sorrow or melancholy in listeners, it has been shown to be associated with positive emotional effects such as regulation of distressing emotions, consolation, and compassion (Taruffi & Koelsch, 2014). Huron and Vuoskoski (2020) discussed this counterintuitive phenomenon in their pleasurable compassion theory.

Self-Reflections

- What title best captures the essence of my playlist?
- Do I observe any changes in my breathing, muscle tension, or heart rate from my playlist's beginning to its end?
- Would I like to share my playlist with a colleague as a supportive gesture?

Group Context

Within a group setting, *Preparing a Playlist* can be carried out as follows to further facilitate a shift in focus to encompass others:

The facilitator can invite participants to prepare a short playlist at home and then share their playlists within the group. Group sessions do not need to focus entirely on the playlists. Each session could include a "playlist sharing" ritual in which one or more participants share their playlists with the group, including their experience of curating their playlists and the personal stories behind the music they selected.

Listening to fellow group members' playlists can invoke compassion in listeners (e.g., McDonald et al., 2022). As participants share their playlists, it opens a window into their world and allows for deeper connections to form. Consequently, listeners are presented with the opportunity to gain insights into their peers' experiences with STS, enabling them to respond with compassion in kind. This compassionate exchange can be facilitated during a group sharing session, enhancing the bonds among participants.

Noticing vs. Overlooking

Practice Orientation and Type:
Various Orientations – Reflection Prompts

Personal Practice

The following practice, adapted from Worline and Dutton (2017),[35] focuses on noticing secondary traumatic stress (STS)-related compassion at work. Additionally, it invites helping professionals to notice any of their own missed opportunities to give and/or receive compassion at work in relation to STS. As such, this practice has the potential not only to bring benefits to your colleagues and yourself but also to serve as a portal toward awakening more compassion within the workplace.

Challenge yourself to notice STS-related compassionate acts that you may have been overlooking at work. Describe what might change or is changing, as you perhaps notice more, even small acts of compassion for STS, and how your heightened awareness of these compassionate acts affects you. Moreover, consider how such compassionate acts create a tapestry of support that enriches your workplace culture.

Additionally, try to notice any of your own missed opportunities to offer and/or receive STS-related compassion at work. What obstacles did you encounter in these instances? Were these missed opportunities potentially caused by feelings of judgment or from being overwhelmed, under pressure, and/or fatigued? Consider such instances when compassion might have been expected but was not forthcoming, and describe what might have changed if such opportunities had been compassionately noticed rather than overlooked.

Regarding the notion of missed opportunities, these are often associated with feelings of regret. Instead, it would rather be beneficial to reframe missed opportunities as evidence that such opportunities exist and to remain receptive toward forthcoming possibilities. Focusing on lessons learned and subsequent successes and accomplishments is therefore recommended.

Self-Reflections

- The term *selective attention* refers to the cognitive process of concentrating on particular stimuli while neglecting the rest (Simons & Chabris, 1999). Relatedly, how might selective attention be impacting my ability to notice compassion related to STS at work?
- As I reflect on recent workdays, were there instances where colleagues may have benefited from STS-related compassion that I may not have fully recognized at the time?

Group Context

Within a group setting, *Noticing vs. Overlooking* can be complemented by the following activity:

The facilitator can guide participants through a three-step mindfulness exercise adapted from Broderick (2021).[36] This exercise is designed to enhance participants' capacity to cultivate a heightened awareness of selective attention:

Step 1: Inattentive Listening

In this step, participants assume comfortable seated positions, preferably with their eyes closed, and engage in 1 minute of unguided silence. Following this quiet interval, they are encouraged to recollect any sounds they may have noticed in their surroundings.

Step 2: Attentive Listening

Next, with their eyes still closed, participants are invited to observe another minute of silence while attentively listening to any sounds present in their surroundings. Following this additional interval, they are again asked to recall any sounds they may have noticed.

Step 3: Comparing Listening Experiences

Finally, participants are encouraged to consider any differences they may have noticed between the first and second steps of this practice and contemplate the possible relevance of this exercise to their capacity to notice compassion related to STS within their work environments. Sharing sessions in pairs, small groups, and/or the whole group can complete this activity.

Practicing Tonglen

Practice Orientation and Type:
Self- to Self-Orientation – Guided Meditation and
Visualization and Breath Awareness

Personal Practice

This practice is based on the Buddhist meditation of *tonglen* (i.e., in Tibetan *tong* means "sending out" and *len* means "taking in;" Chödrön, 2017b). Traditionally, *tonglen* is practiced by visualizing taking in others' suffering (i.e., compassion) with each inhalation and sending others happiness (i.e., loving-kindness) with each exhalation (Rinpoche, 1992).[37] In line with Shonin et al. (2015), however, this traditional *tonglen* practice may not necessarily be advised when one is experiencing secondary traumatic stress (STS) unless one is well-versed in the technique.

Find a comfortable sitting position, close your eyes or lower and soften your gaze, and take several slow, deep breaths to help yourself feel centered and relaxed. This preparatory step sets the stage for the following three-step modified self-*tonglen* practice by creating a sense of calm and receptivity (e.g., Rinpoche, 1992):

Step 1: Focus on breathing in

As you breathe in, imagine that you are breathing in your STS-related challenges and compassionately making room within yourself for these challenges to be acknowledged without judgment.

Step 2: Focus on breathing out

As you breathe out, imagine that you are breathing out happiness and that the happiness is surrounding you and gently embracing you from all sides.[38]

Step 3: Focus on breathing in and out

Continue this practice of breathing in your STS-related challenges while acknowledging them without judgment and breathing out happiness while visualizing the happiness gently embracing you from all sides. Allow this process to be practiced alternately, with these two intentions metaphorically riding in and out with each cycle of breath.

When this practice feels complete, take a few more slow, deep breaths, and then gradually let your breath find its own natural rhythm and depth again. Focus your attention on the sensations of breathing in and out, letting yourself be comforted by the natural rhythm of your breath for a few more moments of silence.

Self-Reflections

• It may be interesting to reflect on how this modified version of *tonglen* is similar to the function of a wetsuit. Just as a wetsuit's specialized material warms up cold water that enters it through contact with your body's warmth – so, too, this practice provides a layer of warmth embracing you from all sides.

Can I think of additional metaphors for this modified version of *tonglen?*

• The traditional *tonglen* practice, in which one envisions taking in others' suffering (i.e., compassion) with each in-breath and sending out happiness (i.e., loving-kindness) with each out-breath, may initially appear counterintuitive. However, this technique aligns with the temperature sensation experienced during each breath cycle. Specifically, each inhalation feels cooler than each exhalation, as each out-breath naturally carries your body's warmth. In this context, when engaging in the traditional *tonglen* practice, it may be beneficial to contemplate that the suffering of others is not retained within you but is instead transformed by the warmth of your compassion.[39]

How might I apply this insight to enhance my capacity for compassion toward others?

Group Context

Within a group setting, *Practicing Tonglen* can be accompanied by the following activity to further facilitate a shift in focus to encompass others:

After individually practicing the modified *tonglen* technique, the group can come together to engage in a collective practice, whereby participants who wish to participate visualize themselves compassionately relieving fellow group members from the burdens of STS with each inhalation and breathing out happiness for the entire group with each exhalation. Importantly, in the context of STS, the phrase "relieving others of suffering" in lieu of "taking in others' suffering" has the potential to reshape the emotional tone of this practice, transforming it from a potentially overwhelming experience into one of relief for the benefit of others.

Moreover, as participants are aware that, in this metaphorical exchange, their own STS-related suffering is simultaneously being reciprocally relieved by other group members (i.e., aligning with the term *voluntary reciprocal altruism*; Landry, 2006), it may foster a sense of shared relief within the group.[40] This, in turn, can strengthen group members' sense of interconnectedness and collective ability to cope with STS compassionately. Sharing sessions in pairs, small groups, and/or the whole group can complete this activity.

Cultivating KINTSUGI

Practice Orientation and Type:
Self- and Other-Orientation – Guided Meditation
and Reflection Prompts

Personal Practice

The traditional Japanese art of *kintsugi* (i.e., *kin* means "golden" and *tsugi* means "joinery" or "repair") is an artform whereby broken pottery is mended with golden lacquer so that the pottery cracks are illuminated rather than concealed (e.g., Dobkin, 2022).[41] Drawing inspiration from the symbolism of the golden joinery lines as a representation of compassionate care, this practice underscores the potential for compassionately addressing secondary traumatic stress (STS), acknowledging that STS may be effectively navigated, even if you are feeling "broken" at present.

This practice consists of the following four steps:

Step 1: Embracing a Kintsugi Mindset

Allow yourself to settle into a comfortable sitting position while fully immersing into the embrace of the present moment. Gently close your eyes or lower and soften your gaze, and invite your awareness to turn inward. Gradually, in this still and quiet state, and in line with a *kintsugi* mindset, envision yourself enveloped by a soothing golden light – analogous to the golden *kintsugi* lacquer – symbolizing your capacity to offer yourself STS-related compassionate care.

Step 2: Kintsugi-inspired Dedication

With each inhalation, imagine the golden light gently permeating the areas of your body where you are experiencing distressing STS sensations, offering release from discomfort and bringing comfort and ease. With each exhalation, let go of any residual tension, allowing the distressing sensations to soften and relax gradually. In parallel, honor the dedication you are investing in restoring your wellbeing, drawing inspiration from the intricate craftsmanship of restoration exemplified by *kintsugi*.

Step 3: Embodying Kintsugi Wholeness

As you gently open or raise your eyes, let the golden light of compassionate care accompany you as a guiding presence. Moreover, as you remain attuned to the messages your body conveys, welcome the soothing golden light to continue permeating and illuminating the areas in your body that still feel in need of care. Embrace the profound interconnection between your physical wellbeing and your overall holistic wellness, recognizing how nurturing one aspect can positively impact another.

Step 4: Reflecting on KINTSUGI

Reflecting on the following recommendations for addressing STS, represented by the acronym KINTSUGI (see Table 7), can further enhance your overall sense of wellness. These reflections offer valuable insights and guidance and provide a framework for compassionate care in the face of STS-related challenges.

Table 7. KINTSUGI Reflection Prompts

Letter of Acronym	Reflections
K	*Kindness toward yourself* – Nurture kindness for yourself by recognizing the negative impact of STS and treating yourself kindly. Just as the wisdom of *kintsugi* illuminates the transformative power of repair, recognize that treating yourself kindly can help transform STS-related challenges into opportunities for growth.
I	*Insights for wellbeing* – Compassionately embrace the lessons you are learning through your STS healing journey. Just as *kintsugi* showcases how the golden artistry of the restored pottery's fractures enhances its worth, the insights you are gaining can empower you to skillfully navigate STS as well as possible future exposure to indirect trauma.
N	*Nurturing support system* – Surround yourself with a network of family, friends, and colleagues as a source of STS-related support. Just as the supportive structure in *kintsugi* allows for successful restoration, a nurturing support system creates a safe environment that can promote your holistic wellbeing.

(Continued)

Table 7. (Continued)

Letter of Acronym	Reflections
T	*Time for cultivating virtues* – Dedicate time to the cultivation of virtues, considering it a nonnegotiable priority that contributes to the development of character traits beneficial for addressing STS. Just as *kintsugi* requires patience, embrace the understanding that cultivating virtues such as equanimity, compassion, and wisdom is a long-term commitment.
S	*Self-reflection for self-awareness* – Deepen your self-awareness regarding STS through self-reflection. Just as *kintsugi* artisans carefully examine each fragment, determining the precise angles and placements for repair, self-reflection can reveal areas for personal growth, thereby promoting your self-awareness in the context of STS.
U	*Unplug and recharge* – Take breaks between STS-related compassionate practices, fostering a mindful and sustainable approach. Just as *kintsugi* artisans step away from their work for a period of time, allowing the repaired piece to undergo the necessary processes for the materials to bond and strengthen – offer yourself moments of relaxation and rejuvenation between practices.
G	*Generosity toward others* – Cultivate generosity toward others by offering them compassion. This includes survivors of trauma and colleagues navigating STS. Just as mended *kintsugi* pottery may be offered as a gift, extend compassionate support to others and recognize your compassion as a meaningful gift.
I	*Imperfections as beauty* – Embrace the idea that your STS-related vulnerability can lead to positive psychological outcomes. Just as the golden seams in *kintsugi* add value to the mended pottery, STS-related challenges can enhance your capacity for compassion and lead to vicarious posttraumatic growth (VPTG).

Note. The STS-related KINTSUGI reflections are not listed by significance or recommended order, nor are they necessarily mutually exclusive. "Generosity toward others," however, which entails offering others compassion, can be viewed as a culmination of the groundwork laid by the other recommendations, serving as their ultimate goal.

Self-Reflection

• Similar to artisans skilled in *kintsugi*, who draw upon their skills and materials – what resources can I draw upon to support both my own and others' wellbeing in light of STS?

Group Context

Within a group setting, *Cultivating KINTSUGI* can be accompanied by the following visual arts activity:

The facilitator can invite participants to create a patchwork STS-related quilt inspired by the principles of *kintsugi*. Each participant can be given a fabric square and the freedom to decorate their square with fabric paints/markers, drawing inspiration from the KINTSUGI reflection prompts. Once all the squares are prepared, participants can share their creative experiences, and the squares can be sewn together and connected by a unifying golden border.[42] The quilt can then be hung in a common area, serving as a visual representation of the group's collective compassionate intentions. Sharing sessions in pairs, small groups, and/or the whole group can complete this activity.

golden joinery –
creating a *kintsugi*
compassionate path

Healing Glow

An illuminated candle in kintsugi pottery

Realizing Similarities

Practice Orientation and Type:
Self- to Other-Orientation – Reflection Prompts

Personal Practice

This practice, adapted from the meditation approach of Tan (2018) and Salzberg (2013) to compassionately address secondary traumatic stress (STS),[43] is based on the traditional Buddhist practice of "equalizing and exchanging oneself with others" (Lavelle, 2017). *Equalizing* involves recognizing the fundamental equality of all beings in their desire for happiness and freedom from suffering. *Exchanging* entails mentally and emotionally "placing oneself in others' shoes" and genuinely empathizing with them (e.g., Dunne, 2019).

The following statements are associated with the list of traumatic stress reactions presented in the first part of this resource guide. As a reminder, these reactions are categorized into four distinct areas: (a) *intrusive*, (b) *avoidance*, (c) *negative alterations in mood and thinking*, and (d) *hyperarousal and reactivity* symptoms (APA, 2022). Please personalize the upcoming statements to focus on the categories and specific reactions that resonate with your experience, and keep in mind that the statements are meant for internal rather than spoken reflection.

Kindly repeat the statements in the first phase of this practice three times as you focus sequentially on close, neutral, and challenging colleagues (i.e., a colleague whom you appreciate or admire, a colleague for whom you have no strong positive or negative feelings, and a colleague whom you perceive as challenging in some way, respectively). Subsequently, during the second phase, allow heartfelt wishes for the wellbeing of these colleagues to surface collectively. Also, feel free to replace the words "my colleague(s)" in the following statements with the actual name(s) of your colleague(s).

Find a comfortable seated position, allowing your body to settle into a posture that promotes relaxation and attentiveness. Take a few slow, deep breaths, and then gradually let your breath settle back into its natural rhythm and depth. When you feel ready, bring to mind the previously mentioned colleagues one by one. Inwardly repeat the following scripts to yourself as is or per your preferred modification, pausing at the end of each category of reactions to allow time for reflection.

First Phase

Repeat this phase of the practice three times as you focus sequentially on close, neutral, and challenging colleagues while recognizing that this practice aims to shift the tendency of prioritizing personal wellbeing ahead of the wellbeing of others (Jinpa, 2019):[44]

- "Just like me" statements for *intrusive reactions* associated with indirect exposure to trauma: Just like me, my colleague may be experiencing distressing nightmares, flashbacks, intrusive thoughts, and/or physiological reactions.
- "Just like me" statements for *avoidance reactions* associated with indirect exposure to trauma: Just like me, my colleague may be trying to avoid distressing internal or external reminders, including disturbing memories, thoughts/ruminations, feelings, and/or physical sensations.
- "Just like me" statements for *hyperarousal and reactivity reactions* associated with indirect exposure to trauma: Just like me, my colleague may be experiencing irritable or aggressive behavior, self-destructive, risky or reckless behavior, jumpiness or being quick to startle, hypervigilance, difficulties with concentration, and/or sleep disturbances.
- "Just like me" statements for *negative alterations in mood and thinking reactions* associated with indirect exposure to trauma: (a) negative alterations in *mood*: Just like me, my colleague may be experiencing a persistent bad or sad mood, difficulty feeling positive emotions, loneliness, and/or feeling detached/disconnected from others, and/or (b) negative alterations in *thinking*: Just like me, my colleague may be experiencing difficulties remembering parts of the traumatic events experienced by their clients, persistent exaggerated negative expectations about themselves, others, and/or the world, decreased interest in previously meaningful matters, and/or persistent distorted blame of themselves and/or others.

Second Phase

After the first phase of this practice, consider extending well-wishes to your colleagues, either by using these provided examples or by creating your own well-wishing sentiments:

Just as I wish for myself . . .
So may you successfully navigate STS and experience wellbeing
For the ultimate benefit of survivors of trauma

Self-Reflections

• "Often, we are our own difficult person" (Jinpa, 2015, p. 133). To what degree does self-compassion facilitate my ability to approach my own challenging behaviors with compassion?
• To what extent am I willing to extend compassion for STS toward all my colleagues, regardless of our current relationships?

Group Context

Within a group setting, *Realizing Similarities* can be carried out as follows:

After guiding participants through the personal practice, the facilitator can invite group members to practice the second phase again, letting compassionate wishes emerge for the wellbeing of the entire group. To facilitate this process, the "Compassion-Wish Chain Method" can be employed. With this method, one participant shares a compassionate wish, followed by another participant, and so forth. Such an inclusive exchange of STS-related compassionate wishes has the potential to uplift and inspire the entire group.

altruism's light
shines through "I," "mine," "me," and "my" –
like a star at noon

North Star

A star shining in a light blue sky

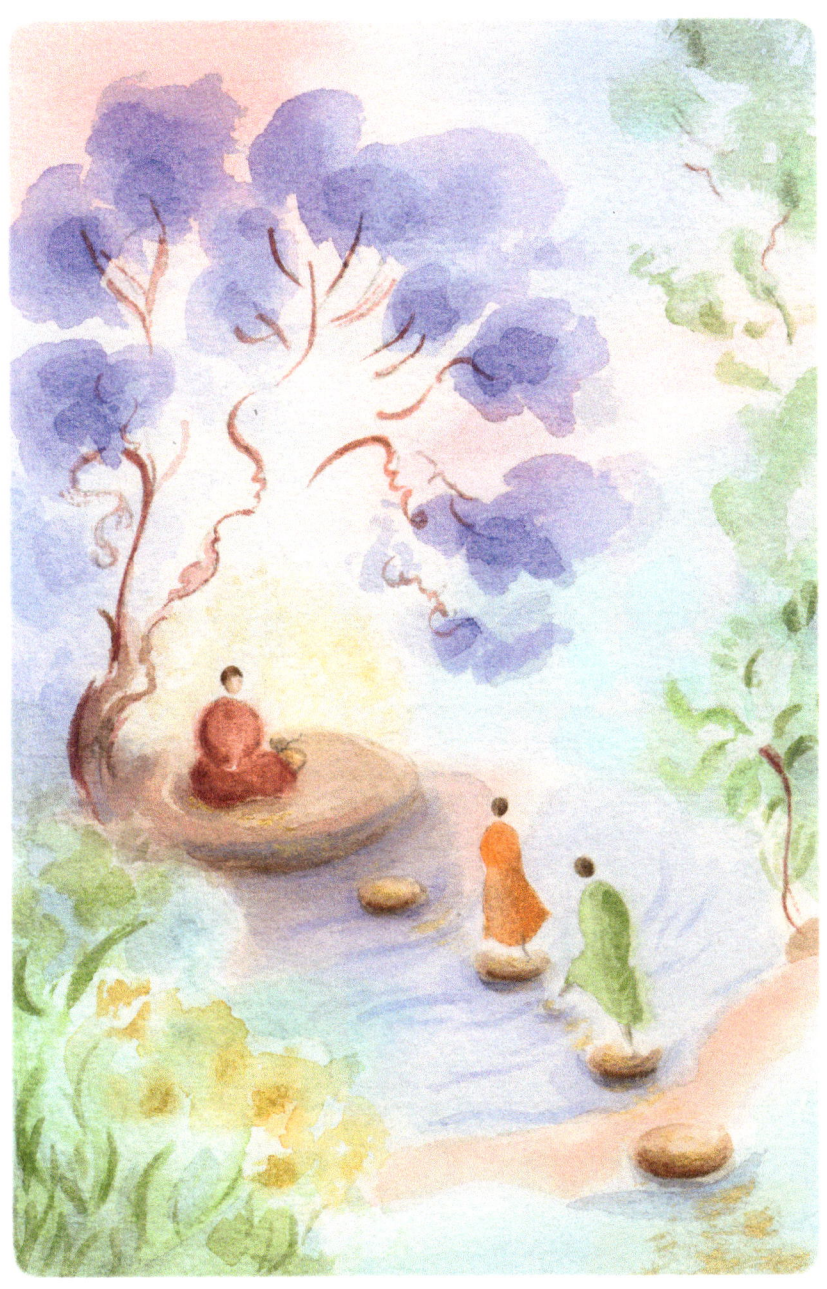

Friends Along the Path

Three figures and a river with stepping stones

Discovering an Oasis

Practice Orientation and Type:
Self- to Self-Orientation – Guided Meditation

Personal Practice

In this practice, adapted from Levine (2010) for compassionately addressing secondary traumatic stress (STS),[45] helping professionals are invited to mindfully shift their attention back and forth between two areas of their body. The chosen areas are distinguished by the presence or absence of a current STS-related physical sensation. In the context of this practice, the area not currently experiencing an STS-related sensation can be considered a compassionate oasis.

Sit comfortably, breathe deeply, and with your eyes preferably closed, direct your awareness to an area of your body that is not currently experiencing an STS-related sensation. For example, an area (even if it is very small) that feels calm, supported, or grounded, or even one that simply feels neutral. Focus your attention on this area of your body and consider greeting it with an inner acknowledgment in the spirit of "Hello, calmness."

Gradually direct your awareness to an area of your body that is experiencing a bodily sensation that you associate with STS (e.g., heaviness, numbness, pain, or tension). You may likewise choose to internally greet this area with an acknowledgment such as "Hello, tension." Note also that if the sensation feels too overwhelming, you can start by focusing on the edges of this sensitive area.[46]

Keep focusing on the chosen two areas of your body with self-compassionate curiosity while slowly and rhythmically shifting your attention from one area to the other. This can help you face distress/discomfort in small doses. Accordingly, this practice can disarm the intensity of STS-related sensations, gradually guiding your nervous system toward increased homeostasis (e.g., Kuhfuss et al., 2021).

Importantly, as you engage in this practice, cultivate equanimity throughout the process. Equanimity involves maintaining even-mindedness, regardless of whether what is perceived is pleasant, neutral, or unpleasant. As you shift your awareness between the previously mentioned two areas of your body, try, therefore, to do so with equanimity, remembering that the goal is not necessarily to eliminate sensations that are perceived as unpleasant. Rather, the goal is to cultivate equanimity, which is key to compassion (e.g., Weber, 2017).[47]

Self-Reflections

- Can the awareness of impermanence become a resource when I experience STS sensations? If so, in what way?
- How might embracing self-compassion in this way hold the potential to benefit the wellbeing of others indirectly?

Group Context

Within a group setting, *Discovering an Oasis* can be accompanied by the following expressive movement activity to further facilitate a shift in focus to encompass others:

The facilitator can invite participants to explore their somatic sensations in pairs via a variation of the body-based technique called *authentic movement* (Adler, 2002; Goldhahn, 2022; Hyatt, 2020).[48] In line with this modified version of the technique, participants work in pairs, with one partner moving while the other partner serves as a compassionate "witness."

"Movers" are encouraged to close their eyes and allow for unscripted movement to unfold without relying on predetermined choreography as they shift their attention between their STS and nonSTS-related sensations.[49] Meanwhile, "witnesses" observe the movement in a compassionately receptive and nonjudgmental way while remaining mindful of their own internal experiences of sensation and meaning. "Movers" and "witnesses" are then encouraged to switch roles (Barkai, 2022).[50]

Following each movement session, "movers" are the first to share their experience verbally. Sharing first gives "movers" the opportunity to express their experiences without the influence of external feedback or interpretations. Also, by listening attentively to the "movers" sharing, "witnesses" can develop their skills of deep listening and nonjudgmental compassionate response.

Significantly, the interplay between the concepts of *witness* and *withness*, denoting the state of being close or connected with someone

(Merriam-Webster, 2024c), underscores the profound sense of interconnectedness inherent in this practice, as reflected in this haiku:

> authentic movement,
> pond reflects a cloudless sky –
> witness and withness

Sharing sessions in pairs and/or with the whole group can complete this activity.

Planning a Vision Board

Practice Orientation and Type:
Self- and Other-Orientation – Visual Arts Expression

Personal Practice

This practice involves creating a vision board as a visual representation of helping professionals' altruistic self-care goals in light of secondary traumatic stress (STS). By practicing altruistic self-care in the context of STS, helping professionals not only compassionately safeguard their own wellbeing but also help ensure that they can continue to provide compassionate care to those who rely on their support. It is important to recognize that the distinction between self-care and altruistic self-care lies in the underlying intention for practicing rather than in the actual self-care practices in and of themselves (e.g., Bhalla & DiCuirci, 2023; Burton & Lent, 2016).[51]

With an altruistic mindset, consider a range of relevant STS-related self-care activities. These can encompass physical, emotional, intellectual, social, spiritual, environmental, and financial practices. For example: practicing yoga, developing a relaxing evening ritual, reading a book, spending quality time with family and friends, meditating, gardening, and incorporating expenses for leisure activities (e.g., Burton & Lent, 2016; Hydon et al., 2015). Essentially, the invitation is to choose self-care practices that can help sustain your work as a helping professional over the long term (e.g., Fuller, 2018).

The following five steps can assist you in creating your altruistic self-care vision board for addressing STS. Arranged alphabetically, from A to E, these steps underscore the interconnection between your own wellbeing and your capacity to support and care for others effectively:

Step 1: Affirm Your Intention

Begin by settling into a comfortable seated position with your back, neck, and head in alignment. Placing your hands comfortably on your lap and gently closing your eyes or lowering and softening your gaze is likewise recommended. Gradually, bring your attention to the movement of your breath at your heart center. Let your breath flow naturally while trying to maintain full awareness from the beginning of each inhalation to the end of each exhalation. As you inhale, affirm your altruistic intention for this practice. As you exhale, metaphorically release any barriers or obstacles that may hinder the fulfillment of your intention.

Step 2: Brainwrite altruistic self-care activities for your vision board[52]

Make a list of as many altruistic self-care ideas as you can for addressing STS. Be compassionate toward yourself and be creative, allowing yourself to include new and potentially helpful ideas. Incorporate activities that align with your values and that will empower you to "pass compassion forward." Also, consider matching specific activities with particular individuals in your care, colleagues who may be in need of support, and/or care settings.

Step 3: Collect images and/or words/phrases for your vision board

Look for images and/or words/phrases that relate to your chosen altruistic self-care activities and that motivate you. You can do so by browsing uplifting websites, flipping through inspiring magazines, and/or creating your own images and self-affirmations.[53]

Step 4: Decide how to assemble and display your vision board

Allow yourself to be creatively playful and intuitive with your arrangement. Also, feel free to add additional images as well as words/phrases as time passes. Your vision board may change over time – it is a dynamic expression of your altruistic self-care priorities in addressing STS.

Step 5: Embody your vision

To embody your STS-related vision, mindfully notice the sensations in your body as you reflect on your vision board. Similarly, as you set a clear and conscious intention to act in alignment with your vision, remain attuned to the dynamic interplay between your mind and body. Embrace your commitment to take steps, both big and small, that support the realization of your goals – navigating your internal landscape with equanimity as you move forward.

Self-Reflections

• What altruistic self-care practice(s) will I continue practicing, or begin practicing today, to create a more compassionate tomorrow?
• If my team or organization were to establish a shared vision board, what ideas could I contribute to support the practice of altruistic self-care at work?[54]

Group Context

Within a group setting, *Planning a Vision Board* can be accompanied by the following activity:

The facilitator can invite participants to create a group vision board centering on their collegial and/or organization-wide STS-related goals. This is important as the responsibility for addressing STS should not solely rest on individual self-care. Group goals can include activities that promote compassionate communication at work, nurture teamwork, and cultivate a caring environment for all members. Specifically, participants can be guided to direct their focus to both proximal (i.e., short-term) and distal (i.e., long-term) STS-related goals for the ultimate benefit of those in their care (e.g., Ekman, 2021; Ekman & Ekman, 2017). A sharing session with the whole group can complete this activity.

Building a Toolkit

Practice Orientation and Type:
Self- to Other-Orientation – Reflection Prompts

Personal Practice

Helping professionals can benefit from developing a compassionate toolkit tailored to secondary traumatic stress (STS), consisting of recommendations they can employ when assisting colleagues navigating STS. To cultivate such a toolkit, initial ideas can involve one or more of the following suggestions, adapted from the Compassion Resilience Toolkit (n.d.),[55] to foster an environment of enhanced compassion for STS within the workplace.

In pursuit of this objective, helping professionals are encouraged to prioritize genuine compassion over what is referred to as the "compassion credential." This term alludes to the display of compassionate behavior primarily for the purpose of enhancing one's self-image as a compassionate person (Lief, 2001). Through the adoption of an authentic approach, a compassionate workplace environment can be cultivated, nurturing a sense of interconnectedness and shared growth.

The following suggestions are provided for your consideration:

- Listen in an embodied way to your colleague's STS-related narrative and compassionately reflect back on what you notice while listening. This includes noticing and reflecting back nonverbal aspects of what your colleague is expressing (e.g., "I noticed you shed a tear" or "I couldn't help but notice a tinge of sadness in your voice").
- Redirect your focus from "What's wrong with my colleague?" to "What happened to my colleague?" and "How might what happened be affecting them?" By redirecting your focus in this way, you can potentially foster a more compassionate approach (e.g., "It seems as if something is troubling you"). Notably, Winfrey and Perry (2021) suggested exploring the question: "What happened to you?" with a holistic perspective. This involves taking into account not only individual factors

but also broader influences such as family, community, and cultural factors.

- Refer to a similar challenge in the past and how it was overcome (e.g., "Is there something that would be helpful for you to remember now about how you dealt with a similar challenge in the past?").
- Identify strengths that may be helpful for addressing STS (e.g., "I hear how challenging this is for you. I've also had the opportunity to observe your strengths. How can you build on your strengths to address STS successfully?").
- Focus on your colleague's desire to address STS (e.g., "This sounds challenging, and I also hear your wish for a positive change," "What are the drawbacks for not addressing STS?" and "What could be the benefits of addressing this challenge?").
- Concentrate on actionable steps that can be taken now in approaching STS with compassion (e.g., "What do you think/feel will help you now?" and "Is there anything I can help with today"?).
- Ask for permission before offering suggestions for addressing STS. Also, instead of assuming what your colleague may need, provide them with options to choose from. This approach will allow your colleague to exercise their autonomy and actively participate in decisions that impact their wellbeing (e.g., "May I offer some suggestions to help you generate your own solutions?").

Furthermore, remember that you can be helpful, even if you cannot change large elements of your colleagues' STS-related circumstances, as incremental change can lead to transformational change. For illustration, Pearson (2006) noted that compassionate acts are often "invisible" as they can be profound even if they are "simple not clever, basic not exquisite, (and) peripheral not central" (p. 22).

Moreover, a compassionate response can be regarded as such, regardless of whether it actually alleviates suffering or not (e.g., Lilius et al., 2008), as referred to also by Wiklund-Gustin and Wagner (2013), who stated that compassion is indeed "related more to caring rather than curing" (pp. 175–176). This perspective underscores the intrinsic value of compassionate responses, irrespective of their immediate outcomes.

Simmer-Brown (2023, p. 2349) similarly stated that "one cannot be assured of saving beings from their suffering, but compassion carries with it an imperative to try." At times, therefore, "compassion is not the alleviation or prevention of pain, but the wise navigation into it and learning from it" (Gilbert et al., 2019, p. 2262). Aligning with this perspective, Feldman and Kuyken (2011, p. 144) suggested that "Compassion is the acknowledgment that not all pain can be 'fixed' or 'solved' but all suffering is made more approachable in a landscape of compassion."

Self-Reflections

- Pessi stated that "when it comes to compassion – small is all" (Pessi as cited in Worline & Dutton, 2017, p. 32). What are my beliefs about this statement?
- What will help me keep in mind that even though I cannot necessarily help *everyone* in need, I may be able to help *someone* in need?

Group Context

Within a group setting, *Building a Toolkit* can be accompanied by the following role-playing activity:

The facilitator can encourage participants to integrate the use of validating statements into their STS-related compassionate toolkit. To do so, participants can be invited to pair up and engage in a role-playing activity. In this activity, one partner shares an STS-related challenge while the other partner practices compassionate listening and responding in a validating way (see Table 8). The premise of this practice is that participants have strengths within them and that a validating interaction can help them turn toward their internal resources. Sharing sessions in pairs, small groups, and/or the whole group can complete this activity.

Table 8. Validating vs. Invalidating Statements

Validating Statements	Invalidating Statements
That sounds challenging	You should not feel like that
I can tell how difficult this is for you	Get over it
What can help you during this time?	You are being too sensitive
Expressing your feelings about this requires courage	I would not speak about this if I were you

Note. Validation can likewise include reflecting back on what you heard, acknowledging the emotions expressed, and inquiring further about colleagues' STS-related experiences (e.g., Call et al., 2022).

Asking SMARTEST

Practice Orientation and Type:
Self- and Other-Orientation – Journaling Prompts[56]

Personal Practice

Helping professionals dealing with secondary traumatic stress (STS) are encouraged to seek support to navigate the challenges they are facing effectively. Inspired by Rubin (2002),[57] the following recommendations, listed according to the SMARTEST acronym, work together to create a pathway for requesting support. As an additional benefit, helping professionals embodying the SMARTEST recommendations may serve as inspiring role models for others to emulate.[58] Notably, the SMARTEST acronym diverges from its conventional goal-setting interpretation found in the SMART and SMARTER acronyms (e.g., **S**pecific, **M**easurable, **A**ttainable, **R**elevant, and **T**imely), aligning with what Rubin (2002) referred to as "acronym drift."

Consider compassionate support that you would appreciate receiving in light of STS and one or more individuals whom you could ask. To guide your request, refer to Table 9 to align with the SMARTEST recommendations:

Table 9. Practicing SMARTEST

Letter of Acronym	SMARTEST Recommendations
S	Seek support mindfully, staying fully present in the interaction. This mindful approach involves being aware of your bodily sensations, thoughts, and feelings as you communicate your needs and seek assistance. It invites you to immerse yourself fully in the moment, recognizing the subtle shifts in your internal landscape. Practicing mindfulness throughout the support-seeking process can also aid in managing possible stress linked to communication, thereby enhancing your overall effectiveness in conveying your message.

(Continued)

Table 9. (Continued)

Letter of Acronym	SMARTEST Recommendations
M	Maintain equanimity regardless of whether the person you ask for support can provide it or not. When you approach someone for assistance, it is important to recognize that their ability to provide support may vary and that their decision is not a reflection of your worth. Maintaining equanimity means accepting the uncertainty of the outcome without allowing it to disrupt your inner balance. Even if the person cannot provide support now, your equanimity may leave a positive impression, leading to potential support or collaboration in the future.
A	Approach the process of asking for support with an altruistic mindset, foreseeing that the help you receive will help you sustain the help you offer others. An altruistic approach to seeking support has the potential to create positive ripple effects that extend beyond your personal needs. By recognizing that the assistance you receive serves a larger purpose, you align your actions with a sense of responsibility and contribution to the greater good.
R	Remain open to diverse forms of assistance, embracing skillful solutions. This collaborative and holistic approach holds value because it encourages a support-seeking process that embodies flexibility, inclusivity, and a strong commitment to effective problem-solving. Moreover, it empowers you to "think outside the box" and consider innovative and creative ways of addressing challenges.
T	Trust in interconnectedness and the potential for mutual benefit. Interconnectedness reminds you that you are not alone in your struggles. When you ask for support, you tap into the web of connections that can provide assistance during challenging times. This sense of not being isolated in your challenges can give you the confidence to reach out for help. It may also be helpful to remember that the person providing support can likewise benefit from the interaction. This benefit might include the satisfaction of helping someone, strengthening the relationship, or gaining a sense of purpose and interconnectedness themselves.
E	Embody virtues such as equanimity, compassion, and wisdom, allowing them to shine through in your interactions. These virtues enable you to: (a) articulate your needs in a balanced way that reflects your ability to engage constructively in finding solutions, (b) show consideration for the challenges the person you are seeking support from may be facing, and (c) maintain an optimistic outlook, understanding that the challenges you are dealing with are impermanent.

(Continued)

Table 9. (Continued)

Letter of Acronym	SMARTEST Recommendations
S	Sustain humility and patience, fostering more harmonious interactions. Approaching others with humility opens the door for collaboration and acknowledges the expertise and support that others can provide. Demonstrating patience in your communication allows you to listen attentively and provide necessary information without pressure. These qualities also help reduce potential conflicts that can arise when seeking support, preventing impatience and promoting a sense of equality and mutual respect.
T	Transform challenges into opportunities for growth, viewing them as stepping stones on your path. This is relevant when asking for support because it conveys a mindset and attitude that can positively influence the support-seeking process in several ways: (a) it demonstrates a resilient and proactive approach to addressing challenges, (b) it fosters a positive outlook, which can be "contagious," and (c) it invites the other person to join you on your journey, creating a sense of partnership (i.e., instead of approaching support passively, you are signaling your willingness to actively engage in finding solutions).

Note. The SMARTEST recommendations are not listed by significance or recommended order.

Self-Reflections

• Reflecting on a time when I asked for support, STS-related or otherwise, which SMARTEST recommendations did I intuitively incorporate into my request and did these recommendations help shape the nature of the support I received?
• When I offer STS-related support to others, can I leverage the SMARTEST recommendations into my approach?

Group Context

Within a group setting, *Asking SMARTEST* can be accompanied by the following activity:

After the SMARTEST recommendations are presented by the facilitator, participants can be encouraged to add additional recommendations. This is important as the acronym, "SMARTEST," should not constrain participants from exploring other such valuable alternatives. Participants can then be guided by the facilitator to form small groups and consider a hypothetical scenario whereby a helping professional is seeking support to navigate STS-related challenges. The scenario can be designed to encompass a range of relevant issues commonly faced by helping professionals. Participants in each group then collaboratively work together to consider how they might best assist the helping professional in the scenario. A sharing session with the whole group can complete this activity.

Witnessing Compassion Flow

Practice Orientation and Type:
Other- to Other-Orientation – Reflection Prompts and
Various Creative Expressions

Personal Practice

Research suggests that witnessing or hearing about a compassionate inter-action can create a state of elevation (Haidt, 2002). That is, a heightened emotional state characterized as feeling "uplifted," "inspired," or "moved" (Sparks et al., 2019). Data likewise suggest that experiencing such elevation can motivate individuals to help others compassionately – thereby initiat-ing a compassionate chain reaction. This implies a prosocial contagion effect, signifying "a process whereby witnessing a prosocial act leads to acting prosocially" (Haidt, 2002; Seppälä, 2013; Sparks et al., 2019, p. 1).

Consider a time when you witnessed compassion being offered or heard about a compassionate action, gesture, or word. Explicitly, consider what specifically made it meaningful. How could you incorporate such meaning-ful aspects into your practice of embodying and extending secondary trau-matic stress (STS)-related compassion to both yourself and others? Take some time to consider this, and if you wish, express your reflections by incorporating one or more creative modalities.

For example, through journaling, you can capture the essence of your reflections and delve into their significance. Drawing, on the other hand, can allow you to visually represent your experience, unlocking the potential to convey insights in an artistic way. Embracing expressive movement can likewise enrich your reflective process by offering an embodied and kines-thetic approach to self-reflection. All in all, the diverse range of creative modalities referred to in this context can provide a holistic approach to witnessing compassion and its application in STS-related compassionate support of yourself and others.

Self-Reflections

• Can I identify any internal barriers/judgments associated with witnessing or hearing about compassionate interactions in the context of STS?
• To what extent can the elements that made the witnessed compassion meaningful be applied when I offer STS-related compassionate support to myself and others?

Group Context

Within a group setting, *Witnessing Compassion Flow* can be accompanied by the following activity:

The facilitator can encourage participants to form pairs or small groups, where they can discuss their experiences of witnessing compassion and explore how it can be applied to STS. In addition, participants can be invited to share their creative expressions with each other. Since witnessing compassionate encounters at work can also enhance participants' appreciation for their colleagues' actions, participants can likewise be prompted to share their reflections in this respect.

Throughout this process, the facilitator can underscore the significance of mindful and generous listening by encouraging group members to (a) mindfully observe both their own embodied responses and the nonverbal cues of those who are sharing, and (b) generously listen to what is true to others (i.e., this does not necessarily entail fully understanding "why the other person feels the way they do . . .. What matters is what's true for this person and you simply receive it and respect it" Remen, 2012, 1:47).[59] A sharing session with the whole group can complete this activity.

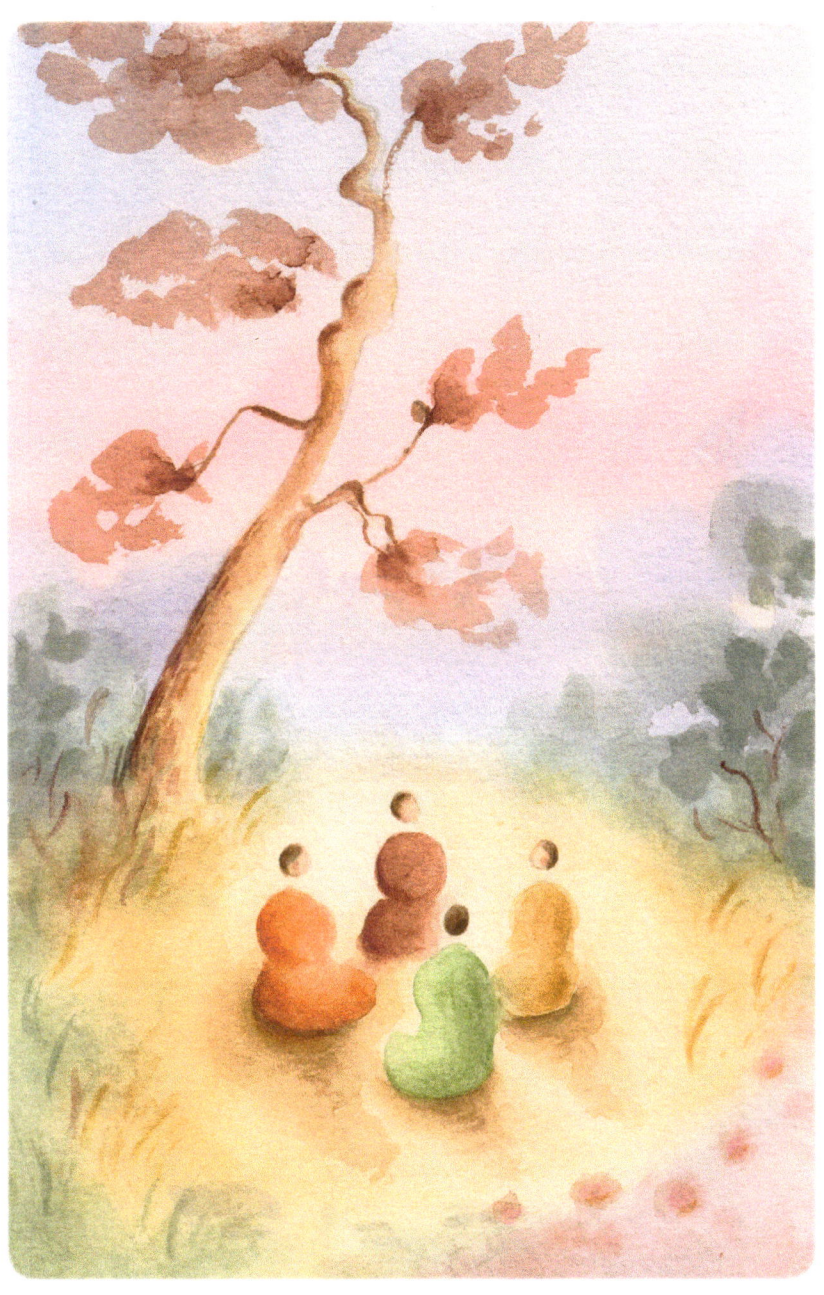

Circle of Support

Four figures meditating together

Advancing Multilevel Thinking

Practice Orientation and Type:
Various Orientations – Reflection Prompts

Personal Practice

The following multilevel items provide valuable considerations for compassionately addressing secondary traumatic stress (STS). Their purpose is to encourage thoughtful reflection and exploration of topics pertinent to fostering compassionate responses across various levels, ultimately joining forces to address STS. Please consider the personal-level items with an altruistic perspective, placing emphasis on interconnectedness. This involves viewing your wellbeing as intimately tied to that of others and self-compassion as a component of a holistic pedagogy encompassing both self- and other-oriented compassionate care (e.g., Anālayo & Dhammadinnā, 2021).

Spanning personal, collegial, organizational, and extra-organizational levels, the following items are listed here for your ongoing reflection:

On a *personal* level, what will help you?

- Develop greater self-awareness to recognize when you are experiencing STS.
- Cultivate your ability to be fully present when you are experiencing STS, and allow your presence to become more self-compassionate.
- Identify and address barriers that may prevent you from offering yourself compassion for STS.
- Find ways to communicate your STS-related challenges to colleagues while maintaining respectful boundaries and refraining from sharing excessive graphic details.
- Become more comfortable asking for and receiving compassion from colleagues with respect to STS.

On a *collegial* level, what will help you?

- Improve your ability to recognize when colleagues are experiencing STS.
- Cultivate the ability to be fully present with colleagues when they share STS-related challenges.
- Develop the ability to set appropriate boundaries when colleagues share challenges associated with STS in order to maintain a healthy and respectful level of detail-sharing.
- Identify and address obstacles that may prevent you from offering compassion to colleagues experiencing STS.
- Respond compassionately when colleagues ask for support in light of STS.

On an *organizational* level, what will help you?

- Assess how you can contribute to STS-related compassionate efforts at an organizational level.
- Play an active role in fostering a compassionate and STS-informed organizational culture.
- Identify and address barriers that may hinder your ability to engage in organization-wide compassionate action in the context of STS.
- Encourage colleagues to join you in taking compassionate action to address STS and work together to generate and refine organizational resources.
- Promote organizational policies and practices that demonstrate compassionate responses to STS.

On an *extra-organizational* level, what will help you?

- Extend compassionate actions related to STS beyond the workplace, creating a ripple effect that positively impacts the broader community of helping professionals.
- Champion interagency collaborations focused on advancing compassionate policies and practices associated with STS.
- Engage with local educational institutions to establish dialogue on the importance of addressing STS among future helping professionals, encouraging compassionate practices from the outset of their careers.
- Advocate for the incorporation of compassion's benefits into STS awareness, education, and research across multiple platforms such as professional associations, interdisciplinary workshops, and academic conferences.
- Engage with online initiatives that provide a space for trauma-informed sharing of resources, and compassionate support relevant to STS.

Self-Reflection

• Are there additional items that I can add to this multi-level list?

Group Context

Within a group setting, *Advancing Multilevel Thinking* can be incorporated as follows:

Participants can be encouraged to discuss compassionate responses to STS across multiple levels (i.e., personal, collegial, organizational, and extra-organizational) in pairs or small groups. To kickstart this activity, the facilitator can present a hypothetical scenario illustrating an employee's specific situation and associated STS-related experiences, providing essential context. Within their pairs or small groups, participants can then be prompted to brainstorm ideas associated with each of the four levels of responses, followed by a reflective wrap-up session. In this final phase, group members can share their insights regarding the interconnectedness of these response levels and how, when considered collectively, they can create a compassionate network of support. A sharing session with the whole group can complete this activity.

Envisioning a Mission

Practice Orientation and Type:
Self- and Other-Orientation – Reflection and Journaling Prompts

Personal Practice

This practice, adapted from Li et al. (2017) for compassionately addressing secondary traumatic stress (STS), incorporates the INSPIRE framework.[60] This variation of the framework can assist professionals in the helping fields develop and actualize a personal mission statement in the context of STS. By committing to compassionately addressing STS in this way, helping professionals are prioritizing wellbeing by ensuring that their actions are aligned with their intentions.

As mission statements sometimes turn out to be unrealistic, try to "keep it real." Moreover, consider sharing your personal mission statement with a colleague, as having a witness to your intentions can help anchor them in the world. Sharing your mission statement not only fosters personal accountability but also creates space for valuable feedback and support, potentially strengthening and sustaining your capacity to extend compassion to those in your care.

As a prelude to crafting your personal mission statement, find a quiet and comfortable space where you can immerse yourself in this seven-step practice (see Table 10). Begin by taking a few deep, mindful breaths to center yourself, inviting your attention to turn inward. Let this moment of introspection be the bridge to the intention you hold for this practice – may it be grounded in compassion, and may many be served.

Table 10. INSPIRE Reflection and Journaling Prompts

Letter of Acronym	INSPIRE Items
I	Identify compassion as a core value, accompanied by additional values that foster its development and wise application.
N	Name the demographics of survivors of trauma whom you serve.
S	Set forth your compassionate vision for addressing STS.
P	Plan how to fulfill your STS-related compassionate vision (mission).
I	Identify compassion-based practices for addressing STS that align with your mission.
R	Refine your personal mission statement for compassionately addressing STS, through review and revision.
E	Engage colleagues to help you achieve your mission, while inspiring them to craft their own.

Self-Reflections

- Is my STS-related compassionate mission statement both inspiring and actionable?
- The alignment between professionals' personal values and those upheld by their organizations can lead to enhanced wellbeing (e.g., Arieli et al., 2020; Pololi et al., 2015). Professionals should, thereby, not only examine their personal values but also consider the values promoted within their workplaces, assessing the degree of alignment and harmonization between these two sets of values (Arieli et al., 2020).

How do I perceive the relationship between my personal values and the values upheld within my workplace? Does this relationship impact the addressing of STS?

Group Context

Within a group setting, *Envisioning a Mission* can be carried out as follows:

The facilitator can invite participants to utilize the "Prepare-Pair-Share" sequence, adapted from Lyman (1981).[61] According to this modified sequence, participants follow three steps, creating a structured and collaborative process for crafting their personal mission statements while also promoting a sense of shared purpose within the group:

Step 1: Prepare

During this initial step, each participant is provided with dedicated time to prepare their personal mission statement for compassionately addressing STS, aligned with the INSPIRE acronym.

Step 2: Pair

Following the first step, participants form pairs and refine their personal mission statements with each other, thereby providing a valuable opportunity for further refinement, and mutual inspiration and insight.

Step 3: Share

Concluding this process, participants share their experiences of preparing and refining their personal mission statements in a group sharing session, and consider what additional steps are needed to bring their mission statements to fruition.

Giving Gratitude

Practice Orientation and Type:
Self- to Other-Orientation – Guided Meditation

Personal Practice

Gratitude has been defined as the quality of being thankful, "being aware and appreciating good things, particularly another's actions" (Brunzell et al., 2015, p. 9).[62] Through the application of this practice, helping professionals can cultivate gratitude toward colleagues who have offered them compassion in light of secondary traumatic stress (STS). This is significant as cultivating gratitude has been linked with improved mental health and wellbeing and can be a powerful tool for managing trauma-related distress (Kashdan et al., 2006; Tachon et al., 2022).

Find a comfortable sitting posture, allowing any unnecessary tension to soften. Make sure that your back, neck, and head are aligned, and gradually and gently bring awareness to your breath. As you breathe in, be present with breathing in. As you breathe out, be present with breathing out. Try to maintain your focus on each inhalation and exhalation and relax into gratitude for each cycle of breath.

Next, recall a colleague who offered you compassion with respect to one or more past or present STS-related reactions, and be mindful of what arises. Whether the compassion you received was subtle or profound, if feelings of gratitude arise, inwardly thank this individual while also noticing the felt-sense of gratitude as experienced in your body. This may manifest, for example, as sensations of warmth, expansion, and relaxation.

You may likewise choose to place your hand on your heart – a symbolic center of both gratitude and compassion. Gratitude has been eloquently described as "the memory of the heart" (Emmons, 2013, p. 10), while compassion has been likened to "the heart that trembles in the face of suffering" (Feldman & Kuyken, 2011, p. 144). May this practice serve as a heartfelt reminder of all those whose compassionate hearts have been moved to support you in your time of need. Similarly, may you wholeheartedly embrace the opportunity to nurture a sense of gratitude toward yourself for engaging in this practice of being thankful.

Self-Reflections

- As I cultivate gratitude, what associated attendant benefits do I experience?
- Does cultivating gratitude help me more mindfully focus on the present? This is beneficial, as STS is a trauma-associated condition, and mindfully focusing on the present is a recommended practice when dealing with trauma-related reactions (e.g., Polizzi et al., 2023; Zerubavel & Messman-Moore, 2015).
- Did I experience any obstacles or distractions that prevented gratitude from arising during this practice, or did a different emotion take its place?

Group Context

Within a group setting, *Giving Gratitude* can be carried out as follows:

The facilitator can guide participants through the individual practice, encouraging group members to reflect on someone within the group who has shown them compassion for STS. As part of the guidance, the facilitator can emphasize that even small acts of compassion, such as a kind word or a supportive gesture, can have a profound impact. This will help ensure that everyone in the group is acknowledged and thanked, even for the smallest of compassionate gestures.

Specifically, participants can be given the opportunity to: (a) share their experiences of receiving STS-related compassion from someone in the group, (b) acknowledge the positive impact of the compassion they received, and (c) express gratitude to the group member who showed them compassion. This practice may be particularly relevant during the concluding sessions of the group, as it provides a meaningful opportunity for participants to convey gratitude to their peers.

Significantly, it is often assumed that recipients of compassion will benefit more from the interaction compared to those who offer compassion. However, cultivating compassion can engender many benefits for those who offer compassion, whereas there is no guarantee that the recipients of compassion will ultimately benefit (Dalai Lama, 2007). As a result, participants who are thanked may, in turn, feel grateful for the chance to have been of assistance, creating a reciprocal cycle of appreciation.

Passing Compassion Forward

Practice Orientation and Type:
Self- to Other-Orientation – Reflection Prompts

Personal Practice

The parable of the raft, in Buddhism, is a multifaceted and profound teaching that is also relevant to the compassionate sharing of one's knowledge. The parable likens Buddhist teachings to a raft that a traveler constructs to cross a river. This raft serves as a means to an end, allowing the traveler to reach the other shore. However, once the traveler safely reaches the far shore, the parable emphasizes that the traveler should lay it down, as its purpose has been fulfilled. Moreover, the raft may be of assistance to others (Epstein, 2013).

In this spirit, reflect on the compassion-based practices that have held the most relevance for you in addressing secondary traumatic stress (STS), and consider sharing these practices with others. Consider both individual and group practices, as well as any adaptations you may have developed to align the practices more closely with your specific needs, preferences, circumstances, and worldview. As you engage in this reflection, please also contemplate what would be most beneficial for those with whom you intend to share these practices.

Significantly, "passing it forward" style activities have demonstrated positive effects not only for those who receive but also for those who give (Pressman et al., 2014). A systematic review and meta-analysis conducted by Curry et al. (2018), for example, revealed that engaging in acts of kindness enhances the wellbeing of individuals who extend such acts. These findings reinforce the overarching notion that, as social beings, we are equipped with psychological mechanisms that motivate us to assist others, ultimately leading to a sense of fulfillment through our compassionate acts.

Find a comfortable seated posture that promotes relaxation and wakefulness. As you settle into your seat, close your eyes or lower your gaze, allowing your mind to let go of external distractions. After settling in, contemplate the STS-related compassion-based practices that have potentially inspired, motivated, or influenced you in a positive way. As you contemplate, consider sharing the practice(s) that you believe might most benefit others.

To assist you, review the STS-related compassion-based practices with a variation of the GLAD acronym (Altman, 2014).[63] This acronym refers to practices that you: (a) are Grateful for receiving, (b) Learned, (c) found to be Affirmative, and (d) Do to offer yourself and others compassion in light of STS. This reflective framework can guide you in identifying the practices that have been particularly meaningful and transformative.

Self-Reflection

• Might reflecting on meaningful practices that others have generously shared with me serve as inspiration for me to reciprocate by sharing meaningful practices with others?

Group Context

Within a group setting, *Passing Compassion Forward* can transition into the following activity that incorporates the visual arts:

After participants select a practice that is particularly meaningful for them, using the GLAD acronym, they can convey their experience using visual arts. This creative expression allows group members to translate their experiences into a tangible form. Whether through painting, drawing, sculpture, or any other artistic outlet, this process empowers participants to communicate the impact of their chosen practice through visual storytelling. As participants present their visual creations to one another in pairs and/or small groups, they provide a window into their world, which, in turn, can serve as a catalyst for dialogue and mutual inspiration. A sharing session with the whole group can complete this activity.

PRACTICES FOR PROMOTING VICARIOUS POSTTRAUMATIC GROWTH (VPTG)

DOI: 10.4324/9781003381747-9

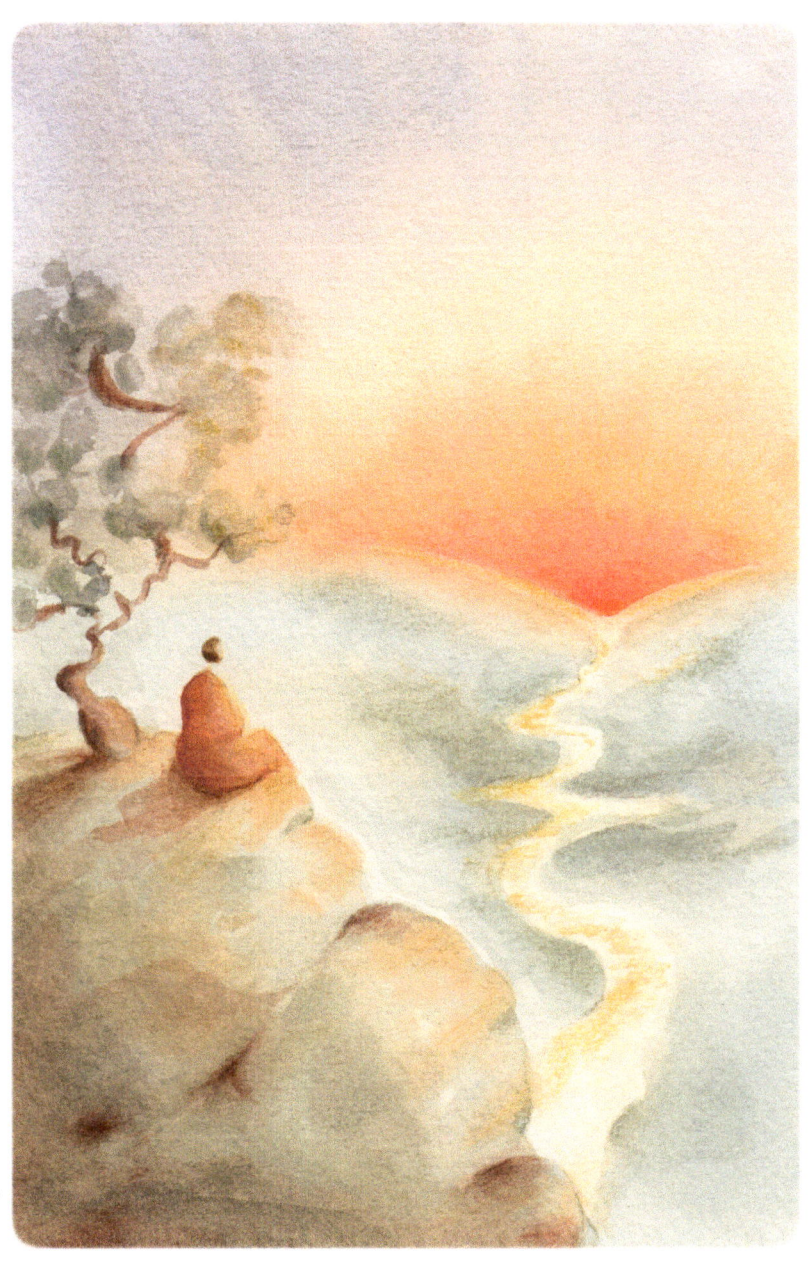

The Compassionate Path

Figure overlooking an illuminated path

Rising Strengths

Practice Orientation and Type:
Self- to Self-Orientation – Reflection Prompts

Personal Practice

As an introduction to the topic of vicarious posttraumatic growth (VPTG), this practice, presented via the acronym RISE, offers a perspective on secondary traumatic stress (STS)-related strengths. "To rise" encompasses several relevant and inspiring definitions, including: (a) *applying oneself to meet a challenge*, aligning with efforts to overcome the complexities of STS, (b) *assuming an upright position*, reflecting resilience in the face of adversity, (c) *responding warmly,* suggesting a supportive approach both toward oneself and others, (d) *becoming heartened*, representing a positive change in one's emotional state, and (e) *appearing above the horizon*, symbolizing a new beginning, much like the dawn of a new day (Merriam Webster, 2024d).

In a comfortable upright sitting position, deepen the quality of your presence by scanning your body with your awareness. Soften any unnecessary tension as you pay attention to the changing dance of sensations in your body. Letting a slight smile lift the corners of your mouth and eyes is likewise recommended as you relax and re-relax any lingering tension with each cycle of breath.[1] Relatedly, Hạnh (2002b, p. 22) referred to smiling as a practice in and of itself and to a smile as "mouth yoga."[2]

When you feel ready, consider the following self-reflection prompts presented via the acronym RISE:

- **Step 1: R**eflect on the strengths you had prior to experiencing STS and how they supported you in addressing it.
- **Step 2: I**lluminate how integrating compassion-based practices allowed you to harness these strengths to address STS.
- **Step 3: S**hine a light on the emerging new strengths that you have developed as a result of compassionately addressing STS.
- **Step 4: E**mpower yourself to engage in forward-looking actions that further promote the development of your strengths, serving as a resilient buffer against STS in the future.

Self-Reflection

• In what ways can I leverage my strengths to empower and support others who are navigating STS?

Group Context

Within a group setting, *Rising Strengths* can be carried out as follows to further facilitate a shift in focus to encompass others:

The facilitator can offer participants the opportunity to consider their group-related strengths and how compassion-based practices have helped them build on these strengths to address STS collectively. Participants can likewise be given time to reflect on possible relevant new strengths they may be developing as a group, and whether there are still areas in which they would like to make adjustments in this respect. Furthermore, participants can be motivated to take proactive steps that foster the continued development of their strengths as a group, serving as a resilient buffer against STS in the future. A sharing session with the whole group can complete this activity.

Evaluating VPTG

Practice Orientation and Type:
Self- and Other-Orientation – Reflection Prompts

Personal Practice

This practice, adapted from Tedeschi and Calhoun (1996),[3] is based on the *Posttraumatic Growth Inventory* (PTGI; i.e., PTG refers to transformative positive psychological changes that can result from directly experiencing one or more traumatic events). Within this practice, the provided statements aim to explore the positive transformations helping professionals may undergo through their work with survivors of trauma. This is relevant as the PTGI is often also utilized for evaluating vicarious posttraumatic growth (VPTG) following indirect exposure to trauma (e.g., Manning-Jones et al., 2015; Tsirimokou et al., 2023).

Find a quiet, peaceful space where external distractions are minimized and invite a warm smile to your face, fostering an optimistic mindset. Once you have assumed a comfortable posture that allows you to feel settled and supported, you are encouraged to reflect on the degree to which you identify with the following VPTG-related statements (e.g., from "*not at all*" to "*a very great degree*"). Notably, higher levels of VPTG are associated with a greater degree of alignment with these statements:

• *My work with survivors of trauma has positively influenced my sense of personal strength*

For example, it has positively influenced my ability to rely on myself, handle difficulties, accept outcomes, and/or realize that I am stronger than I anticipated.

• *My work with survivors of trauma has broadened my perception of new possibilities*

For example, it has enhanced my ability to make changes when needed, develop new interests, establish new pathways, recognize new opportunities, and/or accomplish more with my life.

- *My work with survivors of trauma has positively affected my appreciation for life*

For example, it has improved my ability to realign my priorities in life, deepen my appreciation for the value of life, and/or better appreciate each day.

- *My work with survivors of trauma has enhanced my spiritual growth*

For example, it has heightened my sense of spirituality and/or strengthened my faith.

- *My work with survivors of trauma has positively impacted my relationships with others*

For example, it has improved my ability to count on others in times of need, express my emotions, invest more effort into relationships, gain insights into the positive qualities of others, accept needing others, and/or experience more closeness with and compassion for others.

Self-Reflection

- Following my experience of STS, can I recall one or more instances where I have demonstrated increased compassion in my relations with others?

Group Context

Within a group setting, *Evaluating VPTG* can be accompanied by the following activity:

The facilitator can encourage participants to share any insights they may have gained from their personal practice. While seated in a circle, those who wish to share can do so in turns. To facilitate this process, a talking stick can be placed in the circle's center, accessible for participants to hold while speaking. This group sharing session, following the Native American talking stick tradition (e.g., Wolf & Rickard, 2003), encourages active and respectful dialogue, thereby further enhancing the VPTG-related theme of enhanced relationships. Notably, in lieu of a talking stick, inspiring alternatives could include a symbolic object representing compassion, such as a gemstone, a heart, or a lotus.

Embracing the Path

Practice Orientation and Type:
Self- and Other-Orientation – Reflection Prompts

Personal Practice

This practice, adapted from Campbell (2008) to promote vicarious post-traumatic growth (VPTG),[4] invites helping professionals to reflect on the path from secondary traumatic stress (STS) to VPTG (i.e., while STS is recognized as traumatic stress originating from indirect exposure to trauma, VPTG is defined as "the experience of growth as a result of indirect trauma exposure;" Arnold et al., 2005, as cited in Deaton et al., 2023, p. 17; Molnar et al., 2017).[5] By exploring their motivations for setting out on this path, the challenges they have navigated, and the strengths they have cultivated – helping professionals not only gain deeper insights into their own personal growth but also recognize their potential to inspire and provide support to others.

Start your practice by finding a comfortable and relaxed sitting position, letting a slight smile brighten the corners of your mouth and eyes. Take a few moments to center yourself and connect with your breath. Inhale slowly and exhale even more slowly, releasing any lingering stress with each exhalation. This initial step serves as a starting point for the following 11 sentence-starter prompts designed to help guide your reflection process:

1. My call to initiate the path from STS to VPTG was . . .
2. I resisted this call by . . .
3. What I had to let go of was . . .
4. My biggest challenge in addressing STS has been . . .
5. I overcame this challenge by . . .
6. My strongest source of support was . . .
7. I realized that my strengths are . . .
8. What I now believe about myself is . . .

9. The insights I have gained from addressing STS are . . .
10. When setbacks occur, I remind myself to . . .
11. The gifts I can share with others as a result of setting out on this path are . . .

Self-Reflection

• How can I channel the gifts I have gained to support others on their journeys from posttraumatic stress disorder (PTSD) to posttraumatic growth (PTG) and/or from STS to VPTG?[6]

Group Context

Within a group setting, *Embracing the Path* can be extended as follows:

Following the personal practice, participants can be encouraged to take turns sharing their responses to one or more of the sentence-starter prompts, either in pairs or small groups. As participants identify common challenges, shared strengths, and collective insights, this sharing experience can foster meaningful connections and provide a platform for mutual support.

Notably, in alignment with Hambly (2021), since group members may find themselves at different stages along the path, respecting narrative diversity is important. Such differences may encompass a wide spectrum of experiences, perspectives, challenges, and strengths. Embracing diversity can, therefore, contribute to a more tolerant atmosphere and enhance a sense of belonging and inclusivity among participants. A sharing session with the whole group can complete this activity.

Nurturing CARE

Practice Orientation and Type:
Self- to Self-Orientation – Guided Meditation

Personal Practice

This practice, adapted from Hanson (2013, 2020),[7] can assist helping professionals in further deepening their experience of vicarious posttraumatic growth (VPTG).[8] Based on an evolutionary perspective that the human brain has a built-in negativity bias, this practice offers a neuroscience-based practical roadmap that can help you overcome said bias. In effect, paying special attention to your positive VPTG-related experience has the potential to rewire your brain through self-directed neuroplasticity (e.g., Hanson, 2013, 2020; Norris, 2021).

Find a comfortable sitting position that allows you to feel at ease, relaxed, and focused. Close your eyes or gently lower and soften your gaze, and turn your focus inward. To help facilitate an optimistic and receptive mindset, you may also wish to consider allowing a gentle smile to lift the corners of your mouth and brighten your eyes. This simple act of smiling can enhance your overall experience, fostering a positive and open-hearted approach.

The following four steps outline the basics of this transformative practice, employing the acronym CARE (i.e., **C**onnect, **A**bsorb, **R**eflect, and **E**ngage):

Step 1: Connect with a VPTG experience

Notice a pleasant physical sensation, thought, and/or emotion that you are currently experiencing and that you associate with VPTG. If you first notice a VPTG-related thought or feeling, try to tune in to the associated underlying physical sensation as well.

Step 2: Absorb it

Focus on your experience of VPTG, letting it become more nuanced by exploring as many facets of the experience as possible. In a figurative sense, try to feel that you are metaphorically absorbing the experience as if the positive VPTG-related experience is becoming an integral part of your being.

Step 3: Reflect on how VPTG stemmed from secondary traumatic stress (STS)

While keeping your experience of VPTG more prominent, bring to mind one or more aspects of your STS-related experience. For example, you might recall a physical sensation associated with STS or specific situations or encounters that trigger STS reactions. Try, however, to mindfully keep the negative experience of STS in the background while bringing the positive experience of VPTG to the forefront of your awareness.

Step 4: Engage in gratitude

Consider inwardly thanking the process by which VPTG has emerged in your life in a way that resonates with you. This process involved experiencing challenges that ultimately catalyzed positive change. By embracing a perspective that appreciates what has emerged from the challenges you experienced, consider how, in hindsight, these challenges have revealed themselves as opportunities for growth.

Following this four-step practice, you are likewise invited to embrace the reality of impermanence by acknowledging that positive experiences are inherently subject to life's continuous ebb and flow. In doing so, let the current positive experience that you are savoring gently and mindfully flow through you, much like a river's gentle current enriching your inner landscape. By embracing this flow, you are granting yourself the gift of fully immersing in the present moment while creating a trail of cherished moments whose transient nature only serves to enhance their value.

Self-Reflections

• Reflecting on how a glimmer can grow into a glow and how a glow can become even more radiant (e.g., Dana, 2020) – are there additional metaphors that illustrate how absorbing a positive experience in this way can enhance its significance?
• In what ways can the emergence of VPTG from STS serve as an inspiration for me to support others as they navigate their healing journeys?

Group Context

Within a group setting, *Nurturing CARE* can be accompanied by the following visual arts activity to further facilitate a shift in focus to encompass others:

Participants can be invited to artistically convey their experiences of STS and VPTG by incorporating the visual arts. They can achieve this by portraying their VPTG-related experience in the foreground of their artwork and their STS-related experience in the background. Here, foreground and background refer to elements of the artwork that are respectively positioned nearest to and farthest from the viewer. Upon completion, participants can come together in pairs and/or small groups to share and discuss their artwork. A sharing session with the whole group can complete this activity.

Expanding the Circle

Practice Orientation and Type:
Self- and Other-Orientation – Guided Meditation

Personal Practice

Loving-kindness, referred to as *maitrī* in Sanskrit, involves cultivating a feeling of friendliness and the wish for all beings to experience happiness and its causes (e.g., Hao et al., 2021; Shonin et al., 2015).[9] The practice typically begins by recalling a time when you felt truly loved and cared for by someone. With this memory in mind, the idea is to reimagine the experience as if it were happening in the present moment and allow it to evoke the felt-sense and associated positive thoughts and emotions of being loved and treated kindly (Shonin et al., 2015).

From this starting point, the practice then customarily invites you to extend loving-kindness to others in the following progression: (a) someone you love, (b) someone to whom you hold no particularly positive or negative feelings, (c) someone whom you find challenging in some way, and eventually (d) all living beings (Shonin et al., 2015).[10]

In the context of this resource guide, these steps can be adapted to focus specifically on the workplace and on vicarious posttraumatic growth (VPTG). To illustrate, this can be done by extending wishes associated with VPTG first to yourself and then to a series of colleagues with whom you have: (a) a good relationship, (b) a neutral relationship, (c) a challenging relationship, and, finally, (d) the entire staff (e.g., your team, department, and/or organization).

Sitting comfortably and quietly, begin by closing your eyes or lowering and softening your gaze while tuning into the natural rhythm of your breath and accompanying sensations. You might also let the outer corners of your mouth and eyes pull up into a gentle smile. Gradually, inwardly repeat the following suggested wishes, or adapt them as you see fit, focusing on the experience of moving from secondary traumatic stress (STS) to VPTG:

May I continue to grow from STS,
experience positive changes associated with VPTG,
and be safe, healthy, and happy.

In the next sequential steps of this practice, extend these wishes to a series of colleagues with whom you have: (a) a good relationship, (b) a neutral relationship, and (c) a challenging relationship:

> *May you continue to grow from STS,*
> *experience positive changes associated with VPTG,*
> *and be safe, healthy, and happy.*

Finally, extend these wishes to the entire staff:

> *May we continue to grow from STS,*
> *experience positive changes associated with VPTG,*
> *and be safe, healthy, and happy.*[11]

As you gently open or raise your eyes again, consider mindfully exploring your surroundings and allowing your gaze to settle on something pleasant and calming that evokes positivity. This can serve as a smooth transition and aid in the gradual conclusion of this practice.

Self-Reflections

- What images come to mind when I think of "love," "kindness," and the interplay between the two?
- To what extent do I regard my colleagues as equally deserving of happiness and its causes, regardless of the dynamics of our interactions?

Group Context

Within a group setting, *Expanding the Circle* can be extended as follows:

Following the personal practice, participants can be guided to broaden their VPTG-related wishes to encompass the entire group with an all-embracing mindset. To facilitate this process, participants can employ the "VPTG-wish chain method." In line with this approach, one participant voices a VPTG-inspired wish, followed sequentially by others. This creates an inclusive interchange of positive VPTG-related wishes that have the potential to elevate and inspire the entire group.[12]

I can see two hearts,
one for you and one for me:
reflections of love[13]

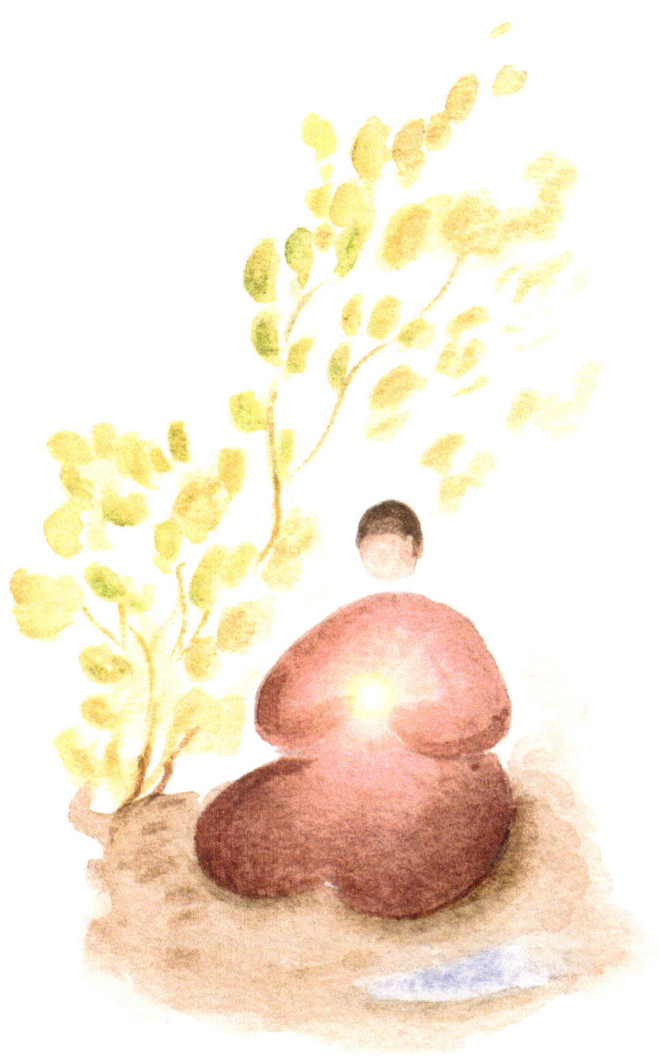

Loving-Kindness

Figure in a meditative posture

Summary of the Practices

Anchored in scientific research in the fields of trauma, secondary traumatic stress (STS), vicarious posttraumatic growth (VPTG), mindfulness, and compassion, the individual and group practices presented herein embrace a rich diversity of techniques. These include contemplative practices such as guided meditations, reflection, and journaling prompts, as well as arts-based creative activities spanning expressive movement, music, role-playing, poetry, and visual arts. Moreover, the practices encompass contemporary adaptations of time-honored Buddhist meditation techniques, extending their relevance to helping professionals from diverse fields engaged in trauma work.

The collections of "Foundational Practices" and "Practices for Promoting VPTG" each include five practices. "Foundational Practices" center on (a) receiving compassion, (b) balancing compassion and equanimity, (c) mindfulness of breathing and bodily sensations, (d) grounding and interconnectedness, and (e) savoring the good within the professional environment. "Practices for Promoting VPTG" focus on (a) acknowledging strengths, (b) evaluating VPTG-related progress, (c) the path from STS to VPTG, (d) nurturing the positive experience of VPTG, and (e) extending VPTG-related wishes to both oneself and others within the workplace.

Following the "Foundational Practices" and leading up to the "Practices for Promoting VPTG," the central theme, titled "Practices for Addressing STS," consists of a collection of 30 practices. These encompass the multifaceted dynamic "flows" of the following STS-related compassionate exchanges: (a) other-to-self (i.e., receiving compassion from others), (b) self-to-self (i.e., offering oneself compassion), (c) self-to-other (i.e., offering others compassion), and (d) other-to-other (i.e., witnessing compassion between others). All of these practices, including those centered on self-compassion, are guided by an altruistic orientation.

It is hoped that helping professionals will discover meaningful benefits within these pages and view the transdiagnostic practices as tools that can be finely tuned to their personal and professional needs and circumstances. The transdiagnostic nature of these practices lies in their ability to be effective across a wide range of clients' traumatic experiences through approaches that are adaptable, flexible, individualized, and attuned to cultural sensitivities and inclusivity. It is likewise hoped that these practices will be generously shared among colleagues, creating a ripple effect of compassionate exchange within the field of trauma care across helping professionals' diverse paths of service.

GUIDANCE FOR GROUP LEADERS

Benefits of Practicing Within a Group Setting

This resource guide offers a versatile group approach that can be tailored to accommodate various group settings, including workforce development training programs. In line with Yalom's (1985) group work curative factors, a list of potential benefits follows for helping professionals engaging in this training program within a group setting. Understanding Yalom's (1985) group work curative factors is important for group leaders, as it provides a foundation for effective group facilitation. These curative factors offer valuable insights into the dynamics of group work and the potential for positive change within a group setting.

- *Instillation of hope* – Engaging in secondary traumatic stress (STS) and vicarious posttraumatic growth (VPTG)-related compassion-based practices within a group setting, while witnessing other group members benefiting from said practices, can foster a sense of optimism among helping professionals regarding the potential benefits they may obtain from these practices.
- *Universality* – When helping professionals engage in group practice, they can gain valuable insights into STS as a shared challenge among their peers. Moreover, members can acknowledge and validate each

DOI: 10.4324/9781003381747-10

other's experiences related to STS, while mutually recognizing the effectiveness of compassion-based practices for addressing STS and promoting VPTG.

• *Imparting information* – A group setting can help empower helping professionals with valuable knowledge pertaining to STS, VPTG, and compassion. This can include psychoeducation about relevant resources that underscore the effectiveness of compassionately addressing STS and promoting VPTG.

• *Helping others* – When helping professionals share their experiences of compassionately addressing STS and promoting VPTG within a group setting, it can serve as a source of inspiration for other group members. This exchange has the potential to enhance helping professionals' belief in their capacity to effectively help others.

• *Development of socializing techniques* – By prioritizing compassionate practices for addressing STS and promoting VPTG within a group setting, helping professionals can refine social skills needed to compassionately connect with others. These improved interpersonal skills, when applied within the group, can contribute to nurturing a compassionate group culture.

• *Imitative behavior* – Group members can serve as inspiring role models for one another by addressing STS and promoting VPTG with compassion. As helping professionals share a common challenge, this dynamic becomes particularly effective, allowing for the modeling of STS and VPTG-related compassionate behaviors.

• *Group cohesiveness* and *interpersonal learning* – A group setting that centers around compassionately addressing STS and promoting VPTG can provide helping professionals with a sense of belonging and social support. The resulting group cohesion can promote mutual learning as members share their insights and coping strategies.

• *Catharsis* – Compassionately addressing STS and promoting VPTG within a group setting can provide helping professionals with a sense of relief and solace. It is beneficial to complement this cathartic experience with self-reflection and introspection as these can enhance self-awareness and create a powerful synergy for healing and wellbeing.

• *Existential factors* – When approaching the conclusion of each group session and, ultimately, the end of the group experience, the awareness of the time-limited nature of the group becomes evident. This existential reality can serve as a powerful motivator for helping professionals to take ultimate responsibility for their reactions to STS and actively pursue VPTG.

Importantly, to enhance the development of the aforementioned benefits, group leaders may wish to incorporate the practice of *appreciative feedback* within the group. Rather than focusing on areas for improvement or critique, this type of feedback intentionally emphasizes positive aspects and reinforces the value of each group member's efforts as well as the efforts of the group as a whole. Namely, appreciative feedback focuses on recognizing and highlighting positive aspects, strengths, qualities, contributions, and achievements. It involves acknowledging and celebrating the progress that is being made, thereby also serving as a valuable tool in building and maintaining positive relationships within group settings (e.g., Applied Compassion Training [ACT], 2021; See Appendix G for additional interpersonal communication recommendations relevant for group facilitators, group members, and helping professionals in general).

Skillful Means Recommendations

"Buddhist thinking has been central in guiding much of the scientific study on compassion and its training" (Lavelle, 2017, as cited in Quaglia, 2023, p. 2431). However, the concept of diversity recognizes that no single perspective encompasses the entire truth (Yong, 2023). As such, the objective, as stated by Yong, is "to skillfully create space to recognize that compassion has many different paths of cultivation, and that the various wisdom traditions have important and nuanced gifts to offer in their own rights" (p. 2369).

Within Buddhist traditions, there are numerous interpretations of the term *skillful means* (Skt. *upāya-kauśalya*; e.g., Schroeder, 2004). These can include how group facilitators skillfully embody compassion while imparting it to a diverse audience. Wisdom can be found within and across diverse positionalities, such as cultural, spiritual, and religious contexts. In this light, facilitators as co-learners in the pursuit of collective wisdom can foster a dynamic learning environment that is conducive to nurturing compassion (Yong, 2023).

Developing skillful means is paramount for facilitators aiming to enhance their ability to promote compassion-based trainings that incorporate principles of East Asian philosophy within interreligious, intercultural, and intersectional contexts (Yong, 2023). The following recommendations encompass such skillful suggestions. Some offer more general, foundational guidance while others delve into specific, nuanced insights that are tailored to the intricacies of this topic. These recommendations, based on Yong (2023), serve as insightful guidelines for facilitators to consider:

• Commence compassion trainings by inviting participants to reflect on their diverse firsthand encounters with receiving compassion. This emphasis on participants' real-life experiences of compassion is important, as it acknowledges that a comprehensive understanding of compassion goes beyond theoretical knowledge. Moreover, it embraces the richness of the various compassionate encounters that individuals from different backgrounds may have experienced.

- Embrace a flexible pace within compassion trainings, prioritizing being fully present with the material at hand. This approach allows time for diverse perspectives to unfold rather than rigidly adhering to pre-defined content. The skillful means of taking time to check in with participants, instead of rushing through the material, fosters a learning environment that embraces and encourages diverse viewpoints. Nonetheless, it remains essential to find a balance between maintaining a flexible pace that respects diverse perspectives and ensuring that essential concepts and objectives are addressed.
- Integrate real-time feedback loops to facilitate participants' reflection throughout compassion trainings, encompassing their dynamic experiences. These feedback loops invite insights, challenges, and suggestions, facilitating immediate adjustments. Posttraining evaluations are likewise encouraged for refinement. Such evaluations are valuable tools for facilitators to gauge the effectiveness of group sessions and gather feedback from participants. This approach not only contributes to the ongoing development and refinement of compassion trainings but also fosters collaborative and responsive learning environments.
- Create a complementary network of resources from diverse wisdom traditions, including resources related to secular compassion education. Curate these resources thoughtfully, making them readily accessible to participants while also inviting participants to add relevant resources that are reflective of their diverse backgrounds. Inviting guest speakers to enrich the collective learning experience can further foster respect for the richness of diverse worldviews.
- Acknowledge the importance of systemic awareness in compassion cultivation, particularly recognizing the significance of systemic suffering, such as racial and collective trauma. This includes acknowledging the possible adverse impacts that such factors may play on the challenges faced by group members (e.g., Jackson-Preston et al., 2023).
- Develop an understanding of participants' diverse backgrounds, especially concerning the intricacies of compassion within these contexts. This understanding enables the facilitation of inclusive discussions and provides informed insights into how compassion is perceived, practiced, and valued across different cultural, philosophical, spiritual, and religious landscapes. This includes highlighting potential intersections with principles found in East Asian philosophy.

Interbeing is …
dependent co-arising:
a stardust *saṅgha*[1]

Rooted in Community

Five figures joining hands in a circle

Call to Compassionate Action

Secondary traumatic stress (STS) serves as a call to action, compelling us to acknowledge the interconnectedness of our human experience and to respond with compassion. The recognition that the suffering endured by individuals who have experienced trauma has the potential to reverberate in those caring for them underscores the significance of compassionate care. This extends not only to individuals directly impacted by trauma but also to their compassionate caregivers, especially considering the interdependence between caregivers' wellbeing and the quality of their service.

This dynamic likewise highlights the necessity of promoting a compassionate ripple effect in the field of trauma care – one that extends beyond individual helping professionals to permeate the broader context in which they provide care. Such a ripple effect would positively contribute not only to helping professionals themselves and to the individuals they serve but also to their colleagues, organizations, and, more broadly, their communities, highlighting compassion's far-reaching potential.

Relatedly, Thích Nhất Hạnh – a Buddhist monk, peace activist, author, and poet – emphasized coming together compassionately in community. To illustrate this point, he offered the image of a raindrop that lands on top of a mountain. For that raindrop to make it all the way down the mountain to the ocean, it needs to be carried by a river (as cited in Desmond, 2015, p. 197). This analogy beautifully encapsulates the idea that our individual efforts are enhanced and carried forward when we come together in compassionate community.

Aligning with this imagery, this resource guide, encompassing the *Compassion for STS* (CSTS) training program, is offered as a compassionate response to the challenges posed by STS. Its aim is to serve as a comprehensive tool that empowers helping professionals and their host organizations to address STS with compassion. Like raindrops collectively flowing together toward the ocean, may we support one another not only in the context of STS but also in the broader context of alleviating suffering and promoting wellbeing. "The wellbeing of 'this' is the wellbeing of 'that,' so we have to do things together" (Hạnh, 1992, p. 86).

thank you, compassion,
thank you, wisdom, and thank you,
gentle ocean breeze

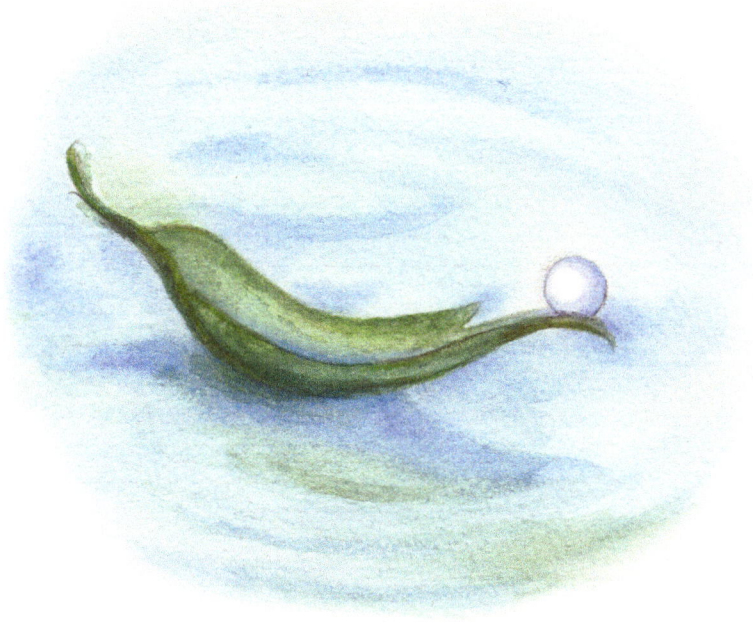

Ocean's Call

A raindrop, a leaf, and a river flowing together

Dedicating the Merits

May whatever merits gained by the creation of this resource guide be dedicated to all those who have experienced trauma, to the compassionate caregivers caring for them, and to a more compassionate world for us all.

Glow of Compassion

An illuminated candle

References

Front Matter

Barclay, H. K., & Barclay, A. C. (2011). Recession compassion: 7 steps on how to treat employees to get the best performance during these global economic times. *Journal of Management Policy and Practice, 12*(1), 21–26.

Brend, D. M., & Sprang, G. (2020). Trauma-informed care in child welfare: An imperative for residential childcare workers. *International Journal of Child and Adolescent Resilience, 7*(1), 154–165. https://doi.org/10.7202/1072595ar

Cleary, E., Curran, D., Dyer, K., Simms, J., & Hanna, D. (2023). Contributing factors to secondary traumatic stress and vicarious posttraumatic growth in therapists. *Journal of Traumatic Stress,* 1–10. https://doi.org/10.1002/jts.22995

Collins. (2023). Ruth. In *Collins online unabridged English dictionary*. https://www.collinsdictionary.com/dictionary/english/ruth

Deaton, J. D., Ohrt, J. H., Linich, K., McCartney, E., & Glascoe, G. (2023). Vicarious posttraumatic growth: A systematic review and thematic synthesis across helping professions. *Traumatology, 29*(1), 17–26. https://doi.org/10.1037/trm0000375

Deaton, J. D., Wymer, B., & Carlson, R. G. (2021). Supervision strategies to facilitate vicarious posttraumatic growth among trauma counselors. *Journal of Counselor Preparation and Supervision, 14*(4), 1–26. https://digitalcommons.sacredheart.edu/jcps/vol14/iss4/12

Diedrich, A., Hofmann, S. G., Cuijpers, P., & Berking, M. (2016). Self-compassion enhances the efficacy of explicit cognitive reappraisal as an emotion regulation strategy in individuals with major depressive disorder. *Behaviour Research and Therapy, 82*, 1–10. https://doi.org/10.1016/j.brat.2016.04.003

Friedman, H. H., & Gerstein, M. (2017). Leading with compassion: The key to changing the organizational culture and achieving success. *Psychosociological Issues in Human Resource Management, 5*(1), 1–22. https://doi.org/10.22381/PIHRM5120175

Gottfried, R., & Bride, B. E. (2018). Trauma–secondary, vicarious, compassion fatigue. In *Encyclopedia of social work*. Oxford University Press. https://doi:10.1093/acrefore/9780199975839.013.1085

Johnson, E. A., & O'Brien, K. A. (2013). Self-compassion soothes the savage ego-threat system: Effects on negative affect, shame, rumination, and depressive symptoms. *Journal of Social and Clinical Psychology, 32*(9), 939–963. https://doi.org/10.1521/jscp.2013.32.9.939

Kanov, J. M., Maitlis, S., Worline, M. C., Dutton, J. E., Frost, P. J., & Lilius, J. M. (2004). Compassion in organizational life. *American Behavioral Scientist, 47*(6), 808–827. https://doi:10.1177/0002764203260211

Karatzias, T., Hyland, P., Bradley, A., Fyvie, C., Logan, K., Easton, P., Thomas, J., Philips, S., Bisson, J. I., Roberts, N. P., Cloitre, M., & Shevlin, M. (2019). Is self-compassion a worthwhile therapeutic target for ICD-11 complex PTSD (CPTSD)? *Behavioural and Cognitive Psychotherapy, 47*(3), 257–269. https://doi.org/10.1017/S1352465818000577

Lown, B. A., Shin, A., & Jones, R. N. (2019). Can organizational leaders sustain compassionate, patient-centered care and mitigate burnout? *Journal of Healthcare Management, 64*(6), 398–412. https://doi:10.1097/JHM-D-18-00023

Lyubomirsky, S., King, L., & Diener, E. (2005). The benefits of frequent positive affect: Does happiness lead to success? *Psychological Bulletin, 131*(6), 803–855. https://doi:10.1037/0033-2909.131.6.803

Malchiodi, C. A. (2020). *Trauma and expressive arts therapy: Brain, body, and imagination in the healing process.* Guilford Publications.

Molnar, B. E., Sprang, G., Killian, K. D., Gottfried, R., Emery, V., & Bride, B. E. (2017). Advancing science and practice for vicarious traumatization/secondary traumatic stress: A research agenda. *Traumatology, 23*(2), 129–142. https://doi.org/10.1037/trm0000122

Mosewich, A. D., Crocker, P. R., Kowalski, K. C., & DeLongis, A. (2013). Applying self-compassion in sport: An intervention with women athletes. *Journal of Sport and Exercise Psychology, 35*(5), 514–524. https://doi.org/10.1123/jsep.35.5.514

Neff, K. D., & Germer, C. K. (2013). A pilot study and randomized controlled trial of the mindful self-compassion program. *Journal of Clinical Psychology, 69*(1), 28–44. https://doi.org/10.1002/jclp.21923

Neff, K. D., & Germer, C. K. (2018). *The mindful self-compassion workbook: A proven way to accept yourself, build inner strength, and thrive* (Kindle ed.). Guilford Publications.

Neff, K. D., Kirkpatrick, K. L., & Rude, S. S. (2007). Self-compassion and adaptive psychological functioning. *Journal of Research in Personality, 41*(1), 139–154. https://doi.org/10.1016/j.jrp.2006.03.004

Odou, N., & Brinker, J. (2015). Self-compassion, a better alternative to rumination than distraction as a response to negative mood. *The Journal of Positive Psychology, 10*(5), 447–457. https://doi.org/10.1080/17439760.2014.967800

Ogińska-Bulik, N., & Juczyński, Z. (2024). Vicarious posttraumatic growth: The benefits of indirect exposure to trauma. In R. Berger (Ed.), *The Routledge international handbook of posttraumatic growth* (Kindle ed., pp. 445–457). Routledge.

Perry, B. D. (2014). *Creative interventions with traumatized children.* Guilford Publications.

Perryman, K., Blisard, P., & Moss, R. (2019). Using creative arts in trauma therapy: The neuroscience of healing. *Journal of Mental Health Counseling, 41*(1), 80–94. https://doi.org/10.17744/mehc.41.1.07

Rushforth, A., Durk, M., Rothwell-Blake, G. A., Kirkman, A., Ng, F., & Kotera, Y. (2023). Self-compassion interventions to target secondary traumatic stress in healthcare workers: A systematic review. *International Journal of Environmental Research and Public Health, 20*(12), 1–14. https://doi.org/10.3390/ijerph20126109

Smeets, E., Neff, K., Alberts, H., & Peters, M. (2014). Meeting suffering with kindness: Effects of a brief self-compassion intervention for female college students. *Journal of Clinical Psychology, 70*(9), 794–807. https://doi.org/10.1002/jclp.22076

Sprang, G. (2018a). Organizational assessment of secondary traumatic stress: Utilizing the secondary traumatic stress informed organizational assessment tool to facilitate organizational learning and change. In V. C. Strand & G. Sprang (Eds.), *Trauma responsive child welfare systems* (pp. 261–270). Springer. https://doi.org/10.1007/978-3-319-64602-2_16

Sprang, G., Lei, F., & Bush, H. (2021). Can organizational efforts lead to less secondary traumatic stress? A longitudinal investigation of change. *American Journal of Orthopsychiatry, 91*(4), 443–453. https://doi.org/10.1037/ort0000546

Unkule, K. (2019). Shoshin. In K. Unkule (Ed.), *Internationalising the university: A spiritual approach* (pp. 121–152). Palgrave Macmillan.

van Dernoot Lipsky, L., & Burk, C. (2010). *Trauma stewardship: An everyday guide to caring for self while caring for others* (Kindle ed.). ReadHowYouWant.com

Winders, S. J., Murphy, O., Looney, K., & O'Reilly, G. (2020). Self-compassion, trauma, and posttraumatic stress disorder: A systematic review. *Clinical Psychology & Psychotherapy, 27*(3), 300–329. https://doi.org/10.1002/cpp.2429

Part I

Acorn, A. E. (2004). *Compulsory compassion: A critique of restorative justice.* UBC Press.

Adams, R. E., Boscarino, J. A., & Figley, C. R. (2006). Compassion fatigue and psychological distress among social workers: A validation study. *American Journal of Orthopsychiatry, 76*(1), 103–108. https://doi.org/10.1037/0002-9432.76.1.103

Alexander, B. N., Greenbaum, B. E., Shani, A. B., Mitki, Y., & Horesh, A. (2021). Organizational posttraumatic growth: Thriving after adversity. *The Journal of Applied Behavioral Science, 57*(1), 30–56. https://doi.org/10.1177/0021886320931119

American Psychiatric Association. (2022). *Diagnostic and statistical manual of mental disorders* (5th ed., text rev.). https://doi.org/10.1176/appi.books.9780890425787

Anālayo, B. (2017). How compassion became painful. *Journal of Buddhist Studies, 14*, 85–113.

Anālayo, B., & Dhammadinnā, B. (2021). From compassion to self-compassion: A text-historical perspective. *Mindfulness, 12*(6), 1350–1360. https://doi.org/10.1007/s12671-020-01575-4

Ash, M., Harrison, T., Pinto, M., DiClemente, R., & Negi, L. T. (2021). A model for cognitively-based compassion training: Theoretical underpinnings and proposed mechanisms. *Social Theory & Health, 19*, 43–67. https://doi.org/10.1057/s41285-019-00124-x

Bachner-Melman, R., & Oakley, B. (2016). Giving 'til it hurts': Eating disorders and pathological altruism. In Y. Latzer & D. Stein (Eds.), *Bio-psycho-social contributions to understanding eating disorders* (pp. 91–103). Springer International Publishing.

Badura, K. L., Grijalva, E., Galvin, B. M., Owens, B. P., & Joseph, D. L. (2020). Motivation to lead: A meta-analysis and distal-proximal model of motivation and leadership. *Journal of Applied Psychology, 105*(4), 331–354. https://doi.org/10.1037/apl0000439

Bartoskova, L. (2017). How do trauma therapists experience the effects of their trauma work, and are there common factors leading to post-traumatic growth? *Counselling Psychology Review, 32*(2), 30–45. https://doi.org/10.53841/bpscpr.2017.32.2.30

Batson, C. D., Batson, J. G., Todd, R. M., Brummett, B. H., Shaw, L. L., & Aldeguer, C. M. (1995). Empathy and the collective good: Caring for one of the others in a social dilemma. *Journal of Personality and Social Psychology, 68*, 619–631. https://doi.org/10.1037/0022-3514.68.4.619

Batson, C. D., Klein, T. R., Highberger, L., & Shaw, L. L. (1995). Immorality from empathy-induced altruism: When compassion and justice conflict. *Journal of Personality and Social Psychology, 68*(6), 1042–1054. https://doi.org/10.1037/0022-3514.68.6.1042

Beck, C. T., Rivera, J., & Gable, R. K. (2017). A mixed-methods study of vicarious posttraumatic growth in certified nurse-midwives. *Journal of Midwifery & Women's Health, 62*(1), 80–87. https://doi.org/10.1111/jmwh.12523

Ben-Porat, A. (2015). Competence of trauma social workers: The relationship between field of practice and secondary traumatization, personal and environmental variables. *Journal of Interpersonal Violence, 32*(8), 1291–1309. https://doi.org/10.1177/0886260515588536

Ben-Porat, A., Gil, L., Brafman, D., Zriker, A., & Levy, D. (2021). Secondary traumatic stress and posttraumatic growth among volunteers at a therapeutic riding center: The role of personal and environmental factors. *Current Psychology*, 1–10. https://doi.org/10.1007/s12144-021-01704-9

Berger, R. (Ed.). (2024). *The Routledge international handbook of posttraumatic growth* (Kindle ed.). Routledge.

Bhalla, T., & DiCuirci, L. (2023). "Me time": Motherhood, reading, and myths of leisure. *Reception: Texts, Readers, Audiences, History, 15*, 41–49. https://doi.org/10.5325/reception.15.1.0041

Blanch, A. (2012). *SAMHSA'S national center for trauma-informed care: Changing communities, changing lives.* https://www.nasmhpd.org/sites/default/files/NCTIC_Marketing_Brochure_FINAL(2).pdf

Bloom, S. L. (2006). *Human service systems and organizational stress: Thinking and feeling our way out of existing organizational dilemmas.* Report for the Trauma Task Force. https://www.researchgate.net/profile/Sandra-Bloom/publication/242222653_Human_Service_Systems_and_Organizational_Stress_Thinking_Feeling_Our_Way_Out_of_Existing_Organizational_Dilemmas/links/55c4551608aebc967df1c0ca/Human-Service-Systems-and-Organizational-Stress-Thinking-Feeling-Our-Way-Out-of-Existing-Organizational-Dilemmas.pdf

Bodhi, B. (2005). *In the Buddha's words: An anthology of discourses from the Pāli Canon.* Wisdom.

Bodhi, B. (2011). What does mindfulness really mean? A canonical perspective. *Contemporary Buddhism, 12*(1), 19–39. https://doi.org/10.1080/14639947.2011.564813

Brach, T. (2004). *Radical acceptance: Embracing your life with the heart of a Buddha.* Bantam.

Brach, T. (2019). *Radical compassion* (Kindle ed.). Penguin Publishing Group.

Braehler, C., & Neff, K. (2020). Self-compassion in PTSD. In M. Tull & N. Kimbrel (Eds.), *Emotion in posttraumatic stress disorder: Etiology, assessment, neurobiology, and treatment* (pp. 567–596). Academic Press. https://doi.org/10.1016/B978-0-12-816022-0.00020-X

Brend, D. M., & Sprang, G. (2020). Trauma-informed care in child welfare: An imperative for residential childcare workers. *International Journal of Child and Adolescent Resilience, 7*(1), 154–165. https://doi.org/10.7202/1072595ar

Brenner, R. E., Vogel, D. L., Lannin, D. G., Engel, K. E., Seidman, A. J., & Heath, P. J. (2018). Do self-compassion and self-coldness distinctly relate to distress and well-being? A theoretical model of self-relating. *Journal of Counseling Psychology, 65*(3), 346–357. https://doi.org/10.1037/cou0000257

Bride, B. E., Sprang, G., Hendricks, A., Walsh, C. R., Mathieu, F., Hangartner, K., Ross, L. A., Fisher, P., & Miller, B. C. (2023). Principles for secondary traumatic stress-responsive practice: An expert consensus approach. *Psychological Trauma: Theory, Research, Practice, and Policy.* Advance online publication. https://doi.org/10.1037/tra0001575

Briere, J. N. (2012). Working with trauma: Mindfulness and compassion. In C. K. Germer & R. D. Siegel (Eds.), *Wisdom and compassion in psychotherapy: Deepening mindfulness in clinical practice* (Kindle ed., pp. 265–279). Guilford Press.

Briere, J. N. (2015). Pain and suffering: A synthesis of Buddhist and Western approaches to trauma. In V. M. Follette, J. Briere, D. Rozelle, J. Hopper, & D. I. Rome (Eds.), *Mindfulness-oriented interventions for trauma: Integrating contemplative practices* (Kindle ed., pp. 11–30). Guilford.

Briere, J. N., & Scott, C. (2006). *Principles of trauma therapy: A guide to symptoms, evaluation, and treatment* (1st ed.). Sage Publications.

Bronfenbrenner, U. (1989). Ecological systems theory. In R. Vasta (Ed.), *Annals of child development* (Vol. 6, pp. 187–249). JAI Press.

Burris, E. R., Detert, J. R., & Romney, A. C. (2013). Speaking up vs. being heard: The disagreement around and outcomes of employee voice. *Organization Science, 24*(1), 22–38. https://doi.org/10.1287/orsc.1110.0732

Burris, E. R., Rockmann, K. W., & Kimmons, Y. S. (2017). The value of voice to managers: Employee identification and the content of voice. *Academy of Management Journal, 60*(6), 2099–2125. https://doi.org/10.5465/amj.2014.0320

Casas, J. B., & Benuto, L. T. (2022). Work-related traumatic stress spillover in first responder families: A systematic review of the literature. *Psychological Trauma: Theory, Research, Practice, and Policy, 14*(2), 209–217. https://doi.org/10.1037/tra0001086

Centers for Disease Control and Prevention Foundation. (2023). *What is public health?* https://www.cdcfoundation.org/what-public-health

Cha, J. E., Serlachius, A. S., Kirby, J. N., & Consedine, N. S. (2023). What do (and don't) we know about self-compassion? Trends and issues in theory, mechanisms, and outcomes. *Mindfulness, 14*(11), 2657–2669. https://doi.org/10.1007/s12671-023-02222-4

Cheng, F. K. (2014). Overcoming "sentimental compassion": How Buddhists cope with compassion fatigue. *Journal of the Oxford Centre for Buddhist Studies, 7,* 56–97.

Chierchia, G., & Singer, T. (2017). The neuroscience of compassion and empathy and their link to prosocial motivation and behavior. In J.-C. Dreher & L. Tremblay (Eds.), *Decision neuroscience* (pp. 247–257). Academic Press. https://doi.org/10.1016/B978-0-12-805308-9.00020-8

Choi, E. Y., Choi, S. H., & Lee, H. (2021). Development and evaluation of a screening scale for indirect trauma caused by media exposure to social disasters. *International Journal of Environmental Research and Public Health, 18*(2), 1–17. https://doi.org/10.3390/ijerph18020698

Choi, G. Y. (2011). Organizational impacts on the secondary traumatic stress of social workers assisting family violence or sexual assault survivors. *Administration in Social Work, 35*(3), 225–242. https://doi:10.1080/03643107.2011.575333

Cieslak, R., Shoji, K., Douglas, A., Melville, E., Luszczynska, A., & Benight, C. C. (2013). A meta-analysis of the relationship between job burnout and secondary traumatic stress among workers with indirect exposure to trauma. *Psychological Services, 11*(1), 175–186. https://doi.org/10.1037/a0033798

Cloitre, M., Hyland, P., Bisson, J., Brewin, C., Roberts, N., Karatzias, T., & Shevlin, M. (2019). ICD-11 posttraumatic stress disorder and complex posttraumatic stress disorder in the United States: A population-based study. *Journal of Traumatic Stress, 32*(6), 833–842. https://doi.org/10.1002/jts.22454

Compassion Resilience Toolkit. (n.d.). *What is compassion resilience?* https://eliminatestigma.org/compassion-resilience-toolkit/health-and-human-services/what-is-compassion-resilience/

Condon, M., Bloomfield, M. A., Nicholls, H., & Billings, J. (2023). Expert international trauma clinicians' views on the definition, composition and delivery of reintegration interventions for complex PTSD. *European Journal of Psychotraumatology, 14*(1), 2165024. https://doi.org/10.1080/20008066.2023.2165024

Condon, P., & Makransky, J. (2023). Compassion and skillful means: Cultural adaptation, psychological science, and creative responsiveness. *Mindfulness, 14*(10), 2331–2341. https://doi.org/10.1007/s12671-022-01866-y

Cooperrider, D. L., & Fry, R. (2012). Mirror flourishing and the positive psychology of sustainability. *Journal of Corporate Citizenship, 46*(1), 3–12. http://www.jstor.com/stable/jcorpciti.46.3

Cozart, D., & Shields, J. M. (Eds.). (2018). *The Oxford handbook of Buddhist ethics.* Oxford University Press.

Craun, S. W., Bourke, M. L., Bierie, D. M., & Williams, K. S. (2014). A longitudinal examination of secondary traumatic stress among law enforcement. *Victims & Offenders, 9*(3), 299–316. https://doi.org/10.1080/15564886.2013.848828

Dalai Lama, X. I. V. (1995). *The power of compassion.* Harper Collins.

Dalai Lama, X. I. V., & Chodron, B. T. (2017). *Buddhism: One teacher, many traditions.* Simon and Schuster.

Dana, D. (2020). *Polyvagal exercises for safety and connection: 50 client-centered practices (Norton series on interpersonal neurobiology)* (Kindle ed.). W.W. Norton & Company.

D'Angelo, S. (2022). *Polyvagal informed embodied mindfulness: An online program* [Mindfulness Studies theses]. https://digitalcommons.lesley.edu/mindfulness_theses/60

Deaton, J. D., Ohrt, J. H., Linich, K., McCartney, E., & Glascoe, G. (2023). Vicarious posttraumatic growth: A systematic review and thematic synthesis across helping professions. *Traumatology, 29*(1), 17–26. https://doi.org/10.1037/trm0000375

Deaton, J. D., Wymer, B., & Carlson, R. G. (2021). Supervision strategies to facilitate vicarious posttraumatic growth among trauma counselors. *Journal of Counselor Preparation and Supervision, 14*(4), 12. https://digitalcommons.sacredheart.edu/jcps/vol14/iss4/12

DeCandia, C. J., Guarino, K., & Clervil, R. (2014). *Trauma-informed care and trauma-specific services: A comprehensive approach to trauma intervention.* American Institutes for Research. https://www.air.org/sites/default/files/downloads/report/Trauma-Informed%20Care%20White%20Paper_October%202014.pdf

DeDecker, J. (2020). "Compassion fatigue" is a misnomer: How compassion can increase quality of life. *Creative Nursing, 26*(4), 246–252. https://doi:10.1891/CRNR-D-19-00086

Dekel, R., Siegel, A., Fridkin, S., & Svetlitzky, V. (2018). The double-edged sword: The role of empathy in military veterans' partners' distress. *Psychological Trauma: Theory, Research, Practice, and Policy, 10*(2), 216–224. https://doi.org/10.1037/tra0000265

Delaney, M. C. (2018). Caring for the caregivers: Evaluation of the effect of an eight-week pilot mindful self-compassion (MSC) training program on nurses' compassion fatigue and resilience. *PLoS One, 13*(11), e0207261. https://doi.org/10.1371/journal.pone.0207261

Dewar, B., Pullin, S., & Tocheris, R. (2011). Valuing compassion through definition and measurement. *Nursing Management, 17*(9), 32–37.

Dodson, S. J., & Heng, Y. T. (2022). Self-compassion in organizations: A review and future research agenda. *Journal of Organizational Behavior, 43*(2), 168–196. https://doi.org/10.1002/job.2556

Donald, J. N., Ciarrochi, J., Parker, P. D., Sahdra, B. K., Marshall, S. L., & Guo, J. (2018). A worthy self is a caring self: Examining the developmental relations between self-esteem and self-compassion in adolescents. *Journal of Personality, 86*(4), 619–630. https://doi.org/10.1111/jopy.12340

Dowling, T. (2018). Compassion does not fatigue! *The Canadian Veterinary Journal, 59*(7), 749–750. https://pubmed.ncbi.nlm.nih.gov/30026620

Drigas, A., & Papoutsi, C. (2023). A new pyramid model of empathy: The role of ICTs and robotics on empathy. *International Journal of Online & Biomedical Engineering, 19*(2). https://doi.org/10.3991/ijoe.v19i02.33591

Driver, M. (2007). Meaning and suffering in organizations. *Journal of Organizational Change Management, 20*(5), 611–632. https://doi.org/10.1108/09534810710779063

Duckworth, D. (2023). Two dimensions of a bodhisattva. *International Journal of Transpersonal Studies Advance Publication Archive.* https://digitalcommons.ciis.edu/advance-archive/56

Duffy, E., Avalos, G., & Dowling, M. (2015). Secondary traumatic stress among emergency nurses: A cross-sectional study. *International Emergency Nursing, 23*(2), 53–58. https://doi.org/10.1016/j.ienj.2014.05.001

Dunne, J. D., & Manheim, J. (2023). Compassion, self-compassion, and skill in means: A Mahāyāna perspective. *Mindfulness, 14*(10), 2374–2382. https://doi.org/10.1007/s12671-022-01864-0

Dutton, J. E., Workman, K. M., & Hardin, A. E. (2014). Compassion at work. *Annual Review of Organizational Psychology and Organizational Behavior, 1*(1), 277–304. https://www.annualreviews.org/doi/abs/10.1146/annurev-orgpsych-031413-091221

Eastwood, C., & Ecklund, K. (2008). Compassion fatigue risk and self-care practices among residential treatment center childcare workers. *Residential Treatment for Children & Youth, 25*(2), 103–122. https://doi.org/10.1080/08865710802309972

Eisler, R. (2017). A conversation with Monica Worline and Jane Dutton: Compassion in the work place. *Interdisciplinary Journal of Partnership Studies, 4*(2), 1–10. https://doi.org/10.24926/ijps.v4i2.161

Ekman, P., & Ekman, E. (2017). Is global compassion achievable? In E. M. Seppälä, E. Simon-Thomas, S. L. Brown, M. Worline, C. D. Cameron, & J. R. Doty (Eds.), *The Oxford handbook of compassion science* (pp. 41–49). Oxford University Press.

Encyclopedia of Buddhism. (2024). *Pratityasamutpada.* https://encyclopediaofbuddhism.org/wiki/Pratityasamutpada

Epstein, M. (2001). *Going on being.* Broadway Books.

Eriksson, T., Germundsjö, L., Åström, E., & Rönnlund, M. (2018). Mindful self-compassion training reduces stress and burnout symptoms among practicing psychologists: A randomized controlled trial of a brief web-based intervention. *Frontiers in Psychology, 9,* 23–40. https://doi.org/10.3389/fpsyg.2018.02340

Everly, G. S., Jr. (2020). Psychological first aid to support healthcare professionals. *Journal of Patient Safety and Risk Management, 25*(4), 159–162. https://doi.org/10.1177/2516043520944637

Fernando, J. (2018). Trauma and the zero process: Clinical illustrations. *Psychoanalysis, 29*(3), 37–45. https://doi.org/10.18529/psychoanal.2018.29.3.37

Figley, C. R. (1995). Compassion fatigue: Toward a new understanding of the costs of caring. In B. H. Stamm (Ed.), *Secondary traumatic stress: Self-care issues for clinicians, researchers, and educators.* Sidran Press.

Figley, C. R. (1999). Compassion fatigue: Toward a new understanding of the costs of caring. In B. H. Stamm (Ed.), *Secondary traumatic stress: Self-care issues for clinicians, researchers, & educators* (2nd ed., pp. 3–28). Sidran Press.

First, M. B., Yousif, L. H., Clarke, D. E., Wang, P. S., Gogtay, N., & Appelbaum, P. S. (2022). DSM-5-TR: Overview of what's new and what's changed. *World Psychiatry, 21*(2), 218–219. https://doi:10.1002/wps.20989

Franco, P. L., & Christie, L. M. (2021). Effectiveness of a one-day self-compassion training for pediatric nurses' resilience. *Journal of Pediatric Nursing, 61,* 109–114. https://doi.org/10.1016/j.pedn.2021.03.020

Garavan, M. (2012). *Compassionate activism – an exploration of integral social care.* Lang A&G International Academic Publishers.

Garcia, A. C. M., Silva, B. D., da Silva, L. C. O., & Mills, J. (2021). Self-compassion in hospice and palliative care: A systematic integrative review. *Journal of Hospice & Palliative Nursing, 23*(2), 145–154. https://doi:10.1097/NJH.0000000000000727

Garfield, J. L. (2022). *Losing ourselves: Learning to live without a self* (Kindle ed.). Princeton University Press.

Garfin, D. R., Silver, R. C., & Holman, E. A. (2020). The novel coronavirus (COVID-2019) outbreak: Amplification of public health consequences by media exposure. *Health Psychology, 39*(5), 355–357. https://doi.org/10.1037/hea0000875

Gerdes, K. (2019). Trauma, trigger warnings, and the rhetoric of sensitivity. *Rhetoric Society Quarterly, 49*(1), 3–24. https://doi.org/10.1080/02773945.2018.1479767

Germer, C. K. (2005). Mindfulness: What is it? What does it matter? In C. K. Germer, R. D. Siegel, & P. R. Fulton (Eds.), *Mindfulness and psychotherapy* (pp. 3–27). Guilford.

Germer, C. K., & Neff, K. (2019). *Teaching the mindful self-compassion program: A guide for professionals* (Kindle ed.). Guilford Press.

Gethin, R. (1998). *The foundations of Buddhism* (Kindle ed.). Oxford University Press.

Gethin, R. (2015). Buddhist conceptualizations of mindfulness. In K. W. Brown, J. D. Creswell, & R. M. Ryan (Eds.), *Handbook of mindfulness: Theory, research, and practice* (pp. 9–41). Guilford Press.

Gil, S., & Weinberg, M. (2015). Secondary trauma among social workers treating trauma clients: The role of coping strategies and internal resources. *International Social Work, 58*(4), 551–561. https://doi.org/10.1177/0020872814564705

Gilbert, P. (2014). The origins and nature of compassion focused therapy. *British Journal of Clinical Psychology, 53*(1), 6–41. https://doi.org/10.1111/bjc.12043

Gilbert, P. (2020a). Compassion: From its evolution to a psychotherapy. *Frontiers in Psychology, 11,* 1–31. https://doi.org/10.3389/fpsyg.2020.586161

Gilbert, P. (2020b). The evolution of prosocial behavior: From caring to compassion. In L. Workman, W. Reader, & J. H. Barkow (Eds.), *Cambridge handbook of evolutionary perspectives on human behavior* (pp. 419–435). Cambridge University Press.

Gilbert, P., Catarino, F., Duarte, C., Matos, M., Kolts, R., Stubbs, J., Ceresatto, L., Duarte, J., Pinto-Gouveia, J., & Basran, J. (2017). The development of compassionate engagement and action scales for self and others. *Journal of Compassionate Health Care, 4*(1), 1–24. https://doi.org/10.1186/s40639-017-0033-3

Gilbert, P., & Mascaro, J. (2017). Compassion: Fears, blocks, and resistances: An evolutionary investigation. In E. M., Seppälä, E. Simon-Thomas, S. L., Brown, M. Worline, C. D. Cameron, & J. R. Doty (Eds.), *The Oxford handbook of compassion science* (pp. 399–420). Oxford University Press.

Gilboa, A., & Ben-Shetrit, S. (2009). Sowing seeds of compassion: The case of a music therapy integration group. *The Arts in Psychotherapy, 36*(4), 251–260. https://doi.org/10.1016/j.aip.2009.06.001

Giusti, L., Mammarella, S., Salza, A., Ussorio, D., Bianco, D., Casacchia, M., & Roncone, R. (2021). Heart and head: Profiles and predictors of self-assessed cognitive and affective empathy in a sample of medical and health professional students. *Frontiers in Psychology, 12*, 1–13. https://doi.org/10.3389/fpsyg.2021.632996

Goetz, J. L., Keltner, D., & Simon-Thomas, E. (2010). Compassion: An evolutionary analysis and empirical review. *Psychological Bulletin, 136*(3), 351–374. https://doi:10.1037/a0018807

Goleman, D., Bennett, L., & Barlow, Z. (2012). *Ecoliterate: How educators are cultivating emotional, social, and ecological intelligence*. John Wiley & Sons.

Gottfried, R., & Bride, B. E. (2018). Trauma–secondary, vicarious, compassion fatigue. In *Encyclopedia of social work*. Oxford University Press. https://doi:10.1093/acrefore/9780199975839.013.1085

Grabbe, L., & Miller-Karas, E. (2018). The trauma resiliency model: A "bottom-up" intervention for trauma psychotherapy. *Journal of the American Psychiatric Nurses Association, 24*(1), 76–84. https://doi:10.1177/1078390317745133

Green, P. (2009). Reconciliation and forgiveness in divided societies: A path of courage, compassion, and commitment. In A. Kalayjian & R. F. Paloutzian (Eds.), *Forgiveness and reconciliation: Psychological pathways to conflict transformation and peace building* (pp. 251–268). Springer.

Gross, J. J. (1998). The emerging field of emotion regulation: An integrative review. *Review of General Psychology, 2*(3), 271–299. https://doi.org/10.1037/1089-2680.2.3.271

Grossman, S., Cooper, Z., Buxton, H., Hendrickson, S., Lewis-O'Connor, A., Stevens, J., Wong, L-Y., & Bonne, S. (2021). Trauma-informed care: Recognizing and resisting re-traumatization in health care. *Trauma Surgery & Acute Care Open, 6*(1), e000815. http://doi:10.1136/tsaco-2021-000815

Gusler, S., Sprang, G., Hood, C., Eslinger, J., Whitt-Woosley, A., Kinnish, K., & Wozniak, J. (2023). Untangling secondary traumatic stress and vicarious traumatization: One construct or two? *Psychological Trauma: Theory, Research, Practice, and Policy*, 1–11. Advanced online publication. https://doi.org/10.1037/tra0001604

Haans, A., & Balke, N. (2018). Trauma-informed intercultural group supervision. *The Clinical Supervisor, 37*(1), 158–181. https://doi.org/10.1080/07325223.2017.1399495

Haase, L., Stewart, J. L., Youssef, B., May, A. C., Isakovic, S., Simmons, A. N., Johnson, D. C., Potterat, E. G., & Paulus, M. P. (2016). When the brain does not adequately feel the body: Links between low resilience and interoception. *Biological Psychology, 113*, 37–45. https://doi.org/10.1016/j.biopsycho.2015.11.004

Halifax, J. (2018). *Standing at the edge: Finding freedom where fear and courage meet* (Kindle ed.). Flatiron Books.

Handran, J. (2015). Trauma-informed systems of care: The role of organizational culture in the development of burnout, secondary traumatic stress, and compassion satisfaction. *Journal of Social Welfare and Human Rights, 3*(2), 1–22. https://doi.org/10.15640/jswhr.v3n2a1

Hạnh, T. N. (1987). *Interbeing: Fourteen guidelines for engaged Buddhism*. Parallax Press.

Hạnh, T. N. (2006). *True love: A practice for awakening the heart*. Shambhala Publications.

Hạnh, T. N. (2008). Foreword. In P. R. Ward & L. Ward (Eds.), *Love's garden: A guide to mindful relationships* (Kindle ed., pp. 52–131). Parallax Press.

Hạnh, T. N. (2014). *No mud, no lotus: The art of transforming suffering* (Kindle ed.). Parallax Press.

Hanson, R. (2020). *Neurodharma: New science, ancient wisdom, and seven practices of the highest happiness* (Kindle ed.). Harmony.

Hargovan, H. (2007). Restorative approaches to justice: "Compulsory compassion" or victim empowerment? *Acta Criminologica: African Journal of Criminology & Victimology, 20*(3), 113–123. https://hdl.handle.net/10520/EJC28939

Harris, D. L. (2023). Spheres of compassionate engagement and response. In D. L. Harris & A. H. Y. Ho (Eds.), *Compassion-based approaches in loss and grief* (pp. 64–71). Routledge. http://doi:10.4324/9781003204121-8

Harris, M., & Fallot, R. D. (2001). Envisioning a trauma-informed service system: A vital paradigm shift. *New Directions for Mental Health Services, 89*, 3–22. https://doi.org/10.1002/yd.23320018903

Harris, S. E. (2014). Suffering and the shape of well-being in Buddhist ethics. *Asian Philosophy, 24*(3), 242–259. https://doi.org/10.1080/09552367.2014.952931

Harvey, P. (2013). *An introduction to Buddhism: Teachings, history and practices* (Kindle ed.). Cambridge University Press.

Haslam, N. (2016). Concept creep: Psychology's expanding concepts of harm and pathology. *Psychological Inquiry, 27*(1), 1–17. https://doi.org/10.1080/1047840X.2016.1082418

Hatfield, E., Bensman, L., Thornton, P. D., & Rapson, R. L. (2014). New perspectives on emotional contagion: A review of classic and recent research on facial mimicry and contagion. *Interpersonal: An International Journal on Personal Relationships, 8*(2), 159–179. http://doi10.5964/ijpr.v8i2.162

Heim, M. (2019). *Buddhist ethics.* Cambridge University Press.

Hensel, J. M., Ruiz, C., Finney, C., & Dewa, C. S. (2015). Meta-analysis of risk factors for secondary traumatic stress in therapeutic work with trauma victims. *Journal of Traumatic Stress, 28*(2), 83–91. https://doi.org/10.1002/jts.21998

Henshaw, L. A. (2022). Building trauma-informed approaches in higher education. *Behavioral Sciences, 12*(10), 368. https://doi.org/10.3390/bs12100368

Henson, C., Truchot, D., & Canevello, A. (2021). What promotes post traumatic growth? A systematic review. *European Journal of Trauma & Dissociation, 5*(4), 100195. https://doi.org/10.1016/j.ejtd.2020.100195

Herman, J. L. (1992a). Complex PTSD: A syndrome in survivors of prolonged and repeated trauma. *Journal of Traumatic Stress, 5*(3), 377–391. https://doi.org/10.1002/jts.2490050305

Herman, J. L. (1992b). *Trauma and recovery: From domestic abuse to political terror.* Basic Books.

Hinton, D. E., & Good, B. J. (Eds.). (2016). *Culture and PTSD: Trauma in global and historical perspective* (Kindle ed.). University of Pennsylvania Press.

Ho, S. M., & Cheng, C. T. (2024). Illusory versus constructive posttraumatic growth in cancer. In R. Berger (Ed.). *The Routledge international handbook of posttraumatic growth* (Kindle ed., pp. 21–28). Routledge.

Hofmeyer, A., Kennedy, K., & Taylor, R. (2020). Contesting the term 'compassion fatigue': Integrating findings from social neuroscience and self-care research. *Collegian, 27*(2), 232–237. https://doi.org/10.1016/j.colegn.2019.07.001

Hopper, E. K., Bassuk, E. L., & Olivet, J. (2010). Shelter from the storm: Trauma-informed care in homeless service settings. *The Open Health Services and Policy Journal, 3*, 80–100. https://doi:10.2174/1874924001003010080

Horesh, D. (2016). The reconstruction of Criterion A in DSM-5: Is it a true incorporation of secondary traumatization into the PTSD diagnosis? *Journal of Loss and Trauma, 21*(5), 345–349. https://doi.org/10.1080/15325024.2015.1072016

Horwitz, E. B., Heinonen, T., Birgitta, A., & Worline, M. (2023). Compassion embodied – the particular power of the arts. In E. Bos & E. Huss (Eds.), *Using art for social transformation: International perspective for social workers, community workers and art therapists* (Kindle ed., pp. 143–155). Routledge Advances in Social Work, Taylor and Francis.

Hruska, B., Patterson, P. D., Doshi, A. A., Guyette, M. K., Wong, A. H., Chang, B. P., Suffoletto, M. L., & Pacella-LaBarbara, M. L. (2023). Examining the prevalence and health impairment associated with subthreshold PTSD symptoms (PTSS) among frontline healthcare workers during the

COVID-19 pandemic. *Journal of Psychiatric Research, 158*, 202–208. https://doi.org/10.1016/j.jpsychires.2022.12.045

Isobel, S., & Angus-Leppan, G. (2018). Neuro-reciprocity and vicarious trauma in psychiatrists. *Australasian Psychiatry, 26*(4), 388–390. https://doi.org/10.1177/1039856218772223

Jackson, H. J., & Haslam, N. (2022). Ill-defined: Concepts of mental health and illness are becoming broader, looser, and more benign. *Australasian Psychiatry, 30*(4), 490–493. https://doi.org/10.1177/10398562221077898

Jackson-Preston, P., Brown, G. C., Garnett, T., Sanchez, D., Fagbamila, E., & Graham, N. (2023). "I am never enough": Factors contributing to secondary traumatic stress and burnout among black student services professionals in higher education. *Trauma Care, 3*(2), 93–107. https://doi.org/10.3390/traumacare3020010

Jayawickreme, E., Infurna, F. J., Alajak, K., Blackie, L. E., Chopik, W. J., Chung, J. M., Dorfman, A., Fleeson, W., Forgeard, M. J. C., Frazier, P., Furr, R. M., Grossmann, I., Heller, A. S., Laceulle, O. M., Lucas, R. E., Luhmann, M., Luong, G., Meijer, L., McLean, K. C., … Zonneveld, R. (2021). Post-traumatic growth as positive personality change: Challenges, opportunities, and recommendations. *Journal of Personality, 89*(1), 145–165. https://doi.org/10.1111/jopy.12591

Jennings, P. A., & Min, H. H. (2023). Transforming empathy-based stress to compassion: Skillful means to preventing teacher burnout. *Mindfulness, 14*, 2311–2322. https://doi.org/10.1007/s12671-023-02115-6

Jinpa, T. (2015). *A fearless heart* (Kindle ed.). Penguin Publishing Group.

Jones, P. J., Bellet, B. W., & McNally, R. J. (2020). Helping or harming? The effect of trigger warnings on individuals with trauma histories. *Clinical Psychological Science, 8*(5), 905–917. https://doi:10.1177/2167702620921341

Kabat-Zinn, J. (2003). Mindfulness-based interventions in context: Past, present, and future. *Clinical Psychology: Science and Practice, 10*(2), 144–156. https://doi.org/10.1093/clipsy.bpg016

Kaiser Permanente. (2021). *Healing from collective trauma.* https://about.kaiserpermanente.org/total-health/health-tips/healing-from-collective-trauma

Karatzias, T., & Cloitre, M. (2019). Treating adults with complex posttraumatic stress disorder using a modular approach to treatment: Rationale, evidence, and directions for future research. *Journal of Traumatic Stress, 32*(6), 870–876. https://doi.org/10.1002/jts.22457

Kelleher, A. (2004). Third-wave public health? Compassion, community, and end-of-life care. *International Journal of Applied Psychoanalytic Studies, 1*(4), 313–323. https://doi.org/10.1002/aps.83

Keltner, D., Marsh, J., & Smith, J. A. (Eds.). (2010). *The compassionate instinct: The science of human goodness.* W.W. Norton & Company.

Kemp, A., & Vidakovic, D. (2023). Students' understanding and development of the definition of circle in Taxicab and Euclidean geometries: An APOS perspective with schema interaction. *Educational Studies in Mathematics, 112*(3), 567–588. https://doi.org/10.1007/s10649-022-10180-2

Kerig, P. K. (2018). Enhancing resilience among providers of trauma-informed care: A curriculum for protection against secondary traumatic stress among non-mental health professionals. *Journal of Aggression, Maltreatment & Trauma, 28*(5), 613–630. https://doi.org/10.1080/10926771.2018.1468373

Khong, B. S. L. (2009). Expanding the understanding of mindfulness: Seeing the tree and the forest. *The Humanistic Psychologist, 37*(2), 117–136. https://doi.org/10.1080/08873260902892006

Killian, K., Hernandez-Wolfe, P., Engstrom, D., & Gangsei, D. (2017). Development of the vicarious resilience scale (VRS): A measure of positive effects of working with trauma survivors. *Psychological Trauma: Theory, Research, Practice, and Policy, 9*(1), 23–31. https://doi.org/10.1037/tra0000199

Kilpatrick, D. G., Resnick, H. S., Milanak, M. E., Miller, M. W., Keyes, K. M., & Friedman, M. J. (2013). National estimates of exposure to traumatic events and PTSD prevalence using DSM-IV and DSM-5 criteria. *Journal of Traumatic Stress, 26*(5), 537–547. https://doi.org/10.1002/jts.21848

Kim, J. J., Cunnington, R., & Kirby, J. N. (2020). The neurophysiological basis of compassion: An fMRI meta-analysis of compassion and its related neural processes. *Neuroscience & Biobehavioral Reviews, 108*, 112–123. https://doi.org/10.1016/j.neubiorev.2019.10.023

King, S. B. (2023). Mindfulness, compassion and skillful means in engaged Buddhism. *Mindfulness, 14*(10), 2516–2531. https://doi.org/10.1007/s12671-022-01847-1

Kira, I. A., Fawzi, M. H., & Fawzi, M. M. (2013). The dynamics of cumulative trauma and trauma types in adult patients with psychiatric disorders: Two cross-cultural studies. *Traumatology, 19*(3), 179–195. https://doi.org/10.1177/1534765612459892

Kira, I. A., Shuweikh, H., Al-Huwailiah, A., El-Wakeel, S. A., Waheep, N. N., Ebada, E. E., & Ibrahim, E. S. R. (2022). The direct and indirect impact of trauma types and cumulative stressors and traumas on executive functions. *Applied Neuropsychology: Adult, 29*(5), 1078–1094. https://doi.org/10.1080/23279095.2020.1848835

Kirby, J. N., Day, J., & Sagar, V. (2019). The 'flow' of compassion: A meta-analysis of the fears of compassion scales and psychological functioning. *Clinical Psychology Review, 70*, 26–39. https://doi.org/10.1016/j.cpr.2019.03.001

Klimecki, O. M., Leiberg, S., Lamm, C., & Singer, T. (2013). Functional neural plasticity and associated changes in positive affect after compassion training. *Cerebral Cortex, 23*(7), 1552–1561. https://doi.org/10.1093/cercor/bhs142

Klimecki, O. M., & Singer, T. (2011). Empathic distress fatigue rather than compassion fatigue? Integrating findings from empathy research in psychology and social neuroscience. In B. Oakley, A. Knafo, G. Madhavan, & D. S. Wilson (Eds.), *Pathological altruism* (pp. 1–23). Oxford University Press.

Knight, C. (2015). Trauma-informed social work practice: Practice considerations and challenges. *Clinical Social Work Journal, 43*(1), 25–37. https://doi:10.1007/s10615-014-0481-6

Koloroutis, M., & Pole, M. (2021). Trauma-informed leadership and posttraumatic growth. *Nursing Management, 52*(12), 28–34. http://doi:10.1097/01.NUMA.0000800336.39811.a3

Koloroutis, M., & Trout, M. (2012). *See me as a person: Creating therapeutic relationships with patients and their families*. Creative Health Care Management.

Kornfeld, J. (2009). *The wise heart: A guide to the universal teachings of Buddhist psychology*. Bantam.

Kraus, S., & Sears, S. (2009). *Self-other four immeasurables scale (SOFI)* [*database record*]. APA PsycTests. https://doi.org/10.1037/t57250-000

Krippner, S., & Barrett, D. (2019). Transgenerational trauma. *The Journal of Mind and Behavior, 40*(1), 53–62. https://www.jstor.org/stable/26740747

Kumar, A. (2023). What exactly does Ahiṃsā in the Indian tradition connote? *International Journal of Sanskrit Research, 9*(2), 74–76. https://doi.org/10.22271/23947519.2023.v9.i2b.2036

Lamb, S. (2002). Women, abuse, and forgiveness: A special case. In S. Lamb & J. G. Murphy (Eds.), *Before forgiving: Cautionary views of forgiveness in psychotherapy* (pp. 155–171). Oxford University Press.

Lampert, K. (2005). *Traditions of compassion: From religious duty to social activism*. Springer.

Lanaj, K., Jennings, R. E., Ashford, S. J., & Krishnan, S. (2022). When leader self-care begets other care: Leader role self-compassion and helping at work. *Journal of Applied Psychology, 107*(9), 1543–1560. https://doi.org/10.1037/apl0000957

Landers, A. L., Dimitropoulos, G., Mendenhall, T. J., Kennedy, A., & Zemanek, L. (2020). Backing the blue: Trauma in law enforcement spouses and couples. *Family Relations, 69*(2), 308–319. https://doi.org/10.1111/fare.12393

Lawson, H., Caringi, J., Gottfried, R., Bride, E. B., & Hydon, S. (2019). Secondary traumatic stress, student trauma, and the need for trauma literacy. *Harvard Educational Review, 89*(3), 421–447. https://doi.org/10.17763/1943-5045-89.3.421

Leana, C. R., & Rousseau, D. M. (Eds.). (2000). *Relational wealth: The advantages of stability in a changing economy.* Oxford University Press.

Lee, K. C., & Oh, A. (2019). Introduction to compassionate view intervention: A Buddhist counseling technique based on Mahāyāna Buddhist teachings. *Journal of Spirituality in Mental Health, 21*(2), 132–151.

Lefebvre, J. I., Montani, F., & Courcy, F. (2020). Self-compassion and resilience at work: A practice-oriented review. *Advances in Developing Human Resources, 22*(4), 437–452. https://doi.org/10.1177/1523422320949145

Levenson, J. (2017). Trauma-informed social work practice. *Social Work, 62*(2), 105–113. https://doi.org/10.1093/sw/swx001

Levine, P. A. (2010). *Healing trauma: A pioneering program for restoring the wisdom of your body* (Kindle ed.). Sounds True.

Lilius, J. M., Worline, M. C., Dutton, J. E., Kanov, J. M., & Maitlis, S. (2011). Understanding compassion capability. *Human Relations, 64*(7), 873–899. http://doi:10.1177/0018726710396250

Lilius, J. M., Worline, M. C., Maitlis, S., Kanov, J., Dutton, J. E., & Frost, P. (2008). The contours and consequences of compassion at work. *Journal of Organizational Behavior, 29*(2), 193–218. https://doi.org/10.1002/job.508

Linley, P. A., & Joseph, S. (2004). Positive change following trauma and adversity: A review. *Journal of Traumatic Stress: Official Publication of the International Society for Traumatic Stress Studies, 17*(1), 11–21. https://doi.org/10.1023/B:JOTS.0000014671.27856.7e

Little, B. W. (2020). *A self-care protocol for hospice chaplains facing compassion fatigue, burnout, and secondary traumatic stress disorder* [Unpublished doctoral dissertation]. Southeastern Baptist Theological Seminary. https://www.proquest.com/docview/2392031540?pq-origsite=gscholar&fromopenview=true

Lockhart, E. A. (2016). Why trigger warnings are beneficial, perhaps even necessary. *First Amendment Studies, 50*(2), 59–69. https://doi.org/10.1080/21689725.2016.1232623

Long, B., & Smith, R. (2017). Attuning, wondering, following, and holding as self-care. In M. Koloroutis & D. Abelson (Eds.), *Advancing relationship-based cultures* (pp. 35–48). Creative Health Care Management.

López, A., Sanderman, R., Ranchor, A. V., & Schroevers, M. J. (2018). Compassion for others and self-compassion: Levels, correlates, and relationship with psychological well-being. *Mindfulness, 9*(1), 325–331. https://doi:10.1007/s12671-017-0777-z

Louchakova-Schwartz, O. (2020). Non-religious mindfulness, phenomenology, and intersubjectivity. In S. K. Dhiman (Ed.), *The Routledge companion to mindfulness at work.* Routledge.

Luo, X., Che, X., Lei, Y., & Li, H. (2021). Investigating the influence of self-compassion-focused interventions on posttraumatic stress: A systematic review and meta-analysis. *Mindfulness, 12*(12), 2865–2876. https://doi.org/10.1007/s12671-021-01732-3

Luskin, F. (2002). *Forgive for good: A proven prescription for health and happiness* (Kindle ed.). Harper.

Luyten, P., & Fonagy, P. (2019). Mentalizing and trauma. In A. Bateman & P. Fonagy (Eds.), *Handbook of mentalizing in mental health practice* (pp. 79–99). American Psychiatric Association Publishing.

Macy, J. (2022). What radical compassion means to activist Joanna Macy. *Yoga Journal.* https://www.yogajournal.com/teach/what-radical-compassion-means-to-author-and-activist-joanna-macy/

Magruder, K. M., McLaughlin, K. A., & Elmore Borbon, D. L. (2017). Trauma is a public health issue. *European Journal of Psychotraumatology, 8*(1), 1375338. https://doi.org/10.1080/20008198.2017.1375338

Mahood, E., Shahid, M., Gavin, N., Rahmann, A., Tadakamadla, S. K., & Kroon, J. (2023). Theories, models, frameworks, guidelines, and recommendations for trauma-informed oral healthcare services: A scoping review. *Trauma, Violence, & Abuse, 25*(2), 869–884. https://doi.org/10.1177/15248380231165699

Maitlis, S. (2020). Posttraumatic growth at work. *Annual Review of Organizational Psychology and Organizational Behavior, 7*, 395–419. https://doi.org/10.1146/annurev-orgpsych-012119-044932

Makransky, J. (2012). Compassion in Buddhist psychology. In K. C. Germer & R. D. Siegel (Eds.), *Wisdom and compassion in psychotherapy: Deepening mindfulness in clinical practice* (Kindle ed., pp. 61–74). Guilford Press.

Makransky, J. (2016). Confronting the "sin" out of love for the "sinner": Fierce compassion as a force for social change. *Buddhist-Christian Studies, 36*(1), 87–96. https://doi:10.1353/bcs.2016.0009

Malchiodi, C. (2021). *Understanding fight, flight, freeze, and the feign response.* https://www.cathymalchiodi.com/2021/07/28/understanding-fight-flight-freeze-and-the-feign-response/

Malchiodi, C. (2022). *Trauma-informed expressive arts therapy.* Sussex.

Manning-Jones, S., de Terte, I., & Stephens, C. (2017). The relationship between vicarious posttraumatic growth and secondary traumatic stress among health professionals. *Journal of Loss and Trauma, 22*(3), 256–270. https://doi.org/10.1080/15325024.2017.1284516

Manyena, B., O'Brien, G., O'Keefe, P., & Rose, J. (2011). Disaster resilience: A bounce back or bounce forward ability? *Local Environment: The International Journal of Justice and Sustainability, 16*(5), 417–424. https://doi.org/10.1080/13549839.2011.583049

Marshall, R. D., Olfson, M., Hellman, F., Blanco, C., Guardino, M., & Struening, E. L. (2001). Comorbidity, impairment, and suicidality in subthreshold PTSD. *American Journal of Psychiatry, 158*(9), 1467–1473. https://doi:10.1176/appi.ajp.158.9.1467

Marshall, S. L., Ciarrochi, J., Parker, P. D., & Sahdra, B. K. (2020). Is self-compassion selfish? The development of self-compassion, empathy, and prosocial behavior in adolescence. *Journal of Research on Adolescence, 30*, 472–484. https://doi.org/10.1111/jora.12492

Maslach, C., Schaufeli, W. B., & Leiter, M. P. (2001). Job burnout. *Annual Review of Psychology, 52*(1), 397–422. https://doi.org/10.1146/annurev.psych.52.1.397

Maté, G. (2022). *The myth of normal: Trauma, illness, and healing in a toxic culture* (Kindle ed.). Penguin.

Mathieu, F. (2012). *The compassion fatigue workbook: Creative tools for transforming compassion fatigue and vicarious traumatization (psychosocial stress series)* (Kindle ed.). Taylor and Francis.

Matto, H. C., Strolin-Goltzman, J., & Ballan, M. (2013). *Neuroscience for social work: Current research and practice.* Springer.

Melinte, B. M., Turliuc, M. N., & Măirean, C. (2023). Secondary traumatic stress and vicarious posttraumatic growth in healthcare professionals: A meta-analysis. *Clinical Psychology: Science and Practice.* Advance online publication. https://doi.org/10.1037/cps0000159

Miech, E. J., Rattray, N. A., Flanagan, M. E., Damschroder, L., Schmid, A. A., & Damush, T. M. (2018). Inside help: An integrative review of champions in healthcare-related implementation. *SAGE Open Medicine, 6*, http://doi:10.1177/2050312118773261

Mitra, J. L., & Greenberg, M. T. (2016). The curriculum of right mindfulness: The relational self and the capacity for compassion. In R. E. Purser, D. Forbes, & A. Burke (Eds.), *Handbook of mindfulness: Culture, context, and social engagement* (pp. 411–424). Springer International Publishing.

Molnar, B. E., Sprang, G., Killian, K. D., Gottfried, R., Emery, V., & Bride, B. E. (2017). Advancing science and practice for vicarious traumatization/secondary traumatic stress: A research agenda. *Traumatology, 23*(2), 129–142. https://doi.org/10.1037/trm0000122

Mordeno, I. G., Go, G. P., & Yangson-Serondo, A. (2017). Examining the dimensional structure models of secondary traumatic stress based on DSM-5 symptoms. *Asian Journal of Psychiatry, 25*, 154–160. https://doi.org/10.1016/j.ajp.2016.10.024

Morland, L. A., Butler, L. D., & Leskin, G. A. (2008). Resilience and thriving in a time of terrorism. In S. Joseph & P. A. Linley (Eds.), *Trauma, recovery, and growth: Positive psychological perspectives on posttraumatic stress* (pp. 39–61). Wiley.

Munger, T., Savage, T., & Panosky, D. M. (2015). When caring for perpetrators becomes a sentence: Recognizing vicarious trauma. *Journal of Correctional Health Care, 21*(4), 365–374. https://doi.org/10.1177/1078345815599976

Muris, P., Meesters, C., Pierik, A., & de Kock, B. (2016). Good for the self: Self-compassion and other self-related constructs in relation to symptoms of anxiety and depression in non-clinical youths. *Journal of Child and Family Studies, 25*, 607–617. https://doi:10.1007s10826-015-0235-2

Muris, P., & Petrocchi, N. (2017). Protection or vulnerability? A meta-analysis of the relations between the positive and negative components of self-compassion and psychopathology. *Clinical Psychology & Psychotherapy, 24*(2), 373–383. https://doi.org/10.1002/cpp.2005

Nair, M. (2022). Ensuring emotional fitness of healthcare workers through employee champion role of human resource management. *Asia Pacific Journal of Health Management, 17*(3), 173–187. https://doi.org/10.24083/apjhm.v17i3.1521

National Child Traumatic Stress Network. (2018). *Complex trauma.* https://www.nctsn.org/what-is-child-trauma/trauma-types/complex-trauma

Neff, K. D. (2003a). Self-compassion: An alternative conceptualization of a healthy attitude toward oneself. *Self and Identity, 2*(2), 85–101. https://doi.org/10.1080/15298860309032

Neff, K. D. (2003b). The development and validation of a scale to measure self-compassion. *Self and Identity, 2*(3), 223–250. https://doi.org/10.1080/15298860309027

Neff, K. D. (2021). *Fierce self-compassion: How women can harness kindness to speak up, claim their power, and thrive.* Harper Collins.

Neff, K. D. (2022). The differential effects fallacy in the study of self-compassion: Misunderstanding the nature of bipolar continuums. *Mindfulness, 13,* 572–576. https://doi.org/10.1007/s12671-022-01832-8

Neff, K. D. (2023). Self-compassion: Theory, method, research, and intervention. *Annual Review of Psychology, 74,* 193–218. https://doi.org/10.1146/annurev-psych-032420-031047

Neff, K. D., & Germer, C. (2018). *The mindful self-compassion workbook: A proven way to accept yourself, build inner strength, and thrive* (Kindle ed.). Guilford Publications.

Neff, K. D., & Pommier, E. (2013). The relationship between self-compassion and other-focused concern among college undergraduates, community adults, and practicing meditators. *Self and Identity, 12,* 1–17. https://doi:10.1007/s12671-017-0777-z

Neff, K. D., & Tóth-Király, I. (2022). Self-compassion scale (SCS). In O. N., Medvedev, C. U. Krägeloh, R. J. Siegert, & N. N. Singh (Eds.), *Handbook of assessment in mindfulness research* (pp. 1–22). Springer International Publishing.

Nielsen, K., Taris, T. W., & Cox, T. (2010). The future of organizational interventions: Addressing the challenges of today's organizations. *Work and Stress, 24*(3), 219–233. https://doi.org/10.1080/02678373.2010.519176

North, C. S., Surís, A. M., Smith, R. P., & King, R. V. (2016). The evolution of PTSD criteria across editions of DSM. *Annals of Clinical Psychiatry, 28*(3), 197–208.

Nussbaum, M. C. (2003). Compassion & terror. *Daedalus, 132*(1), 10–26. https://www.jstor.org/stable/20027819

Ogińska-Bulik, N., & Juczyński, Z. (2024). Vicarious posttraumatic growth: The benefits of indirect exposure to trauma. In R. Berger (Ed.), *The Routledge international handbook of posttraumatic growth* (Kindle ed., pp. 445 457). Routledge.

Olendzki, A. (2012). Wisdom in Buddhist psychology. In C. K. Germer & R. D. Siegel (Eds.), *Wisdom and compassion in psychotherapy: Deepening mindfulness in clinical practice* (Kindle ed., pp. 7–34). Guilford Press.

O'Malley, M., Robinson, Y. A., Hydon, S., Caringi, J., & Hu, M. (2019). *Organizational resilience: Reducing the impact of secondary trauma on front line human services staff.* SAMHSA ReCAST Issue Brief. https://selcenter.wested.org/resource/organizational-resilience-reducing-the-impact-of-secondary-traumatic-stress-on-front-line-human-services-staff/

Owens-King, A. P. (2019). Secondary traumatic stress and self-care inextricably linked. *Journal of Human Behavior in the Social Environment, 29*(1), 37–47. https://doi.org/10.1080/10911359.2018.1472703

Papa, A., & Robinson, K. (2023). Leadership and trauma-informed care: Working to support staff and teams. *Journal of Emergency Nursing, 49*(2), 172–174. https://doi.org/10.1016/j.jen.2022.11.001

Parry, S., Cox, N., Andriopoulou, P., Oldfield, J., Roscoe, S., Palumbo-Haswell, J., & Collins, S. (2023). Mechanisms to enhance resilience and post-traumatic growth in residential care: A narrative review. *Adversity and Resilience Science, 4*(1), 1–21. https://doi.org/10.1007/s42844-022-00074-w

Pearlman, L. A., & MacIan, P. S. (1995). Vicarious traumatization: An empirical study of the effects of trauma work on trauma therapists. *Professional Psychology: Research and Practice, 26*(6), 558–565. https://doi.org/10.1037/0735-7028.26.6.558

Pearlman, L. A., & Saakvitne, K. W. (1995). Treating therapists with vicarious traumatization and secondary traumatic stress disorders. In C. R. Figley (Ed.), *Compassion fatigue: Coping with secondary traumatic stress disorder in those who treat the traumatized* (Kindle ed., pp. 150–177). Brunner/Mazel.

Pelden, K. (2007). *The nectar of Manjushri's speech: A detailed commentary on Shantideva's way of the bodhisattva* (Kindle ed.). Shambhala Publications.

Poli, A., Gemignani, A., & Woodruff, C. C. (2022). Self-compassion: From neuroscience to clinical setting. *Frontiers in Psychology, 13*, 96373. https://doi:10.3389/fpsyg.2022.963738

Porges, S. W. (1995). Orienting in a defensive world: Mammalian modifications of our evolutionary heritage. A polyvagal theory. *Psychophysiology, 32*(4), 301–318. https://doi.org/10.1111/j.1469-8986.1995.tb01213.x

Porges, S. W. (2011). *The polyvagal theory: Neurophysiological foundations of emotions, attachment, communication, and self-regulation (Norton series on interpersonal neurobiology)* (Kindle ed.). W.W. Norton & Company.

Porges, S. W. (2017). Vagal pathways: Portals to compassion. In E. M., Seppälä, E. Simon-Thomas, S. L. Brown, M. Worline, C. D., Cameron, & J. R. Doty (Eds.), *The Oxford handbook of compassion science* (pp. 41–49). Oxford University Press.

Porges, S. W. (2021). Polyvagal theory: A biobehavioral journey to sociality. *Comprehensive Psychoneuroendocrinology, 7*, 100069. https://doi.org/10.1016/j.cpnec.2021.100069

Potocky, M., & Guskovict, K. L. (2020). *Addressing secondary traumatic stress: Models and promising practices*. Grantmakers Concerned with Immigrants and Refugees. https://www.gcir.org/sites/default/files/resources/final_Addressing%20Secondary%20Traumatic%20Stress%20Final%20Report%20%28Sept%202020%29_0.pdf

Price, M. (2018). Change through curiosity in the 'insight approach to conflict'. *Revista de Mediación, 11*(1), 2340–9754.

Pryce, J. G., Shackelford, K. K., & Pryce, D. H. (2007). *Secondary traumatic stress and the child welfare professional*. Lyceum Books.

Purkey, E., Patel, R., & Phillips, S. P. (2018). Trauma-informed care: Better care for everyone. *Canadian Family Physician, 64*(3), 170–172.

Quaglia, J. T. (2023). One compassion, many means: A big two analysis of compassionate behavior. *Mindfulness, 14*(10), 2430–2442. https://doi.org/10.1007/s12671-022-01895-7

Quaglia, J. T., Cigrand, C., & Sallmann, H. (2021). Caring for you, me, and us: The lived experience of compassion in counselors. *Psychotherapy*. Advance online publication. https://doi.org/10.1037/pst0000412

Quaglia, J. T., & Simmer-Brown, J. (2023). Compassion and skillful means: Diverse views, novel insights, and extended applications for compassion science and training. *Mindfulness, 14*, 2293–2298. https://doi.org/10.1007/s12671-023-02223-3

Quaglia, J. T., Soisson, A., & Simmer-Brown, J. (2021). Compassion for self versus other: A critical review of compassion training research. *The Journal of Positive Psychology, 16*(5), 675–690. https://doi.org/10.1080/17439760.2020.1805502

Raes, F., Pommier, E., Neff, K. D., & Van Gucht, D. (2011). Construction and factorial validation of a short form of the self-compassion scale. *Clinical Psychology & Psychotherapy, 18*(3), 250–255. https://doi.org/10.1002/cpp.702

Raja, S., Rabinowitz, E. P., & Gray, M. J. (2021). Universal screening and trauma informed care: Current concerns and future directions. *Families, Systems, & Health, 39*(3), 526–534. https://doi.org/10.1037/fsh0000585

Reniers, R. L., Corcoran, R., Drake, R., Shryane, N. M., & Völlm, B. A. (2011). The QCAE: A questionnaire of cognitive and affective empathy. *Journal of Personality Assessment, 93*(1), 84–95. https://doi.org/10.1080/00223891.2010.528484

Rigas, N., Soldatou, A., Dagla, M., Nanou, C., & Antoniou, E. (2023). The risk of the development of secondary post-traumatic stress disorder among pediatric health care providers: A systematic review. *Reports, 6*(1), 1–11. https://doi.org/10.3390/reports6010009

Rizzolatti, G., Sinigaglia, C., & Andersen, F. (2023). *Mirroring brains: How we understand others from the inside.* Oxford University Press.

Roberts, F., Teague, B., Lee, J., & Rushworth, I. (2021). The prevalence of burnout and secondary traumatic stress in professionals and volunteers working with forcibly displaced people: A systematic review and two meta-analyses. *Journal of Traumatic Stress, 34*(4), 773–785. https://doi.org/10.1002/jts.22659

Roberts, N. P., Lotzin, A., & Schäfer, I. (2022). A systematic review and meta-analysis of psychological interventions for comorbid post-traumatic stress disorder and substance use disorder. *European Journal of Psychotraumatology, 13*(1), 2041831. https://doi.org/10.1080/20008198.2022.2041831

Roxas, M. M., David, A. P., & Aruta, J. J. B. R. (2019). Compassion, forgiveness and subjective well-being among Filipino counseling professionals. *International Journal for the Advancement of Counselling, 41,* 272–283. https://doi.org/10.1007/s10447-019-09374-w

Royle, L., Keenan, P., & Farrell, D. (2009). Issues of stigma for first responders accessing support for post-traumatic stress. *International Journal of Emergency Mental Health, 11*(2), 79–86.

Rushforth, A., Durk, M., Rothwell-Blake, G. A., Kirkman, A., Ng, F., & Kotera, Y. (2023). Self-compassion interventions to target secondary traumatic stress in healthcare workers: A systematic review. *International Journal of Environmental Research and Public Health, 20*(12), 1–14. https://doi.org/10.3390/ijerph20126109

Russell, M., & Brickell, M. (2015). The "double-edge sword" of human empathy: A unifying neurobehavioral theory of compassion stress injury. *Social Sciences, 4*(4), 1087–1117. https://doi.org/10.3390/socsci4041087

Sacco, T. L., & Copel, L. C. (2018). Compassion satisfaction: A concept analysis in nursing. *In Nursing Forum, 53*(1), 76–83. https://doi:10.1111/nuf.12213

Sahdra, B. K., Ciarrochi, J., Fraser, M. I., Yap, K., Haller, E., Hayes, S. C., Hofmann, S. G., & Gloster, A. T. (2023). The compassion balance: Understanding the interrelation of self-and other-compassion for optimal well-being. *Mindfulness, 14*(8), 1997–2013. https://doi.org/10.1007/s12671-023-02187-4

Salanova, M., Bakker, A., & Llorens, S. (2006). Flow at work: Evidence for a gain spiral of personal and organizational resources. *Journal of Happiness Studies, 7,* 1–22. https://doi.org/10.1007/s10902-005-8854-8

Salzberg, S. (2013). *Real happiness at work: Meditations for accomplishment, achievement, and peace* (Kindle ed.). Workman Publishing.

Sambrook, S. (2012). Human and resource development is hard. *Human Resource Development International, 15*(2), 135–139. https://doi.org/10.1080/13678868.2012.663189

Samuel, G. (2015). The contemporary mindfulness movement and the question of non-self. *Transcultural Psychiatry, 52*(4), 485–500. https://doi.org/10.1177/1363461514562061

Śāntideva. (n.d.). *The Bodhicaryavatara* (P. Williams, Ed., K. Crosby & A. Skilton, Trans., 1st ed.). Oxford University Press. (Original work published 7th–8th century).

Scheeringa, M. (2022). *PTSD for children 6 years and younger.* https://www.ptsd.va.gov/professional/treat/specific/ptsd_child_under6.asp

Schippert, A. C. S. P., Grove, E. K., Dahl-Michelsen, T., Silvola, J., Sparboe-Nilsen, B., Danielsen, S. O., Lie, I., & Bjørnnes, A. K. (2023). Re-traumatization of torture survivors during treatment in somatic healthcare services: A mapping review and appraisal of literature presenting clinical guidelines and recommendations to prevent re-traumatization. *Social Science & Medicine*, 115775. https://doi.org/10.1016/j.socscimed.2023.115775

Scott, C. F., Marcu, G., Anderson, R. E., Newman, M. W., & Schoenebeck, S. (2023). *Trauma-informed social media: Towards solutions for reducing and healing online harm*. Proceedings of the 2023 CHI Conference on Human Factors in Computing Systems (CHI '23), April 23–28, 2023, Hamburg, Germany and New York, NY, USA, ACM, 20 pages. https://doi.org/10.48550/arXiv.2302.05312

Sharp, S., McAllister, M., & Broadbent, M. (2016). The vital blend of clinical competence and compassion: How patients experience person-centered care. *Contemporary Nurse, 52*(2–3), 300–312. https://doi.org/10.1080/10376178.2015.1020981

Shaver, P., Schwartz, J., Kirson, D., & O'Connor, C. (1987). Emotion knowledge: Further exploration of a prototype approach. *Journal of Personality and Social Psychology, 52*(6), 1061–1086.

Shea, C. M. (2021). A conceptual model to guide research on the activities and effects of innovation champions. *Implementation Research and Practice, 2*, 1–13. https://doi.org/10.1177/2633489521990443

Shonin, E., Van Gordon, W., & Griffiths, M. D. (2014). Changing paradigms: Buddhist insight in Western psychological treatments. *Psy-PAG Quarterly, 92*, 35–39.

Shuck, B., Alagaraja, M., Immekus, J., Cumberland, D., & Honeycutt-Elliott, M. (2019). Does compassion matter in leadership? A two-stage sequential equal status mixed method exploratory study of compassionate leader behavior and connections to performance in human resource development. *Human Resource Development Quarterly, 30*(4), 537–564. https://doi.org/10.1002/hrdq.21369

Siegel, D. J. (1999). *The developing mind: Towards a neurobiology of interpersonal experience*. Guilford Press.

Siegel, R. D., & Germer, C. K. (2012). Wisdom and compassion: Two wings of a bird. In C. K. Germer & R. D. Siegel (Eds.), *Wisdom and compassion in psychotherapy: Deepening mindfulness in clinical practice* (Kindle ed., pp. 7–34). Guilford Press.

Silver, R. C., Holman, E. A., Andersen, J. P., Poulin, M., McIntosh, D. N., & Gil-Rivas, V. (2013). Mental-and physical-health effects of acute exposure to media images of the September 11, 2001 attacks and the Iraq War. *Psychological Science, 24*(9), 1623–1634. https://doi:10.1177/0956797612460406

Simmer-Brown, J. (2023). Activity of the armless mother: Applications of compassion and skillful means from Indo-Tibetan Buddhism. *Mindfulness, 14*, 2342–2353. https://doi.org/10.1007/s12671-022-01868-w

Simpson, A. V., Farr-Wharton, B., & Reddy, P. (2020). Cultivating organizational compassion in healthcare. *Journal of Management & Organization, 26*(3), 340–354. https://doi.org/10.1017/jmo.2019.54

Singer, T., & Klimecki, O. M. (2014). Empathy and compassion. *Current Biology, 24*(18), R875–R878. https://doi.org/10.1016/j.cub.2014.06.054

Spence, J. (2021). *Trauma-informed yoga: A toolbox for therapists: 47 practices to calm balance and restore the nervous system* (Kindle ed.). PESI Publishing, Inc.

Sprang, G. (2018a). Organizational assessment of secondary traumatic stress: Utilizing the secondary traumatic stress informed organizational assessment tool to facilitate organizational learning and change. In V. C. Strand & G. Sprang (Eds.), *Trauma responsive child welfare systems* (pp. 261–270). Springer. https://doi.org/10.1007/978-3-319-64602-2_16

Sprang, G. (2018b). *Secondary traumatic stress core competencies for trauma-informed support and supervision, mental health version*. University of Kentucky Center on Trauma and Children. Publication #180123-1. https://ctac.uky.edu/projects-and-programs/sts-practice-laboratory/sts-lab-translational-tools#:~:text=Secondary%20Traumatic%20Stress%20Informed-Organizational%20Assessment%20The%20STSI-OA%20is,impact%20of%20secondary%20traumatic%20stress%20in%20the%20workplace.

Sprang, G. (2022). *Supervisory competencies for trauma informed supervision self-rating tool, cross disciplinary version*. University of Kentucky Center on Trauma and Children, #220830-1. https://www.nctsn.org/resources/secondary-traumatic-stress-core-competencies-in-trauma-informed-supervision-cross-disciplinary-self-rating-tool

Sprang, G., & Craig, C. (2015). An inter-battery exploratory factor analysis of primary and secondary traumatic stress: Determining a best practice approach to assessment. *Best Practices in Mental Health, 11*(1), 1–13. http://ezproxy.uky.edu/login?url=https://www-proquest-com.ezproxy.uky.edu/scholarly-journals/inter-battery-exploratory-factor-analysis-primary/docview/1679872314/se-2?accountid=11836

Sprang, G., Eslinger, J., Gottfried, R., & Gusler, S. (2022a). *The secondary traumatic stress policy analysis tool.* University of Kentucky Center on Trauma and Children publication #22-STSPL-01. https://ctac.uky.edu/projects-and-programs/sts-practice-laboratory/sts-lab-translational-tools

Sprang, G., Eslinger, J, Gottfried, R., & Gusler, S. (2022b). *The secondary traumatic stress policy analysis tool implementation guide.* University of Kentucky Center on Trauma and Children publication #22-STSPL-02. https://uky.az1.qualtrics.com/WRQualtricsControlPanel/File.php?F=F_6LLG5Jifl8SgL3g

Sprang, G., Ford, J., Kerig, P., & Bride, B. (2019). Defining secondary traumatic stress and developing targeted assessments and interventions: Lessons learned from research and leading experts. *Traumatology, 25*(2), 72–81. https://doi.org/10.1037/trm0000180

Sprang, G., Lei, F., & Bush, H. (2021). Can organizational efforts lead to less secondary traumatic stress? A longitudinal investigation of change. *American Journal of Orthopsychiatry, 91*(4), 443–453. https://doi.org/10.1037/ort0000546

Sprang, G., Miech, E. J., & Gusler, S. (2023). The role of secondary traumatic stress breakthrough champions in reducing worker trauma and improving organizational health using a configurational analysis approach. *Implementation Research and Practice, 4,* 1–13. https://doi.org/10.1177/26334895231164582

Sprang, G., Ross, L., Blackshear, K., Miller, B., Vrabel, C., Ham, J., Henry, J., & Caringi, J. (2014). *The secondary traumatic stress informed organization assessment (STSI-OA) tool.* University of Kentucky Center on Trauma and Children. https://ctac.uky.edu/projects-and-programs/sts-practice-laboratory/sts-lab-translational-tools#:~:text=Secondary%20Traumatic%20Stress%20Informed-Organizational%20Assessment%20The%20STSI-OA%20is,impact%20of%20secondary%20traumatic%20stress%20in%20the%20workplace.

Sprang, G., & Steckler, Z. (2022). Traumatic stress symptom expression following indirect exposure: A multidisciplinary investigation. *Traumatology. Advance Online Publication.* https://doi.org/10.1037/trm0000388

Sprang, G., Whitt-Woosley, A., & Eslinger, J. (2022). Diagnostic and translational utility of the secondary traumatic stress clinical algorithm (STS-CA). *Journal of Interpersonal Violence, 37*(21–22), NP19811-NP19826. https://doi.org/10.1177/08862605211044961

Stamm, B. H. (2010). *The concise ProQOL manual* (2nd ed.). ProQOL.org. https://www.researchgate.net/publication/340033923_The_Concise_ProQOL_Manual_The_concise_manual_for_the_Professional_Quality_of_Life_Scale_2_nd_Edition

Stevens, F. L., & Taber, K. (2021). The neuroscience of empathy and compassion in pro-social behavior. *Neuropsychologia, 159,* 107925. https://doi.org/10.1016/j.neuropsychologia.2021.107925

Stevens, L., & Benjamin, J. (2018). The brain that longs to care for others: The current neuroscience of compassion. In G. L. Stevens & C. C. Woodruff (Eds.), *The neuroscience of empathy, compassion, and self-compassion* (pp. 53–89). Academic Press.

Strand, V. C., & Sprang, G. (Eds.). (2018). *Trauma responsive child welfare systems.* Springer International Publishing.

Strauss, C., Taylor, B. L., Gu, J., Kuyken, W., Baer, R., Jones, F., & Cavanagh, K. (2016). What is compassion and how can we measure it? A review of definitions and measures. *Clinical Psychology Review, 47,* 15–27. https://doi.org/10.1016/j.cpr.2016.05.004

Strolin-Goltzman, J., Breslend, N., Hemenway Deaver, A., Wood, V., Woodside-Jiron, H., & Krompf, A. (2020). Moving beyond self-care: Exploring the protective influence of interprofessional collaboration, leadership, and competency on secondary traumatic stress. *Traumatology.* Advance online publication. https://doi.org/10.1037/trm0000244

Study Group on Buddhist Sanskrit Literature. (2006). *Vimalakīrtinirdeśa: A Sanskrit edition based upon the manuscript newly found at the Potala Palace*. The Institute for Comprehensive Studies of Buddhism. Taisho University Press. https://www2.hf.uio.no/polyglotta/index.php?page=person&bid=2&vid=112&entity=112&kid=112

Substance Abuse and Mental Health Services Administration (2014). *SAMHSA's concept of trauma and guidance for a trauma-informed approach. HHS publication no. (SMA) 14-4884*. Substance Abuse and Mental Health Services Administration. https://ncsacw.samhsa.gov/userfiles/files/SAMHSA_Trauma.pdf

Szoke, D., Putnam, A., & Hazlett-Stevens, H. (2022). Mindfulness-based interventions for traumatic stress. In H. Hazlett-Stevens (Ed.), *Biopsychosocial factors of stress, and mindfulness for stress reduction* (pp. 177–200). Springer. https://doi.org/10.1007/978-3-030-81245-4_8

Tedeschi, R. G. (2020). Growth after trauma. *Harvard Business Review*. https://hbr.org/2020/07/growth-after-trauma

Tedeschi, R. G., & Calhoun, L. G. (2004). Posttraumatic growth: Conceptual foundations and empirical evidence. *Psychological Inquiry, 15*(1), 1–18. https://doi.org/10.1207/s15327965pli1501_01

Thera, N. (1962). *The heart of Buddhist meditation*. Weiser.

Tirado, J. M. (2008). The Buddhist notion of emptiness and its potential contribution to psychology and psychotherapy. *International Journal of Transpersonal Studies, 27*(1), 74–79. https://doi.org/10.24972/ijts.2008.27.1.74

Tosone, C. (2012). Shared trauma. In C. Figley (Ed.), *Encyclopedia of trauma: An interdisciplinary guide* (pp. 625–628). SAGE Publications, Inc.

Tosone, C., Solomon, E., Barry, R., Beinart, E., Bellas, K. K., Blaker, E. C., Capasse, N., Colby, M. D., Corcoran, M., Delaney, A., Doyle, K., Elfo, S., Gilzene, T.-A. P., Kadriovski, A., Kim, R., Lavoie, M., Lempel, R., Linn, C., Liu, C., … Wei, Z. (2021). Shared trauma: Group reflections on the COVID-19 pandemic. In C. Tosone (Ed.), *Shared trauma, shared resilience during a pandemic* (pp. 347–353). Springer.

Trauma-Informed Oregon. (2018). *Trauma-informed care screening tool*. https://traumainformedoregon.org/wp-content/uploads/2018/12/Trauma-Informed-Care-Screening-Tool.jpg

Treleaven, D. A. (2018). *Trauma-sensitive mindfulness: Practices for safe and transformative healing* (Kindle ed.). W.W. Norton & Company.

Trzeciak, S., Mazzarelli, A., & Booker, C. (2019). *Compassionomics: The revolutionary scientific evidence that caring makes a difference*. Studer Group.

Tsirimokou, A., Kloess, J. A., & Dhinse, S. K. (2023). Vicarious post-traumatic growth in professionals exposed to traumatogenic material: A systematic literature review. *Trauma, Violence & Abuse, 24*(3), 1848–1866. https://doi:10.1177/15248380221082079

Tsur, N., & Talmon, A. (2023). Post-traumatic orientation to bodily signals: A systematic literature review. *Trauma, Violence, & Abuse, 24*(1), 174–188. https://doi:10.1177/15248380211025237

Tzohar, R. (2019). Where the self and other meet: Early Indian Yogācāra Buddhist approaches to intersubjectivity. In J. Tuske (Ed.), *Indian epistemology and metaphysics* (Kindle ed., pp. 319–334). Bloomsbury Publishing.

van der Kolk, B. A. (1994). The body keeps the score: Memory and the evolving psychobiology of posttraumatic stress. *Harvard Review of Psychiatry, 1*(5), 253–265. https://doi.org/10.3109/10673229409017088

van der Kolk, B. A. (2002). Beyond the talking cure: Somatic experience and subcortical imprints in the treatment of trauma. In F. Shapiro (Ed.), *EMDR as an integrative psychotherapy approach: Experts of diverse orientations explore the paradigm prism* (pp. 57–83). American Psychological Association. https://doi.org/10.1037/10512-003

van der Kolk, B. A. (2014). *The body keeps the score: Mind, brain and body in the transformation of trauma* (Kindle ed.). Penguin.

van Knippenberg, D. (2020). Meaning-based leadership. *Organizational Psychology Review, 10*(1), 6–28. https://doi.org/10.1177/2041386619897618

Varela, F., Thompson, E., & Rosch, E. (1991). *The embodied mind: Cognitive science and human experience.* MIT Press.

Vavrichek, S. (2012). *The guide to compassionate assertiveness: How to express your needs and deal with conflict while keeping a kind heart.* New Harbinger Publications.

Wallace, B. A. (2001). Intersubjectivity in Indo-Tibetan Buddhism. *Journal of Consciousness Studies, 8*(5–6), 209–230.

Watson, P. (2019). PTSD as a public mental health priority. *Current Psychiatry Reports, 21*, 1–12. https://doi.org/10.1007/s11920-019-1032-1

Watson, V. S. (2016). *Re-traumatization of sexual trauma in women's reproductive health care* [Unpublished Master's thesis, University of Tennessee]. https://trace.tennessee.edu/utk_chanhonoproj/1950

Wemmers, J. A., Parent, I., & Lachance Quirion, M. (2023). Restoring victims' confidence: Victim-centered restorative practices. *International Review of Victimology, 29*(3), 466–486.

Wiklund-Gustin, L., & Wagner, L. (2013). The butterfly effect of caring–clinical nursing teachers' understanding of self-compassion as a source to compassionate care. *Scandinavian Journal of Caring Sciences, 27*(1), 175–183. https://doi.org/10.1111/j.1471-6712.2012.01033.x

Williams, J. W., & Allen, S. (2015). Trauma-inspired prosocial leadership development. *Journal of Leadership Education, 14*(3), 86–103. http://doi:10.12806/V14/I3/R6

Winders, S. J., Murphy, O., Looney, K., & O'Reilly, G. (2020). Self-compassion, trauma, and posttraumatic stress disorder: A systematic review. *Clinical Psychology & Psychotherapy, 27*(3), 300–329. https://doi.org/10.1002/cpp.2429

Winfrey, O., & Perry, B. (2021). *What happened to you? Conversations on trauma, resilience, and healing* (Kindle ed.). Flatiron Books.

Witvliet, C. V., Blank, S. L., & Gall, A. J. (2022). Compassionate reappraisal and rumination impact forgiveness, emotion, sleep, and prosocial accountability. *Frontiers in Psychology, 13*, 992768. https://doi.org/10.3389/fpsyg.2022.992768

Wong, D. B. (2015). Growing virtue: The theory and science of developing compassion from a Mencian perspective. In B. Bruya (Ed.), *The philosophical challenge from China* (pp. 23–58). The Massachusetts Institute of Technology Press.

Worline, M., & Dutton, J. (2017). *Awakening compassion at work: The quiet power that elevates people and organizations* (Kindle ed.). Berrett-Koehler Publishers. https://www.naca.org/JCAPS/Documents/Killam_Book_Review_JCAPS_Fall_2020.pdf

Wu, B. W. Y., Gao, J., Leung, H. K., & Sik, H. H. (2019). A randomized controlled trial of awareness training program (ATP), a group-based Mahayana Buddhist intervention. *Mindfulness, 10*, 1280–1293. https://doi.org/10.1007/s12671-018-1082-1

Xie, W., Wang, J., Zhang, Y., Zuo, M., Kang, H., Tang, P., Zeng, L., Jin, M., Ni, W., & Ma, C. (2021). The levels, prevalence and related factors of compassion fatigue among oncology nurses: A systematic review and meta-analysis. *Journal of Clinical Nursing, 30*(5–6), 615–632. http://doi:10.1111/jocn.15565

Yong, A. G. (2023). Skillful means in interreligious compassion education. *Mindfulness, 14*(10), 2365–2373. https://doi.org/10.1007/s12671-023-02197-2

Yuan, F. (2022). Sensemaking and creativity at work when employees are coping with traumatic life experiences: Implications for positive organizational change. *The Journal of Applied Behavioral Science, Volume Online First, 59*(3), 1–23. https://doi.org/10.1177/00218863221113319

Zerach, G., Horesh, D., & Solomon, Z. (2022). Secondary posttraumatic stress symptom trajectories and perceived health among spouses of war veterans: A 12-year longitudinal study. *Psychology & Health, 37*(6), 675–691. https://doi.org/10.1080/08870446.2021.1879807

Zhang, M., Murphy, B., Cabanilla, A., & Yidi, C. (2021). Physical relaxation for occupational stress in healthcare workers: A systematic review and network meta-analysis of randomized controlled trials. *Journal of Occupational Health, 63*(1), e12243. https://doi.org/10.1002/1348-9585.12243

Zhou, L., Min, T., Bian, X., Dong, Y., Zhang, P., & Wen, Y. (2022). Rational design of intelligent and multifunctional dressing to promote acute/chronic wound healing. *ACS Applied Bio Materials, 5*(9), 4055–4085. https://doi.org/10.1021/acsabm.2c00500

Part II

Adler, J. (2002). *Offering from the conscious body: The discipline of authentic movement* (Kindle ed.). Simon and Schuster.

Agapi, A. A. (2021). A Buddhist-informed conceptual framework for compassion fatigue prevention. http://doi:10.15760/honors.1011

Akira, S. (2024). Śāntideva. In J. A. Silk (Ed.), *Brill's encyclopedia of Buddhism online*. Brill. https://doi.org/10.1163/2467-9666_enbo_COM_2057

Allen, R. (2015). The health benefits of nose breathing. *Nursing in General Practice*, 40–42. http://hdl.handle.net/10147/559021

Altman, D. (2014). *The mindfulness toolbox: 50 practical tips, tools & handouts for anxiety, depression, stress & pain* (Kindle ed.). PESI Publishing and Media.

American Psychiatric Association. (2022). *Diagnostic and statistical manual of mental disorders* (5th ed., text rev.). https://doi.org/10.1176/appi.books.9780890425787

Anālayo, B. (2019). Immeasurable meditations and mindfulness. *Mindfulness, 10*(12), 2620–2628. https://doi.org/10.1007/s12671-019-01237-0

Anālayo, B., & Dhammadinnā, B. (2021). From compassion to self-compassion: A text-historical perspective. *Mindfulness, 12*(6), 1350–1360. https://doi.org/10.1007/s12671-020-01575-4

Antonelli, M., Donelli, D., Carlone, L., Maggini, V., Firenzuoli, F., & Bedeschi, E. (2022). Effects of forest bathing (shinrin-yoku) on individual well-being: An umbrella review. *International Journal of Environmental Health Research, 32*(8), 1842–1867. https://doi.org/10.1080/09603123.2021.1919293

Applied Compassion Training (ACT). (2021). http://ccare.stanford.edu/education/applied-compassion-training/

Arieli, S., Sagiv, L., & Roccas, S. (2020). Values at work: The impact of personal values in organisations. *Applied Psychology, 69*(2), 230–275. https://doi.org/10.1111/apps.12181

Atkins, P. W., Wilson, D. S., & Hayes, S. C. (2019). *Prosocial: Using evolutionary science to build productive, equitable, and collaborative groups* (Kindle ed.). New Harbinger Publications.

Barkai, Y. (2022). On the authentic movement model: A space for creation – a place to be. *American Journal of Dance Therapy, 44*(1), 4–20. https://doi.org/10.1007/s10465-022-09354-5

Beamish, A. J., Foster, J. J., Edwards, H., & Olbers, T. (2019). What's in a smile? A review of the benefits of the clinician's smile. *Postgraduate Medical Journal, 95*(1120), 91–95. https://doi.org/10.1136/postgradmedj-2018-136286

Benjamin, S., & Kline, C. (2019). How to yes-and: Using improvisational games to improv(e) communication, listening, and collaboration techniques in tourism and hospitality education. *Journal of Hospitality, Leisure, Sport & Tourism Education, 24*, 130–142. https://doi.org/10.1016/j.jhlste.2019.02.002

Bhalla, T., & DiCuirci, L. (2023). "Me time": Motherhood, reading, and myths of leisure. *Reception: Texts, Readers, Audiences, History, 15*, 41–49. https://doi.org/10.5325/reception.15.1.0041

Bhikkhu, B. (1980). *Ānāpānasati: Mindfulness of breathing*. Sublime Life Mission.

Boehme, R., Hauser, S., Gerling, G. J., Heilig, M., & Olausson, H. (2019). Distinction of self-produced touch and social touch at cortical and spinal cord levels. *Proceedings of the National Academy of Sciences, 116*(6), 2290–2299. www.pnas.org/cgi/doi/10.1073/pnas.1816278116

Bowen, S., Chawla, N., Grow, J., & Marlatt, G. A. (2021). *Mindfulness-based relapse prevention for addictive behaviors*. Guilford Publications.

Brach, T. (2019). *Radical compassion* (Kindle ed.). Penguin Publishing Group.

Broderick, P. C. (2021). *Learning to breathe: A mindfulness curriculum for adolescents to cultivate emotion regulation, attention, and performance* (Kindle and 2nd ed.). New Harbinger Publications.

Brown, B. (2017). *Braving the wilderness: The quest for true belonging and the courage to stand alone* (Kindle ed.). Random House.

Brunzell, T., Waters, L., & Stokes, H. (2015). Teaching with strengths in trauma-affected students: A new approach to healing and growth in the classroom. *American Journal of Orthopsychiatry, 85*(1), 3–9. https://doi.org/10.1037/ort0000048

Burton, L., & Lent, J. (2016). The use of vision boards as a therapeutic intervention. *Journal of Creativity in Mental Health, 11*(1), 52–65. https://doi.org/10.1080/15401383.2015.1092901

Call, M., Mai, T., & Whitlock, M. J. (2022). *Using emotion coaching to build a peer support culture.* University of Utah. https://accelerate.uofuhealth.utah.edu/resilience/using-emotion-coaching-to-build-a-peer-support-culture

Campbell, J. (2008). *The hero with a thousand faces.* New World Library.

Cassie, K. M., & DuBose, E. M. (2023). An exploratory examination of the effect of self-care practices on job satisfaction and organizational commitment. *Journal of Evidence-Based Social Work, 20*(2), 258–271. https://doi.org/10.1080/26408066.2022.2156832

Chesner, A. (2020). Psychodrama and healing the traumatic wound. In A. Chesner & S. Lykou (Eds.), *Trauma in the creative and embodied therapies: When words are not enough* (pp. 69–80). Routledge.

Chödrön, P. (2017a). *The compassion book: Teachings for awakening the heart* (Kindle ed.). Shambhala Publications.

Chödrön, P. (2017b). *Tonglen: Bad in, good out.* https://www.lionsroar.com/tonglen-bad-in-good-out-september-2010/

Clark, K. R., & Sonsiadek, J. S. (2023). Trauma-informed care in medical imaging and radiation therapy to reduce retraumatization. *Radiologic Technology, 95*(1), 26–35.

Compassion Resilience Toolkit. (n.d.). *What is compassion resilience?* https://eliminatestigma.org/compassion-resilience-toolkit/health-and-human-services/what-is-compassion-resilience/

Condon, P., & Feldman Barrett, L. (2013). Conceptualizing and experiencing compassion. *Emotion, 13*(5), 817–821. https://doi.org/10.1037/a0033747

Condon, P., & Makransky, J. (2020a). Recovering the relational starting point of compassion training: A foundation for sustainable and inclusive care. *Perspectives on Psychological Science, 15*(6), 1346–1362. https://doi.org/10.1177/1745691620922200

Condon, P., & Makransky, J. (2020b). Sustainable compassion training: Integrating meditation theory with psychological science. *Frontiers in Psychology, 11*, 2249. https://doi.org/10.3389/fpsyg.2020.02249

Condon, P., & Makransky, J. (2023). Compassion and skillful means: Cultural adaptation, psychological science, and creative responsiveness. *Mindfulness, 14*(10), 2331–2341. https://doi.org/10.1007/s12671-022-01866-y

Curry, O. S., Rowland, L. A., Van Lissa, C. J., Zlotowitz, S., McAlaney, J., & Whitehouse, H. (2018). Happy to help? A systematic review and meta-analysis of the effects of performing acts of kindness on the well-being of the actor. *Journal of Experimental Social Psychology, 76*, 320–329. https://doi.org/10.1016/j.jesp.2018.02.014

Cutler, W. J., Shira, A., & Monk, L. (2014). *Writing alone together: Journalling in a circle of women for creativity, compassion and connection* (Kindle ed.). Butterfly Press.

Dalai Lama, X. I. V. (2001). *An open heart.* Hodder and Stoughton.

Dalai Lama, X. I. V. (2007). *How to see yourself as you really are* (J. Hopkins, Trans.). Atria Books.

Dana, D. (2020). *Polyvagal exercises for safety and connection: 50 client-centered practices* (*Norton series on interpersonal neurobiology*) (Kindle ed.). W.W. Norton & Company.

Davis, C. J. (2017). *Safety first: Fostering the neurological experience of safety in dance/movement therapy sessions for survivors of sexual trauma* [Unpublished Master's thesis]. Columbia College Chicago. https://digitalcommons.colum.edu/theses_dmt/84

De Britos, A. (2016). Mother tongue other tongue multilingual project for schools: Add your voice to the poet-tree. *Scottish Languages Review, 31*, 43–52. https://doi.org/10.6084/m9.figshare.3806589

De Tord, P., & Bräuninger, I. (2015). Grounding: Theoretical application and practice in dance movement therapy. *The Arts in Psychotherapy, 43*, 16–22. https://doi.org/10.1016/j.aip.2015.02.001

Dearly, B. (2019). Restoring the wholeness of being: Working with trauma from the focusing-oriented experiential therapy perspective. *Psychotherapy and Counselling Journal of Australia, 7*(2), 1–18.

Deaton, J. D., Ohrt, J. H., Linich, K., McCartney, E., & Glascoe, G. (2023). Vicarious posttraumatic growth: A systematic review and thematic synthesis across helping professions. *Traumatology, 29*(1), 17–26. https://doi.org/10.1037/trm0000375

Desmond, T. (2015). *Self-compassion in psychotherapy: Mindfulness-based practices for healing and transformation* (Kindle ed.). W.W. Norton & Company.

Dobkin, P. L. (2022). Kintsugi mind: How clinicians can be restored rather than broken by the pandemic. *Canadian Family Physician, 68*(4), 252–254. https://doi.org/10.46747/cfp.6804252

Dodson-Lavelle, B. (2015). *Against one method: Toward a critical-constructive approach to the adaptation and implementation of Buddhist-based contemplative programs in the United States* [Unpublished doctoral dissertation, Emory University.] https://etd.library.emory.edu/concern/etds/7h149q77f?locale=es

Doty, J. R. (n.d.). 10 letters to live by: Alphabet of the heart. Excerpted from J. R. Doty (2016). *Into the magic shop: A neurosurgeon's quest to discover the mysteries of the brain and the secrets of the heart*. Penguin. http://intothemagicshop.com/sites/default/files/Alphabet_of_the_Heart-Doty.pdf

Dreisoerner, A., Junker, N. M., Schlotz, W., Heimrich, J., Bloemeke, S., Ditzen, B., & van Dick, R. (2021). Self-soothing touch and being hugged reduce cortisol responses to stress: A randomized controlled trial on stress, physical touch, and social identity. *Comprehensive Psychoneuroendocrinology, 8*, 100091. https://doi.org/10.1016/j.cpnec.2021.100091

Dunne, J. D. (2019). Innate human connectivity and Śāntideva's cultivation of compassion. In J. C. Gold & D. S. Duckworth (Eds.), *Readings of Śāntideva's guide to bodhisattva practice* (pp. 235–251). Columbia University Press.

Dunne, J. D., & Manheim, J. (2023). Compassion, self-compassion, and skill in means: A Mahāyāna perspective. *Mindfulness, 14*(10), 2374–2382. https://doi.org/10.1007/s12671-022-01864-0

Dupasquier, J. R., Kelly, A. C., Moscovitch, D. A., & Vidovic, V. (2018). Practicing self-compassion weakens the relationship between fear of receiving compassion and the desire to conceal negative experiences from others. *Mindfulness, 9*(2), 500–511. https://doi:10.1007/s12671-017-0792-0

Ekman, P. (2021). *Developing global compassion.* https://www.paulekman.com/projects/global-compassion/

Ekman, P., & Ekman, E. (2017). Is global compassion achievable? In E. M. Seppälä, E. Simon-Thomas, S. L., Brown, M. Worline, C. D. Cameron, & J. R. Doty. (Eds.), *The Oxford handbook of compassion science* (pp. 41–49). Oxford University Press.

Emmons, R. A. (2013). *Gratitude works! A 21-day program for creating emotional prosperity.* John Wiley & Sons.

Epstein, M. (2013). *Thoughts without a thinker: Psychotherapy from a Buddhist perspective* (Kindle ed.). Basic Books a Member of Perseus Books Group.

Feldman, C., & Kuyken, W. (2011). Compassion in the landscape of suffering. *Contemporary Buddhism, 12*(1), 143–155. https://doi:10.1080/14639947.2011.564831

Ferry, B. (Ed.). (2017). *The amygdala: Where emotions shape perception, learning and memories.* BoD–Books on Demand.

Fredrickson, B. L. (1998). What good are positive emotions? *Review of General Psychology, 2*(3), 300–319. https://doi.org/10.1037/1089-2680.2.3.300

Freese, J. B. (2023). Towards trauma-informed Buddhist spiritual care: A mutual critical correlation of Vipassana meditation and somatic experiencing. *Pastoral Psychology, 72*, 447–464. https://doi.org/10.1007/s11089-023-01065-z

Fuller, L. K. (2018). In defense of self-care. *Journal of Pastoral Theology, 28*(1), 5–21. https://doi/10.1080/10649867.2018.1459106

Garfield, J. L. (2019). Second persons and the constitution of the first person. *Humana Mente, 12*(36), 42–66. https://scholarworks.smith.edu/phi_facpubs/34

Gendlin, E. (1988). *Focusing*. Bantam Double Day Books.

Gethin, R. (2015). Buddhist conceptualizations of mindfulness. In K. W. Brown, J. D. Creswell, & R. M. Ryan (Eds.), *Handbook of mindfulness: Theory, research, and practice* (pp. 9–41). Guilford Press.

Gibson, D. (2018). A visual conversation with trauma: Visual journaling in art therapy to combat vicarious trauma. *Art Therapy, 35*(2), 99–103. https://doi.org/10.1080/07421656.2018.1483166

Gilbert, P., Basran, J., MacArthur, M., & Kirby, J. N. (2019). Differences in the semantics of prosocial words: An exploration of compassion and kindness. *Mindfulness, 10*(11), 2259–2271. https://doi.org/10.1007/s12671-019-01191-x

Gilbert, P., McEwan, K., Matos, M., & Rivis, A. (2011). Fears of compassion: Development of three self-report measures. *Psychology and Psychotherapy: Theory, Research and Practice, 84*(3), 239–255. https://doi.org/10.1348/147608310X526511

Glennon, A., Pruitt, D. K., & Rouland Polmanteer, R. S. (2019). Integrating self-care into clinical practice with trauma clients. *Journal of Human Behavior in the Social Environment, 29*(1), 48–56. https://doi.org/10.1080/10911359.2018.1473189

Goenka, S. N. (1990). *10-day English discourse – day 7*. https://www.youtube.com/watch?v=Oro4bEM-pCA

Goldberg, L. D., McDonald, S. D., & Perrin, P. B. (2019). Predicting trajectories of posttraumatic growth following acquired physical disability. *Rehabilitation Psychology, 64*(1), 37–49. https://doi.org/10.1037/rep0000247

Goldhahn, E. (2022). Authentic movement: A guide to practice. In E. Goldhahn (Ed.), *Reflections on authentic movement* (Kindle ed., pp. 40–61). Routledge.

Goodman, C. (2016). *Śāntideva*. Stanford Encyclopedia of Philosophy. https://plato.stanford.edu/entries/shantideva/

Graff, M. (2020). *The compassion fatigued organization: Restoring compassion to helping professionals* (Kindle ed.). Cultivating Human Resiliency.

Haidt, J. (2002). The moral emotions. In R. J. Davidson, K. R. Scherer, & H. H. Goldsmith (Eds.), *Handbook of affective sciences* (pp. 852–870). Oxford University Press.

Haiku Society of America. (2004). *Definitions of haiku & related terms*. https://www.hsa-haiku.org/hsa-definitions.html#Senryu

Halifax, J. (2018). *Standing at the edge: Finding freedom where fear and courage meet* (Kindle ed.). Flatiron Books.

Hambly, G. (2021). The not so universal hero's journey. *Journal of Screenwriting, 12*(2), 135–150. https://doi.org/10.1386/josc_00056_1

Hạnh, T. N. (1992). *Peace is every step: The path of mindfulness in everyday life*. Bantam.

Hạnh, T. N. (1998). *The heart of the Buddha's teaching: Transforming suffering into peace, joy & liberation: The four noble truths, the noble eightfold path, and other basic Buddhist teachings*. Random House.

Hạnh, T. N. (2001). *Anger: The wisdom for cooling the flames* (Kindle ed.). Riverhead Books – Penguin Publishing Group.

Hạnh, T. N. (2002a). The fourteen precepts of engaged Buddhism (special feature). *Social Policy, 33*(1), 39–41.

Hạnh, T. N. (2002b). *Be free where you are* (Kindle ed.). Parallax Press.

Hạnh, T. N. (2014). *No mud, no lotus: The art of transforming suffering* (Kindle ed.). Parallax Press.

Hanson, R. (2009). *Buddha's brain: The practical neuroscience of happiness, love, and wisdom*. New Harbinger Publications.

Hanson, R. (2013). *Hardwiring happiness* (Kindle ed.). Harmony/Rodale.

Hanson, R. (2020). *Neurodharma: New science, ancient wisdom, and seven practices of the highest happiness* (Kindle ed.). Harmony.

Hao, J., Liu, C., Feng, S., & Luo, J. (2021). Imagination-based loving-kindness and compassion meditation: A new meditation method developed from Chinese Buddhism. *Journal of Religion and Health, 61*(4), 2753–2769. https://doi.org/10.1007/s10943-021-01409-0

Harvey, P. (2013). *An introduction to Buddhism: Teachings, history and practices* (Kindle ed.). Cambridge University Press.

Hayashi, A., Anzai, E., Saiwaki, N., Sumioka, H., & Shiomi, M. (2022, March). *Does encouraging self-touching behaviors with supportive voices increase stress-buffering effects?* 2022 17th ACM/IEEE International Conference on Human-Robot Interaction (HRI), IEEE, pp. 787–791. http://doi.org/10.1109/HRI53351.2022.9889461

Hayes, S. C. (2020). *A liberated mind: How to pivot toward what matters.* Penguin.

Heslin, P. A. (2009). Better than brainstorming? Potential contextual boundary conditions to brainwriting for idea generation in organizations. *Journal of Occupational and Organizational Psychology, 82*(1), 129–145. https://doi.org/10.1348/096317908X285642

Huron, D., & Vuoskoski, J. K. (2020). On the enjoyment of sad music: Pleasurable compassion theory and the role of trait empathy. *Frontiers in Psychology, 11*, 1060. https://doi.org/10.3389/fpsyg.2020.01060

Husain, A., & Hasan, A. (2021). *Psychology of meditation: A practical guide to self-discovery.* Psycho Information Technologies.

Huseinagić, E., & Hodzić, A. (2008). Stress and techniques of overcoming mental stress. *Sport Scientific and Practical Aspects, 5*(1–2), 75–80.

Hyatt, L. (2020). From compassion fatigue to vitality: Memoir with art response for self-care. *Art Therapy, 37*(1), 46–50. https://doi.org/10.1080/07421656.2019.1677423

Hydon, S., Wong, M., Langley, A. K., Stein, B. D., & Kataoka, S. H. (2015). Preventing secondary traumatic stress in educators. *Child and Adolescent Psychiatric Clinics, 24*(2), 319–333. https://doi.org/10.1016/j.chc.2014.11.003

Jackson-Preston, P., Brown, G. C., Garnett, T., Sanchez, D., Fagbamila, E., & Graham, N. (2023). "I am never enough": Factors contributing to secondary traumatic stress and burnout among black student services professionals in higher education. *Trauma Care, 3*(2), 93–107. https://doi.org/10.3390/traumacare3020010

Jakubiak, B. K., & Feeney, B. C. (2016). Keep in touch: The effects of imagined touch support on stress and exploration. *Journal of Experimental Social Psychology, 65*, 59–67. https://doi.org/10.1016/j.jesp.2016.04.001

Jeebodh-Desai, L., & Dwarika, V. M. (2022). Trauma-sensitive mindfulness for war refugees: Communication of preliminary findings. *Trauma Care, 2*(4), 556–568. https://doi.org/10.3390/traumacare2040046

Jinpa, T. (2015). *A fearless heart* (Kindle ed.). Penguin Publishing Group.

Jinpa, T. (2019). Bodhicaryāvatāra and Tibetan mind training (Lojong). In J. C. Gold & D. S. Duckworth (Eds.), *Readings of Śāntideva's guide to bodhisattva practice* (pp. 146–161). Columbia University Press.

Joyce, E. W. (2010). *"The small space of a pause": Susan Howe's poetry and the spaces between.* Bucknell University Press.

Kalaitzaki, A., Tamiolaki, A., & Tsouvelas, G. (2022). From secondary traumatic stress to vicarious post-traumatic growth amid COVID-19 lockdown in Greece: The role of health care workers' coping strategies. *Psychological Trauma: Theory, Research, Practice, and Policy, 14*(2), 273–280. https://doi.org/10.1037/tra0001078

Kashdan, T. B., Uswatte, G., & Julian, T. (2006). Gratitude and hedonic and eudaimonic well-being in Vietnam war veterans. *Behaviour Research and Therapy, 44*(2), 177–199. https://doi.org/10.1016/j.brat.2005.01.005

Kelsey, J. B. (2020). *What is haiku?* https://thehaikufoundation.org/new-to-haiku-what-is-haiku-2/

Kraybill, O. G. (2015). *Experiential training to address secondary traumatic stress in aid personnel* [Unpublished doctoral dissertation]. Lesley University. https://digitalcommons.lesley.edu/expressive_dissertations/18/

Kuhfuss, M., Maldei, T., Hetmanek, A., & Baumann, N. (2021). Somatic experiencing–effectiveness and key factors of a body-oriented trauma therapy: A scoping literature review. *European*

Journal of Psychotraumatology, 12(1), 1929023. https://doi.org/10.1080/20008198.2021.1929023

Kusala, B. (2020). *The Satipatthana Sutta: A new translation with the Pali and English texts* (2nd ed.). Dhamma Sukha Publications.

Landis-Shack, N., Heinz, A. J., & Bonn-Miller, M. O. (2017). Music therapy for posttraumatic stress in adults: A theoretical review. *Psychomusicology: Music, Mind, and Brain, 27*(4), 334–342. https://doi.org/10.1037/pmu0000192

Landry, D. W. (2006). Voluntary reciprocal altruism: A novel strategy to encourage deceased organ donation. *Kidney International, 69*(6), 957–959. https://doi.org/10.1038/sj.ki.5000280

Latinjak, A. T., Morin, A., Brinthaupt, T. M., Hardy, J., Hatzigeorgiadis, A., Kendall, P. C., Neck, C., Oliver, E., Puchalska-Wasyl, M. M., Tovares, A., & Winsler, A. (2023). Self-talk: An interdisciplinary review and transdisciplinary model. *Review of General Psychology, 27*(4), 355–386. https://doi.org/10.1177/10892680231170263

Lauffenburger, S. K. (2020). 'Something more': The unique features of dance movement therapy/psychotherapy. *American Journal of Dance Therapy, 42*(1), 16–32. https://doi.org/10.1007/s10465-020-09321-y

Lavelle, B. D. (2017). Compassion in context: Tracing the Buddhist roots of secular, compassion-based contemplative programs. In E. M., Seppälä, E. Simon-Thomas, S. L., Brown, M. Worline, C. D., Cameron, & J. R. Doty (Eds.), *The Oxford handbook of compassion science* (pp. 17–26). Oxford University Press.

Le Page, J., & Le Page, L. (2013). *Mudras for healing and transformation* (Kindle ed.). Integrative Yoga Therapy.

Levine, P. A. (2010). *Healing trauma: A pioneering program for restoring the wisdom of your body* (Kindle ed.). Sounds True.

Li, S. T. T., Frohna, J. G., & Bostwick, S. B. (2017). Using your personal mission statement to INSPIRE and achieve success. *Academic Pediatrics, 17*(2), 107–109. https://doi:https://doi.org/10.1016/j.acap.2016.11.010

Lieberman, M. D., Eisenberger, N. I., Crockett, M. J., Tom, S. M., Pfeifer, J. H., & Way, B. M. (2007). Putting feelings into words: Affect labeling disrupts amygdala activity in response to affective stimuli. *Psychological Science, 18*(5), 421–428. https://doi.org/10.1111/j.1467-9280.2007.01916.x

Lief, J. L. (2001). *Making friends with death: A Buddhist guide for encountering mortality*. Shambhala Publications.

Lilius, J. M., Worline, M. C., Maitlis, S., Kanov, J., Dutton, J. E., & Frost, P. (2008). The contours and consequences of compassion at work. *Journal of Organizational Behavior, 29*(2), 193–218. https://doi.org/10.1002/job.508

Lindsay, E. K., & Creswell, J. D. (2014). Helping the self-help others: Self-affirmation increases self-compassion and pro-social behaviors. *Frontiers in Psychology, 5*, 1–9. https://doi.org/10.3389/fpsyg.2014.00421

Loy, D. R. (2019). *Nonduality: In Buddhism and beyond*. Simon and Schuster.

Lutz, A., Jha, A. P., Dunne, J. D., & Saron, C. D. (2015). Investigating the phenomenological matrix of mindfulness-related practices from a neurocognitive perspective. *American Psychologist, 70*(7), 632–658. https://doi.org/10.1037/a0039585

Lyman, F. T. (1981). The responsive classroom discussion: The inclusion of all students. In A. S. Anderson (Ed.), *Mainstreaming digest* (pp. 109–113). University of Maryland Press.

Maddock, A. (2023). The clinically modified Buddhist psychological model for social work practice and self-care. *Clinical Social Work Journal, 51*(1), 54–64. https://doi.org/10.1007/s10615-022-00849-9

Manning-Jones, S. F., de Terte, I., & Stephens, C. (2015). Vicarious posttraumatic growth: A systematic literature review. *International Journal of Wellbeing, 5*(2), 125–139. http://doi:10.5502/ijw.v5i2.8

Martínková, I., & Wang, Q. (2022). Shikantaza–the practice of 'just sitting': Ultimate slowing down and its effect on experiencing. *Sport, Ethics and Philosophy, 16*(2), 221–236. https://doi.org/10.1080/17511321.2022.2045345

Mathieu, F. (2012). *The compassion fatigue workbook: Creative tools for transforming compassion fatigue and vicarious traumatization (psychosocial stress series)* (Kindle ed.). Taylor and Francis.

May Peace Prevail on Earth International. (2020). https://www.worldpeace.org/founder/

McCallie, M. S., Blum, C. M., & Hood, C. J. (2006). Progressive muscle relaxation. *Journal of Human Behavior in the Social Environment, 13*(3), 51–66. https://doi.org/10.1300/J137v13n03_04

McDonald, B., Böckler, A., & Kanske, P. (2022). Soundtrack to the social world: Emotional music enhances empathy, compassion, and prosocial decisions but not theory of mind. *Emotion, 22*(1), 19–29. https://doi.org/10.1037/emo0001036

McHale, L. (2022). *Neuroscience for organizational communication: A guide for communicators and leaders.* Palgrave Macmillan and Springer.

Meekums, B. (2002). *Dance movement therapy: A creative psychotherapeutic approach.* Sage Publications Ltd.

Merriam Webster. (2024a). Afterimage. In *Merriam Webster online unabridged English dictionary.* https://www.merriam-webster.com/dictionary/afterimage

Merriam Webster. (2024b). Ground. In *Merriam Webster online unabridged English dictionary.* https://www.merriam-webster.com/dictionary/ground

Merriam Webster. (2024c). Withness. In *Merriam Webster online unabridged English dictionary.* https://www.merriam-webster.com/dictionary/withness

Merriam Webster. (2024d). Rise. In *Merriam Webster online unabridged English dictionary.* https://www.merriam-webster.com/dictionary/rise

Mintarsih, R. A., & Azizah, B. S. I. (2020, January). *Mirroring exercise: Dance/movement therapy for individuals with trauma.* 5th ASEAN Conference on Psychology, Counselling, and Humanities (ACPCH 2019), Atlantis Press, pp. 132–138. https://doi:10.2991/assehr.k.200120.029

Missouri Department of Mental Health. (2014). *The Missouri model: A developmental framework for trauma-informed approaches.* https://dmh.mo.gov/media/pdf/missouri-model-developmental-framework-trauma-informed-approaches

Mundle, R. G., & Smith, B. (2013). Hospital chaplains and embodied listening: Engaging with stories and the body in healthcare environments. *Illness, Crisis & Loss, 21*(2), 95–108. https://doi.org/10.2190/IL.21.2.b

Murphy, S. K. (2021). *Utilizing blind contour portrait drawing to promote positive emotions and connection during the COVID-19 pandemic* [Unpublished doctoral dissertation]. Notre Dame de Namur University. https://www.proquest.com/docview/2532103824?pq-origsite=gscholar&from openview=true

Musicant, S. (1994). Authentic movement and dance therapy. *American Journal of Dance Therapy, 16,* 91–106. https://doi.org/10.1007/BF02358569

Neff, K. D. (2021). *Fierce self-compassion: How women can harness kindness to speak up, claim their power, and thrive.* Harper Collins.

Neff, K. D. & Germer, C. (2018). *The mindful self-compassion workbook: A proven way to accept yourself, build inner strength, and thrive* (Kindle ed.). Guilford Publications.

Nieuwenhuis, M. (2019). Porous skin: Breathing through the prism of the holey body. *Emotion, Space and Society, 33,* 1–8. https://doi.org/10.1016/j.emospa.2019.100595

Norris, C. J. (2021). The negativity bias, revisited: Evidence from neuroscience measures and an individual differences approach. *Social Neuroscience, 16*(1), 68–82. https://doi.org/10.1080/174709 19.2019.1696225

Papies, E. K. (2016). Mindfulness and health behaviour: Examining the roles of attention regulation and decentering. In J. C. Karremans & E. K. Papies (Eds.), *Mindfulness in social psychology* (pp. 94–108). Routledge.

Patra, S. K. (2017). Physiological effect of kriyas: Cleansing techniques. *International Journal of Yoga-Philosophy, Psychology and Parapsychology, 5*(1), 3–5. https://doi:10.4103/ijny.ijoyppp_31_17

Paulus, M. P., Potterat, E. G., Taylor, M. K., Van Orden, K. F., Bauman, J., Momen, N., Padilla, G. A., & Swain, J. L. (2009). A neuroscience approach to optimizing brain resources for human performance in extreme environments. *Neuroscience & Biobehavioral Reviews, 33*(7), 1080–1088. https://doi.org/10.1016/j.neubiorev.2009.05.003

Pearson, A. (2006). Powerful caring: A simple act by a nurse who 'cared from the heart' has stayed with Alan Pearson. *Nursing Standard, 20*(48), 20–23. https://doi.org/10.7748/NS.20.48.20.S24

Perciavalle, V., Blandini, M., Fecarotta, P., Buscemi, A., Di Corrado, D., Bertolo, L., Fichera, F., & Coco, M. (2017). The role of deep breathing on stress. *Neurological Sciences, 38*(3), 451–458. https://doi:10.1007/s10072-016-2790-8

Polizzi, C. P., Sleight, F. G., Aksen, D. E., McDonald, C. W., & Lynn, S. J. (2023). Mindfulness and COVID-19-related stress: Staying present during uncertain times. *Mindfulness*, 1135–1147. https://doi.org/10.1007/s12671-023-02132-5

Polk, K. L., Schoendorff, B., Webster, M., & Olaz, F. O. (2016). *The essential guide to the ACT Matrix: A step-by-step approach to using the ACT Matrix model in clinical practice* (Kindle ed.). New Harbinger Publications.

Pollak, S. M., Pedulla, T., & Siegel, R. D. (2014). *Sitting together: Essential skills for mindfulness-based psychotherapy* (Kindle ed.). Guilford Press.

Pololi, L. H., Evans, A. T., Civian, J. T., Gibbs, B. K., Coplit, L. D., Gillum, L. H., & Brennan, R. T. (2015). Faculty vitality – surviving the challenges facing academic health centers: A national survey of medical faculty. *Academic Medicine, 90*(7), 930–936. http://doi:10.1097/ACM.0000000000000674

Porges, S. W. (2017). Vagal pathways: Portals to compassion. In E. M., Seppälä, E. Simon-Thomas, S. L. Brown, M. Worline, C. D. Cameron, & J. R. Doty (Eds.), *The Oxford handbook of compassion science* (pp. 41–49). Oxford University Press.

Pressman, S. D., Kraft, T. L., & Cross, M. P. (2015). It's good to do good and receive good: The impact of a 'pay it forward' style kindness intervention on giver and receiver well-being. *The Journal of Positive Psychology, 10*(4), 293–302. https://doi.org/10.1080/17439760.2014.965269

Quaglia, J. T. (2023). One compassion, many means: A big two analysis of compassionate behavior. *Mindfulness, 14*(10), 2430–2442. https://doi.org/10.1007/s12671-022-01895-7

Rakel, D. (2018). *The compassionate connection: The healing power of empathy and mindful listening*. W.W. Norton & Company.

Rand, M. L. (2004). Vicarious trauma and the Buddhist doctrine of suffering. *Annals of the American Psychotherapy Association, 7*(1), 40–42.

Rauch, S., & Foa, E. (2006). Emotional processing theory (EPT) and exposure therapy for PTSD. *Journal of Contemporary Psychotherapy, 36*, 61–65. https://doi:10.1007/s10879-006-9008-y

Reilly, E. B., & Stuyvenberg, C. L. (2023). A meta-analysis of loving-kindness meditations on self-compassion. *Mindfulness, 14*(10), 2299–2310. https://doi.org/10.1007/s12671-022-01972-x

Remen, R. N. (2012). *Generous listening* [video]. https://www.youtube.com/watch?v=UdhP6sR5uvk

Renzenbrink, I. (Ed.). (2011). *Caregiver stress and staff support in illness, dying and bereavement*. Oxford University Press.

Rinpoche, S. (1992). *The Tibetan book of living and dying* (Kindle ed.). Rider.

Rook, J. (2016). *How to create a stress-reducing playlist*. https://www.anxiety.org/music-therapy-stress-reducing-playlist

Rosenthal, C., & Vanderbeke, D. (2015). Introduction. In D. Vanderbeke & C. Rosenthal (Eds.), *Probing the skin: Cultural representations of our contact zone* (pp. 1–10). Cambridge Scholars Publishing.

Rubin, R. S. (2002). Will the real SMART goals please stand up. *The Industrial-Organizational Psychologist, 39*(4), 26–27.

Salzberg, S. (2013). *Real happiness at work: Meditations for accomplishment, achievement, and peace* (Kindle ed.). Workman Publishing.

Śāntideva. (n.d.). *The Bodhicaryavatara* (P. Williams, Ed., K. Crosby & A Skilton, Trans., 1st ed.). Oxford University Press. (Original work published 7th–8th century).

Saraswati, S. B. (2021). *Hollywood to the Himalayas: A journey of healing and transformation* (Kindle ed.). Simon and Schuster.

Saraswati, S. S. (2009). *Yoga Nidra* (4th ed.). Yoga Publication Trust.

Sax, A. (2019). *Understanding trauma: The healing process of poetry*. https://arts.cgu.edu/tufts-poetry-awards/understanding-trauma-the-healing-process-of-poetry/

Schroeder, J. W. (2004). *Skillful means: The heart of Buddhist compassion*. Motilal Banarsidass.

Senthil, K., & Britto, J. (2022). Yoga based ocular exercise (Trataka): The scriptural and scientific review. *Journal of Positive School Psychology, 6*(6), 6231–6240.

Seoane, K. J. (2016). Parenting the self with self-applied touch: A dance/movement therapy approach to self-regulation. *American Journal of Dance Therapy, 38*(1), 21–40. https://doi:10.1007/s10465-016-9207-3

Seppälä, E. M. (2013). The compassionate mind. *Association for Psychological Science Observer, 26*(5). https://www.psychologicalscience.org/observer/the-compassionate-mind?utm_source=buffer&utm_medium=twitter&utm_campaign=Buffer%3A%2BDanGilliland%2Bon%2Btwitter&buffer_share=dd330

Shannon, P. J., Simmelink-McCleary, J., Im, H., Becher, E., & Crook-Lyon, R. E. (2014). Developing self-care practices in a trauma treatment course. *Journal of Social Work Education, 50*(3), 440–453. https://doi.org/10.1080/10437797.2014.917932

Shonin, E., Van Gordon, W., Compare, A., Zangeneh, M., & Griffiths, M. D. (2015). Buddhist-derived loving-kindness and compassion meditation for the treatment of psychopathology: A systematic review. *Mindfulness, 6*(5), 1161–1180. https://doi.org/10.1007/s12671-014-0368-1

Siegel, R. D., & Germer, C. K. (2012). Wisdom and compassion: Two wings of a bird. In C. K. Germer & R. D. Siegel (Eds.), *Wisdom and compassion in psychotherapy: Deepening mindfulness in clinical practice* (Kindle ed., pp. 7–34). Guilford Press.

Simmer-Brown, J. (2023). Activity of the armless mother: Applications of compassion and skillful means from Indo-Tibetan Buddhism. *Mindfulness, 14*, 2342–2353. https://doi.org/10.1007/s12671-022-01868-w

Simons, D., & Chabris, C. (1999). *Selective attention test* [video]. Visual Cognition Laboratory: University of Illinois. http://viscog.beckman.illinois.edu/flashmovie/15.php

Singh, A. N. (2015). Application of yoga therapy to psychosomatic disorders. *International Medical Journal, 22*(4), 277–282.

Sparks, A. M., Fessler, D. M., & Holbrook, C. (2019). Elevation, an emotion for prosocial contagion, is experienced more strongly by those with greater expectations of the cooperativeness of others. *PLoS One, 14*(12), e0226071. https://doi.org/10.1371/journal.pone.0226071

Spence, J. (2021). *Trauma-informed yoga: A toolbox for therapists: 47 practices to calm balance, and restore the nervous system* (Kindle ed.). PESI Publishing, Inc.

Sprang, G., Ford, J., Kerig, P., & Bride, B. (2019). Defining secondary traumatic stress and developing targeted assessments and interventions: Lessons learned from research and leading experts. *Traumatology, 25*(2), 72–81. https://doi.org/10.1037/trm0000180

Strycharczyk, D., Clough, P., & Perry, J. (2021). *Developing mental toughness: Strategies to improve performance, resilience and wellbeing in individuals and organizations* (Kindle ed.). Kogan Page Publishers.

Super, A. (2015). *A year of self-compassion: Finding care, connection and calm in our challenging times*. Troubador Publishing Ltd.

Tachon, G., Rouibah, A., Morgan, B., & Shankland, R. (2022). A prototype analysis of self-gratitude: Towards a broadening of the concept of gratitude. *Journal of Happiness Studies, 23*(5), 1867–1885. https://doi.org/10.1007/s10902-021-00475-1

Tal, M. (2006). *"Re-joining the stream of life" STREAM model: An integrated model of trauma group treatment combining dance movement therapy and somatic experiencing for older women suffering from spouse abuse* [Unpublished doctoral dissertation]. Anglia Ruskin University. https://www.researchgate.net/publication/333479646_Re-joining_the_Stream_of_Life_STREAM_model_An_Integrated_Model_of_Trauma_group_treatment_combining_Dance_Movement_Therapy_and_Somatic_ExperiencingR_for_older_women_suffering_from_spouse_abuse#fullTextFileContent

Tan, C. M. (2018). *Search inside yourself* (Kindle ed.). Bentang Pustaka.

Taruffi, L., & Koelsch, S. (2014). The paradox of music-evoked sadness: An online survey. *PLoS One, 9*(10), e110490. https://doi.org/10.1371/journal.pone.0110490

Taylor, S. E., Klein, L. C., Lewis, B. P., Gruenewald, T. L., Gurung, R. A., & Updegraff, J. A. (2000). Biobehavioral responses to stress in females: Tend-and-befriend, not fight-or-flight. *Psychological Review, 107*(3), 411–429. https://doi.org/10.1037/0033-295X.107.3.411

Tedeschi, R. G., & Calhoun, L. G. (1996). The posttraumatic growth inventory: Measuring the positive legacy of trauma. *Journal of Traumatic Stress, 9*(3), 455–471.

Tedeschi, R. G., & Calhoun, L. G. (2004). Posttraumatic growth: Conceptual foundations and empirical evidence. *Psychological Inquiry, 15*(1), 1–18. https://doi.org/10.1207/s15327965pli1501_01

Theodore, G. (2020). Hermeneutics. In *Stanford encyclopedia of philosophy*. https://plato.stanford.edu/entries/hermeneutics/

Treleaven, D. A. (2018). *Trauma-sensitive mindfulness: Practices for safe and transformative healing* (Kindle ed.). W.W. Norton & Company.

Tsirimokou, A., Kloess, J. A., & Dhinse, S. K. (2023). Vicarious post-traumatic growth in professionals exposed to traumatogenic material: A systematic literature review. *Trauma, Violence & Abuse, 24*(3), 1848–1866. https://doi.org/10.1177/15248380221082079

Vaidya, P. L. (1960). *Bodhicaryāvatāra of Śāntideva with the commentary Pañjika of Prajñākaramati*. Mithila Institute (Buddhist Sanskrit Texts, 12). https://archive.org/details/in.ernet.dli.2015.426132/page/n61/mode/2up?view=theater

Volkan, K. (2013). A psychoanalytic view of the sangha: Group functioning in Mahayana and Tibetan Buddhism. *Asian Journal of Humanities and Social Studies, 1*(02), 47–54.

Wallace, A. B. (2004). *The four immeasurables* (Kindle and 2nd ed.). Snow Lion Publications.

Wang, Y. I. (2022). Ink talks: Processing compassion fatigue through culturally relevant arts-making. *Creative Arts in Education and Therapy, 8*(2), 158–172. https://doi:10.15212/CAET/2022/8/18158-172

Weber, J. (2017). Mindfulness is not enough: Why equanimity holds the key to compassion. *Mindfulness & Compassion, 2*(2), 149–158. https://doi.org/10.1016/j.mincom.2017.09.004

Wheeler, A. J., & McElvaney, R. (2018). Why would you want to do that work? The positive impact on therapists working with child victims of sexual abuse in Ireland: A thematic analysis. *Counselling Psychology Quarterly, 31*(4), 513–527. https://doi.org/10.1080/09515070.2017.1336077

White, M., & Epston, D. (1990). *Narrative means to therapeutic ends*. W.W. Norton & Company.

Wiklund-Gustin, L., & Wagner, L. (2013). The butterfly effect of caring–clinical nursing teachers' understanding of self-compassion as a source to compassionate care. *Scandinavian Journal of Caring Sciences, 27*(1), 175–183. https://doi.org/10.1111/j.1471-6712.2012.01033.x

Wilson-Mendenhall, C. D., Dunne, J. D., & Davidson, R. J. (2023). Visualizing compassion: Episodic simulation as contemplative practice. *Mindfulness, 14*, 2532–2548. https://doi.org/10.1007/s12671-022-01842-6

Winfrey, O., & Perry, B. (2021). *What happened to you? Conversations on trauma, resilience, and healing* (Kindle ed.). Flatiron Books.

Wolf, P. R., & Rickard, J. A. (2003). Talking circles: A Native American approach to experiential learning. *Journal of Multicultural Counseling and Development, 31*(1), 39–43. https://doi.org/10.1002/j.2161-1912.2003.tb00529.x

Worline, M., & Dutton, J. (2017). *Awakening compassion at work: The quiet power that elevates people and organizations* (Kindle ed.). Berrett-Koehler Publishers. https://www.naca.org/JCAPS/Documents/Killam_Book_Review_JCAPS_Fall_2020.pdf

Yalom, I. (1985). *The theory and practice of group psychotherapy* (3rd ed.). Basic Book, Inc.

Yehuda, N. (2011). Music and stress. *Journal of Adult Development, 18*, 85–94. http://doi:10.1007/s10804-010-9117-4

Yong, A. G. (2023). Skillful means in interreligious compassion education. *Mindfulness, 14*(10), 2365–2373. https://doi.org/10.1007/s12671-023-02197-2

Zahavi, D. (2019). Second-person engagement, self-alienation, and group-identification. *Topoi, 38*(1), 251–260. http://doi:10.1007/s11245-016-9444-6

Zerubavel, N., & Messman-Moore, T. L. (2015). Staying present: Incorporating mindfulness into therapy for dissociation. *Mindfulness, 6*, 303–314. https://doi:10.1007/s12671-013-0261-3

Zhang, M., Murphy, B., Cabanilla, A., & Yidi, C. (2021). Physical relaxation for occupational stress in healthcare workers: A systematic review and network meta-analysis of randomized controlled trials. *Journal of Occupational Health, 63*(1), e12243. https://doi.org/10.1002/1348-9585.12243

Appendices

Abdullah, A. (2021). The helpful aspects of digital creative arts therapy during COVID 19 crisis: A qualitative investigation. *International Journal of Innovative Science and Research Technology, 6*(3), 763–767.

American Psychiatric Association. (2022). *Diagnostic and statistical manual of mental disorders* (5th ed., text rev.). https://doi.org/10.1176/appi.books.9780890425787

Amiti, F. (2020). Synchronous and asynchronous e-learning. *European Journal of Open Education and E-Learning Studies, 5*(2), 60–70. https://doi:10.46827/ejoe.v5i2.3313

Baker, W. J., Hunter, M., & Thomas, S. (2016). Arts education academics' perceptions of eLearning & teaching in Australian early childhood and primary ITE degrees. *Australian Journal of Teacher Education, 41*(11), 31–43. https://doi.org/10.14221/ajte.2016v41n11.3

Bride, B. E. (2013). *The secondary traumatic stress scale, DSM 5 revision*. Unpublished manuscript. http://www.srcac.org/wp-content/uploads/2020/07/18_STSS_DSM_5.pdf

Cieslak, R., Benight, C. C., Rogala, A., Smoktunowicz, E., Kowalska, M., Zukowska, K., Yeager, C., & Luszczynska, A. (2016). Effects of internet-based self-efficacy intervention on secondary traumatic stress and secondary posttraumatic growth among health and human services professionals exposed to indirect trauma. *Frontiers in Psychology, 7*, 1–13. https://doi:10.3389/fpsyg.2016.01009

Clark, A. A., & Haddock, L. (2015). Supervision in online counselor and education programs: An account from multiple perspectives. *VISTAS Online, 32*, 1–13. https://www.counseling.org/docs/default-source/vistas/article_325c5c21f16116603abcacf0000bee5e7.pdf?sfvrsn=c24a412c_8

Cutcher, A., & Cook, P. (2016). One must also be an artist: Online delivery of teacher education. *International Journal of Education & the Arts, 17*(13), 1–19. http://www.ijea.org/v17n13/

Dana, D. (2020). *Polyvagal exercises for safety and connection: 50 client-centered practices (Norton series on interpersonal neurobiology)* (Kindle ed.). W.W. Norton & Company.

D'Angelo, S. (2022). *Polyvagal informed embodied mindfulness: An online program* [Mindfulness Studies theses]. https://digitalcommons.lesley.edu/mindfulness_theses/60

Ferrara, K. W. (1994). *Therapeutic ways with words*. Oxford University Press.

Finlay-Jones, A., Kane, R., & Rees, C. (2017). Self-compassion online: A pilot study of an internet-based self-compassion program for psychology trainees. *Journal of Clinical Psychology, 73*(7), 797–816. https://doi.org/10.1002/jclp.22375

Garcia-Medrano, S. (2021). Screen–bridges: Dance movement therapy in online contexts. *Body, Movement and Dance in Psychotherapy, 16*(1), 64–72. https://doi.org/10.1080/17432979.2021.1883741

Kirby, J. N. (2017). Compassion interventions: The programmes, the evidence, and implications for research and practice. *Psychology and Psychotherapy: Theory, Research and Practice, 90*(3), 432–455. https://doi.org/10.1111/papt.12104

Knox, M. C., & Franco, P. L. (2023). Acceptability and feasibility of an online version of the self-compassion for healthcare communities program. *Psychology, Health & Medicine, 28*(7), 1709–1719. https://doi.org/10.1080/13548506.2022.2094428

Korman-Hacohen, S., Regev, D., & Roginsky, E. (2022). Creative arts therapy in the "remote therapeutic response" format in the education system. *Children, 9*(4), 467. https://doi.org/10.3390/children9040467

MacDonald, H. Z., & Neville, T. (2023). Promoting college students' mindfulness, mental health, and self-compassion in the time of COVID-19: Feasibility and efficacy of an online, interactive mindfulness-based stress reduction randomized trial. *Journal of College Student Psychotherapy, 37*(3), 260–278. https://doi.org/10.1080/87568225.2022.2028329

Mallen, M. J., Vogel, D. L., & Rochlen, A. B. (2005). The practical aspects of online counseling: Ethics, training, technology, and competency. *The Counseling Psychologist, 33,* 776–818. https://doi:10.1177/0011000005278625

McCutcheon, K., O'Halloran, P., & Lohan, M. (2018). Online learning versus blended learning of clinical supervisee skills with pre-registration nursing students: A randomised controlled trial. *International Journal of Nursing Studies, 82,* 30–39. https://doi.org/10.1016/j.ijnurstu.2018.02.005

Selič-Zupančič, P., Klemenc-Ketiš, Z., & Onuk Tement, S. (2023). The impact of psychological interventions with elements of mindfulness on burnout and well-being in healthcare professionals: A systematic review. *Journal of Multidisciplinary Healthcare, 16,* 1821–1831. https://doi.org/10.2147/JMDH.S398552

Singh, J., Steele, K., & Singh, L. (2021). Combining the best of online and face-to-face learning: Hybrid and blended learning approach for COVID-19, post vaccine, & post-pandemic world. *Journal of Educational Technology Systems, 50*(2), 140–171. https://doi.org/10.1177/00472395211047865

Sprang, G., Whitt-Woosley, A., & Eslinger, J. (2022). Diagnostic and translational utility of the secondary traumatic stress clinical algorithm (STS-CA). *Journal of Interpersonal Violence, 37*(21–22), NP19811–NP19826. https://doi.org/10.1177/08862605211044961

Villalón, F. J., Moreno, M. I., Rivera, R., Venegas, W., Arancibia C, J. V., Soto, A., & Pemjean, A. (2023). Brief online mindfulness-and compassion-based inter-care program for students during COVID-19 pandemic: A randomized controlled trial. *Mindfulness, 14*(8), 1918–1929. https://doi.org/10.1007/s12671-023-02159-8

Villarreal-Davis, C., Sartor, T. A., & McLean, L. (2021). Utilizing creativity to foster connection in online counseling supervision. *Journal of Creativity in Mental Health, 16*(2), 244–257. https://doi.org/10.1080/15401383.2020.1754989

Wahbeh, H., Lu, M., & Oken, B. (2011). Mindful awareness and non-judging in relation to posttraumatic stress disorder symptoms. *Mindfulness, 2,* 219–227. https://doi:10.1007/s12671-011-0064-3

Wakelin, K. E., Perman, G., & Simonds, L. M. (2023). Feasibility and efficacy of an online compassion-focused imagery intervention for veterinarian self-reassurance, self-criticism and perfectionism. *Veterinary Record, 192*(2), 1–17. https://doi.org/10.1002/vetr.2177

Zubala, A., Kennell, N., & Hackett, S. (2021). Art therapy in the digital world: An integrative review of current practice and future directions. *Frontiers in Psychology, 12,* 595536, 1–20. https://doi.org/10.3389/fpsyg.2021.600070

Appendices

Appendix A

Self-Assessment Scale

STS Domain Scale (STS-DS)

By estimating your levels of secondary traumatic stress (STS) before and after engaging with this resource guide, you can evaluate its effectiveness. Moreover, periodically assessing your levels of STS as you incorporate the practices into your routine can allow you to track and monitor your ongoing progress.[1]

The *STS Domain Scale* (STS-DS) DSM-5-TR version (see Table A1) is adapted from the *STS Scale* (STSS) DSM-5 version (Bride, 2013) and includes 20 items.[2] These items reflect the experiences of practitioners who have been negatively impacted by their work with survivors of trauma. Consider STS reactions that you have encountered in the past month, and indicate how frequently each of the STS-DS items resonates with your own experiences on a scale from 1 to 5 (1 = *never* to 5 = *very often*).

Note that in the scale, the term *client* is used to indicate a person with whom you have been engaged in a helping relationship. You may substitute another word that better represents your work, such as consumer, patient, recipient, or student. Also, the phrasing "client sessions" in item 11 may be adjusted to "interactions with clients" to expand the measure's applicability to a broader range of helping professionals.

Table A1. STS Domain Scale (STS-DS)

In the past month I have found that. . .					
Traumatic Stress Reactions	**Never**	**Rarely**	**Occasionally**	**Often**	**Very Often**
Intrusion Reactions					
1. My heart starts pounding when I think about my work with clients	1	2	3	4	5
2. It seems as if I am reliving the trauma(s) experienced by my client(s)	1	2	3	4	5
3. Reminders of my work with clients upset me	1	2	3	4	5
4. I think about my work with clients when I do not intend to	1	2	3	4	5
5. I have disturbing dreams about my work with clients	1	2	3	4	5
Domain Score:	_____				
Avoidance Reactions					
6. I avoid people, places, or things that remind me of my work with clients	1	2	3	4	5
7. I want to avoid working with some clients	1	2	3	4	5
Domain Score:	_____				

(Continued)

Table A1. (Continued)

In the past month I have found that. . .					
Traumatic Stress Reactions	**Never**	**Rarely**	**Occasionally**	**Often**	**Very Often**
Negative Cognition and Mood Reactions					
8. I feel emotionally numb	1	2	3	4	5
9. I have little interest in being around others	1	2	3	4	5
10. I am less active than usual	1	2	3	4	5
11. I notice gaps in my memory about client sessions	1	2	3	4	5
12. I experience negative emotions	1	2	3	4	5
13. I unrealistically blame others for the cause or consequences of the trauma(s) experienced by my client(s)	1	2	3	4	5
14. I have negative expectations about myself, others, or the world	1	2	3	4	5
Domain Score:	_____				
Hyperarousal and Reactivity Reactions					
15. I have trouble sleeping	1	2	3	4	5
16. I feel jumpy	1	2	3	4	5
17. I have trouble concentrating	1	2	3	4	5

(*Continued*)

Table A1. (Continued)

In the past month I have found that. . .						
Traumatic Stress Reactions		**Never**	**Rarely**	**Occasionally**	**Often**	**Very Often**
18.	I am easily annoyed	1	2	3	4	5
19.	I expect something bad to happen	1	2	3	4	5
20.	I engage in reckless or self-destructive behavior	1	2	3	4	5
Domain Score:		_____				
Total Score		_____				

STS-DS Scoresheet and Scoring Guide

Table A2 provides space to record your STS-DS domain and total scores. Elevated scores correspond to higher levels of STS, with total STS scores ranging from 20 to 100.[3] Domain and total STS scores within the lower ranges indicate enhanced wellbeing. Additionally, space is provided to record your STS and functional impairment levels (B. E. Bride, personal communication, November 30, 2023; Sprang et al., 2022). Notably, regarding STS levels, a clinical cutoff of 39 may be used to differentiate between practitioners who are experiencing clinically significant levels of STS (and may need clinical intervention) and those who are not.

Table A2. STS-DS Scoresheet

Assessment Date: _____

Domain Scores

Domain	Score
Domain 1: Intrusion	
Domain 2: Avoidance	
Domain 3: Negative Cognitions and Mood	
Domain 4: Hyperarousal and Reactivity	

Summary

Metric	Value
Total Score	
STS Level	
Functional Impairment Level	

Instructions

1. **Date**: Enter the date of the assessment.
2. **Domain Scores**: Enter the scores for each domain by summing the items within each domain.
3. **Total Score**: Sum all the domain scores to get the total score.
4. **STS Level**: Use the following ranges to determine the STS level:
   30 and below = Little/No STS
   31–38 = Mild STS
   39–47 = Moderate STS
   48–51 = High STS
   52+ = Severe STS
5. **Functional Impairment Level**: Record the overall level of functional impairment as one of the following categories: None, Mild, Moderate, Severe, or Extreme
6. **Multiple Assessments:** To track multiple assessments over time, replicate these instructions for each new date.

Appendix B

"Compassion for STS" (CSTS) Partner Practice

Helping professionals have the opportunity to regularly engage with the practices presented in this resource guide alongside a trusted colleague. Peer support sessions can be scheduled at a frequency that works best for both individuals, such as weekly, biweekly, monthly, or any other mutually agreed-upon interval. Particularly, these sessions can be conducted in person or through an online platform (with the necessary modifications), with the duration of each session tailored to accommodate the comfort and availability of both colleagues.

In each session, a particular compassion-based practice can take center stage. For enhanced exploration and integration of the benefits of each practice, it is likewise possible to focus on the same practice for more than one session. During sessions, colleagues are encouraged to direct their focus toward challenges tied to secondary traumatic stress (STS). It is important, however, to select challenges that are manageable within the peer-support framework. The sessions then culminate in a reflective debrief, where colleagues can share their experiences in a supportive, nonjudgmental environment, acknowledging any challenges faced constructively and noting valuable insights.

Additional recommendations follow: (a) it is advisable for partners to schedule several sessions in advance, ensuring that they have a consistent and regular meeting schedule, (b) if there is a need to reschedule a session, partners should try their best to notify each other in advance, allowing for ample time to adjust their plans accordingly, (c) starting and ending sessions on time is advised to maximize the efficiency of the peer support system and demonstrate respect for each other's time and commitment, and (d) if at any point, either partner feels the need to end the session or peer-support partnership, their wishes should be honored. Finally, (e) it is preferable that partners recognize that unexpected circumstances may arise that require adjustments to the schedule or session duration. Practicing understanding and flexibility is, therefore, recommended when accommodating such changes while still maintaining a commitment to regular partner meetings.

In cultivating a trauma-informed, person-centered, strengths focused, and appreciative atmosphere (see the section on "Guidance for Group Leaders" for added information on appreciative feedback), partners can promote compassionate handling of STS-related challenges, ensuring accountability toward each other's wellbeing. Significantly, it is important to identify STS-related issues that may require extra attention and support. Indeed, the idea is for partners to understand their role as supporting peers and to be ready to recommend professional assistance if necessary.

bluebirds and blue skies,
a gentle ray of sunshine –
embracing the gold

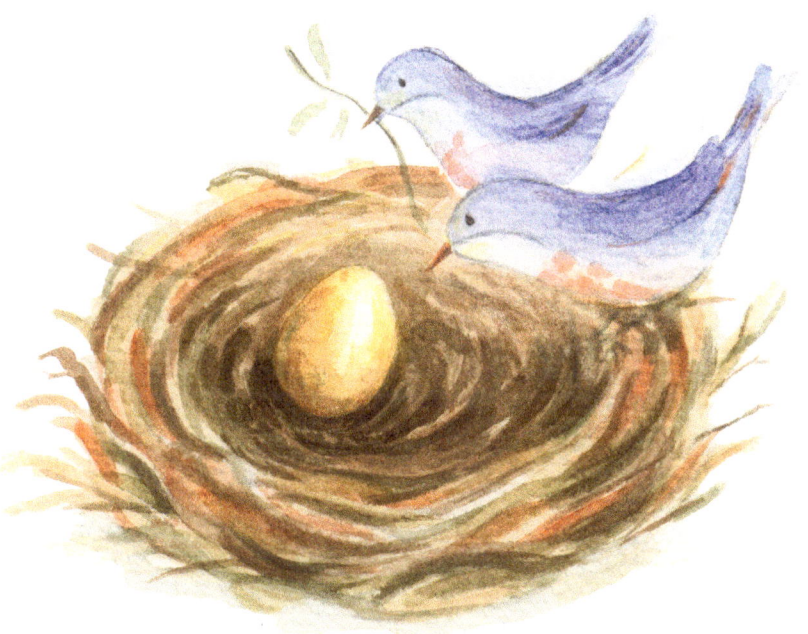

Nurturing Nest

Two birds in a nest with a golden egg

Appendix C

Guide to Sanskrit Pronunciation

The principle applied throughout this resource guide is the use of italics for all Sanskrit words and titles of texts, but not proper names. Capital letters are used for proper names, titles of texts, and for any Sanskrit word found at the beginning of a sentence. Certain words that have gained widespread recognition in the English language, such as "mantra," are left unitalicized. This excludes the word "yoga" in the compound "*yoga-nidrā*" which is italicized since it is part of a larger term.

Also, while most compound words in Sanskrit have been hyphenated for the sake of readability, the decision to split a compound or not was not always straightforward. For instance, "*bodhicitta*" and "*bodhisattva*" are technically compounds, yet since they are well-known and widely recognized Sanskrit compounds, they have been left unhyphenated. Notably, the decision regarding hyphenation can vary and, in some publications, hyphens may still be used to maintain consistency or to emphasize the compound nature of these two terms.

Furthermore, since Sanskrit has more than 26 letters, writing Sanskrit using the English alphabet necessitates the use of diacritical marks. Regarding the pronunciation of these marks, the following basic instructions will help you correctly pronounce the Sanskrit words included in this resource. For the purposes of this guide, all other letters can be pronounced similarly to how they are pronounced in English:

- Vowels appear in two forms, short and long. The short vowels do not have a diacritical mark and can be pronounced similarly to how they are pronounced in English.
- A diacritical dash over a vowel (e.g., ā, ī, and ū) makes it sound twice as long as a short vowel. Also, the letters ī and ū are pronounced, respectively, like the "ee" in beet and the "oo" in moon.
- The Sanskrit vowels "ai" and "au" are respectively pronounced like the "ai" in aisle and the "ow" in vow and are pronounced as long-sounding vowels.
- The vowels "e" and "o" are likewise considered long-sounding vowels.
- c is pronounced like "ch."
- The letter ḥ indicates that the preceding vowel should be pronounced with an aspiration, which involves producing a sound similar to "h" followed by a subtle prolongation of the vowel's echo.
- ñ is pronounced like the "n" in new and is formed by touching the middle of the tongue against the roof of the mouth.
- ṅ appears almost exclusively before the letters "g" or "k" and is, therefore, the nasal sound that is most naturally pronounced before these consonants. As such, the Sanskrit ṅg and ṅk correspond to the English "ng" and "nk," respectively, in words like "bang" and "bank."

- ṁ is a nasal sound that changes (for ease of pronunciation) depending on the immediately following consonant. For example, the ṁ sounds like ñ before c, ṅ before k, and n before t. As this is a bit complex, for general purposes, ṁ can be pronounced as the "n" or "m" sounds in English.
- ś is pronounced like "sh."
- v may be similar to "v" in English when it is at the start of a word or between vowels, but it is pronounced like "w" when it is combined with another consonant.
- When there is a dot beneath a letter (e.g., ṣ, ṇ, ḍ, and ṭ), this indicates that it is a "cerebral" letter. Imagine a dot on the roof of your mouth that you need to touch with the tip of your tongue when pronouncing these letters.
- The consonant "r" is always pronounced with the tip of the tongue touching the roof of the mouth.
- Double consonants (e.g., nn) are pronounced long.
- Aspirated consonants (kh, gh, ch, jh, ṭh, ḍh, th, dh, ph, and bh) are pronounced with a breath-pulse.

While pronouncing Sanskrit terms correctly can seem like a linguistic yoga challenge, it is hoped that their inclusion enhances your reading experience and adds depth to the concepts and ideas explored herein. For consistency, terms in additional languages (e.g., Japanese, Tibetan, and Pāli) are likewise italicized, aligning with the same guidelines. An exception is the Japanese term *haiku*, which, much like the Sanskrit term *mantra*, has achieved widespread recognition in the English language. Lastly, note that the English translations of the Sanskrit terms included in this resource guide are based primarily on the Monier-Williams Sanskrit-English Dictionary.

Appendix D

Practice Orientations

Table A3 lists all personal practices categorized by orientation type, with each orientation's list following the order of the table of contents. While these practices are designed for personal use, they can also be practiced individually within a group setting. Notably, personal practices based on a self- to self-orientation are followed by group practices that expand their orientation to encompass others.

Table A3. Personal Practices Categorized by Orientation

Page	Name of Practice	Orientation Type
70	Seeking REFUGE	Other-to-Self
89	*Lighting the Candle of Compassion	
73	Surfing the Waves	Self-to-Self
75	Finding Equilibrium	
92	Extending a Helping Hand	
101	Transforming Technique	
107	Turning Toward vs. Away	
112	Embodying a Path to Compassion	
120	Identifying Compassionate Words	
123	Letting the Words Sink in	
125	Journaling Journey	
127	Externalizing STS	
130	Composing a Haiku	
134	Preparing a Playlist	
139	Practicing Tonglen	
152	Discovering an Oasis	

(Continued)

Table A3. (Continued)

Page	Name of Practice	Orientation Type
182	Rising Strengths	
188	Nurturing CARE	
147	Realizing Similarities	Self-to-Other
158	Building a Toolkit	
174	Giving Gratitude	
176	Passing Compassion Forward	
77	Grounding Connections	Self-and-Other
81	Recollecting Positivity	
89	*Lighting the Candle of Compassion	
95	Strengthening Inner Resolve	
99	Reciting a Mantra	
104	Inspiring Rituals	
110	Healing Hands	
115	Breathing Compassion	
117	Flowing RIVER	
142	Cultivating KINTSUGI	
155	Planning a Vision Board	
161	Asking SMARTEST	
171	Envisioning a Mission	
184	Evaluating VPTG	

(Continued)

Table A3. (Continued)

Page	Name of Practice	Orientation Type
186	Embracing the Path	
191	Expanding the Circle	
165	Witnessing Compassion Flow	Other-to-Other
137	Noticing vs. Overlooking	Various Orientations
168	Advancing Multilevel Thinking	

Note. The practice marked with an asterisk is associated with more than one orientation type.

Appendix E

Practice Types

Table A4 lists all personal practices categorized by type, with each type's list following the order of the table of contents. While these practices are designed for personal use, they can also be practiced individually within a group setting. Notably, group practices may expand the focus of the personal practices to include additional practice types.

Table A4. Personal Practices Categorized by Type

Page	Name of Practice	Practice Type
75	Finding Equilibrium	Visualization and Breath Awareness
139	*Practicing Tonglen	
115	*Breathing Compassion	
77	*Grounding Connections	Creative Expressions (Journaling/Creative Writing/ Poetry, Movement, Music, Role-Playing, Visual Arts)
92	*Extending a Helping Hand	
107	Turning Toward vs. Away	
112	Embodying a Path to Compassion	
120	*Identifying Compassionate Words	
123	Letting the Words Sink in	
125	Journaling Journey	
130	Composing a Haiku	
134	Preparing a Playlist	
155	Planning a Vision Board	

(Continued)

Table A4. (Continued)

Page	Name of Practice	Practice Type
165	*Witnessing Compassion Flow	
171	*Envisioning a Mission	
73	Surfing the Waves	Guided Meditations
77	*Grounding Connections	
89	Lighting the Candle of Compassion	
92	*Extending a Helping Hand	
95	Strengthening Inner Resolve	
101	Transforming Technique	
110	Healing Hands	
115	*Breathing Compassion	
139	*Practicing Tonglen	
142	*Cultivating KINTSUGI	
152	Discovering an Oasis	
174	Giving Gratitude	
188	Nurturing CARE	
191	Expanding the Circle	
70	Seeking REFUGE	Reflection Prompts
81	Recollecting Positivity	
99	Reciting a Mantra	
104	Inspiring Rituals	

(Continued)

Table A4. (Continued)

Page	Name of Practice	Practice Type
117	Flowing RIVER	
120	*Identifying Compassionate Words	
127	Externalizing STS	
137	Noticing vs. Overlooking	
142	*Cultivating KINTSUGI	
147	Realizing Similarities	
158	Building a Toolkit	
161	Asking SMARTEST	
165	*Witnessing Compassion Flow	
168	Advancing Multilevel Thinking	
171	*Envisioning a Mission	
176	Passing Compassion Forward	
182	Rising Strengths	
184	Evaluating VPTG	
186	Embracing the Path	

Note. Practices marked with an asterisk are associated with more than one practice type.

Practices That Include Creative Expression

Tables A5 and A6 list all personal practices comprising creative expression, with each type's list following the order of the table of contents. While the practices listed in Table A5 are designed for personal use, they can also be practiced individually within a group setting. Notably, the "movement" category in Tables A5 and A6 comprises expressive movement practices as well as stationary practices such as yoga and symbolic hand gestures (Skt. *mudrā*).

Table A5. Personal Practices That Include Creative Expression

Page	Name of Practice	Specific Type of Creative Expression
107	Turning Toward vs. Away	Journaling/Poetry
112	*Embodying a Path to Compassion	
120	*Identifying Compassionate Words	
123	Letting the Words Sink in	
125	Journaling Journey	
130	Composing a Haiku	
165	*Witnessing Compassion Flow	
171	Envisioning a Mission	
77	Grounding Connections	Movement
92	Extending a Helping Hand	
112	*Embodying a Path to Compassion	
165	*Witnessing Compassion Flow	
120	*Identifying Compassionate Words	Music
134	Preparing a Playlist	
155	Planning a Vision Board	Visual arts
165	*Witnessing Compassion Flow	

Note. Practices marked with an asterisk are associated with more than one type of creative expression.

Table A6. Group Practices That Include Additional Types of
　　　　　 Creative Expression

Page	Name of Practice	Specific Type of Creative Expression
99	Reciting a Mantra	Creative writing/Journaling
70	Seeking REFUGE	Movement
77	*Grounding Connections	
110	Healing Hands	
152	Discovering an Oasis	
120	Identifying Compassionate Words	Role-playing
158	Building a Toolkit	
77	*Grounding Connections	Visual Arts
92	Extending a Helping Hand	
112	Embodying a Path to Compassion	
117	Flowing RIVER	
127	Externalizing STS	
142	Cultivating KINTSUGI	
176	Passing Compassion Forward	
188	Nurturing CARE	

Note. The group practices not listed here include either the same types of creative expression as their associated personal practices or do not include the creative arts.

Appendix F

Practicing Online

Although the group context practices offered in this resource guide are designed for implementation in face-to-face settings, the majority of the activities are adaptable for virtual settings. Online training sessions may be synchronous or asynchronous. Synchronous training is conducted at scheduled times and includes real-time interactions.[4] By contrast, asynchronous training enables participants to access training materials at their convenience, without real-time interactions (e.g., common methods used in asynchronous training include recorded lectures, video demonstrations, and discussion forums; Amiti, 2020).

Alternatively, blended or hybrid training programs combine the advantages of face-to-face participation with the benefits of synchronous and/or asynchronous online formats (e.g., McCutcheon et al., 2018). Such programs offer a balanced learning experience that can leverage the strengths of both online and in-person elements, providing participants with diverse opportunities for engagement and skill development. Significantly, synchronous, asynchronous, and blended/hybrid learning methods are continuously evolving, encouraging facilitators to harness innovative technology for improved teaching and learning (e.g., Singh et al., 2021).

Advantages and Challenges of Practicing Online

Online training programs offer numerous advantages. For instance, they save time, as participants can access the training sessions from the comfort of their own homes or offices, eliminating the need for commuting. This contributes to cost-effectiveness as well as to larger-scale access since individuals from different geographical locations can participate. Moreover, online platforms provide opportunities to learn from experts worldwide, fostering a global learning community and expanding cross-cultural networking possibilities. Importantly, online training programs benefit various groups, including individuals with disabilities, by offering accessible and adaptable learning options (Abdullah, 2021; Clark & Haddock, 2015).

However, online training is not without its challenges. One concern is the varying technological proficiency of participants, which can affect their overall experience of engaging with the training. This includes internet connectivity or other hardware/software technical challenges that may disrupt online sessions. Furthermore, online sessions may lack privacy, as there is a possibility of interruptions from family members, housemates, or peers/colleagues. Yet another challenge is the absence of visual cues for monitoring nonverbal communication, which can hinder the understanding of participants' reactions during sessions (Clark & Haddock, 2015; Mallen et al., 2005).

Additional challenges and advantages relate specifically to online training that incorporates the creative arts, which are relevant to the current training program. Among such challenges is the responsibility placed on participants to provide their own visual arts materials (Villarreal-Davis et al., 2021). Baker et al. (2016) and Cutcher and Cook (2016) also expressed concerns that online platforms most likely would not be able to fully replicate the rich, hands-on artistic experiences provided by face-to-face settings.

Conversely, potential advantages include the use of online technology, which may be incorporated to enhance creative expression. Examples are visual art making using digital tools and journaling via a web-based personal diary (Korman-Hacohen et al., 2022; Zubala et al., 2021). In addition, Garcia-Medrano (2021) intriguingly emphasized that virtual spaces may potentially provide an environment wherein group members can explore their embodied experiences, heighten their body awareness, and even cultivate embodied empathy through dance/movement.

Online Training Programs

Online synchronous compassion and/or mindfulness-based training programs have been demonstrated to be effective in various studies. For example, Knox and Franco (2023), Villalón and colleagues (2023), and MacDonald and Neville (2023) reported significant participant wellbeing improvements, with Villalón and colleagues underlining the importance of combining online training with organizational support. Moreover, in their 2023 review, Selič-Zupančič and colleagues confirmed the effectiveness of online psychological interventions incorporating mindfulness practices for professionals and underscored the indirect, positive influence that online interventions can have on patient care.

Asynchronous training programs focusing on compassion have likewise been found to be effective. Finlay-Jones et al. (2017) demonstrated the positive impact of an online self-compassion training course. They noted increased levels of self-compassion and happiness as well as reduced levels of perceived stress and emotional regulation difficulties. Furthermore, Wakelin et al. (2023) examined an asynchronous compassion-based intervention that demonstrated impressive retention, engagement, and promising signs of effectiveness. Lastly, Cieslak et al. (2016) carried out an online intervention for human services professionals and found that professionals who reported increased levels of self-efficacy demonstrated lower STS and higher vicarious posttraumatic growth (VPTG) at the 2-month follow-up point.

Appendix G

"Practicing the Pause" Guidelines

The following recommendations are relevant for group facilitators wishing to help guide group members out of habitual and conditioned ways of interacting and reacting, which may not align with their highest potential. Significantly, these recommendations are also relevant for group members themselves interested in contributing to supportive interpersonal interactions within group settings as well as for helping professionals in general wishing to contribute to positive interactions, including within their teams and organizations.[5]

For your convenience, these recommendations, not listed by significance or recommended order, are presented under two subtitles: "Breathing in pause-itivity" and "Breathing out pause-itivity" – in line with more inward- vs. outward-oriented recommendations, respectively (i.e., the term *pause-itivity* is a fusion of "pause" and "positivity").

Breathing in Pause-itivity

1. Take a moment to quietly form a compassionate intention before speaking. Throughout the conversation, revisit your intention and allow it to positively impact your contribution.
2. Pause to reflect if what you are about to say is: true, helpful, kind, and timely while recognizing that your perception of what constitutes truth, helpfulness, kindness, and timeliness may be a reflection of your subjective perspective.
3. Communicate at a pace that enables you to be present, pausing to reconnect with an anchoring point such as your breath.
4. If you begin to feel overwhelmed in the presence of others, take a moment to consider your body as a container mindfully. This perspective can be valuable, as it allows you to see overwhelming sensations, thoughts, and emotions as being held within the embrace of your physical being.
5. If you become triggered, pause to recognize that in the absence of external triggers, you might not become fully aware of any ingrained, unhelpful tendencies you may have, making it more challenging to reshape them positively.
6. Reduce emotional reactivity by pausing to remind yourself of your interconnectedness with others, even if their views differ from your own.
7. In your interactions, take time to reflect on the differences between objective and subjective value judgments regarding your observations.[6]
8. Try to be like a clear mirror when reflecting back on what others say or do.[7] This may call for suspending/setting aside/bracketing your own

internal dialogue, which includes your own narratives, judgments, agenda, and advice.

9. When you are offered appreciation by others, pause before responding to consider the significance of viewing yourself as a conduit for positivity in their lives. By reframing your achievements in this way, you pay tribute to the benevolence of others who have contributed to your growth and development.

10. Notice when your mind has wandered away from interactions. When you realize your mind has drifted, pause to re-center yourself and re-engage with the interaction at hand.

11. Take as much time as necessary to consider your responses. Giving yourself time to respond demonstrates that the conversation is important to you and that you want to give it the consideration it merits.

12. The art of pausing can help you remain centered, introspective, calm, and collected instead of impulsively reactive to others. If you find yourself overwhelmed, you can politely request to disengage temporarily.

Breathing out Pause-itivity

1. Look for the good in others and explore "the best of what is," taking the time to identify others' strengths, contributions, and areas of excellence as well as how these can be leveraged.

2. Recognize individuals as experts in their own experiences. This implies investing time to understand how experiences are perceived by them, even if their opinions are different from your own.

3. Pause to perceive what others need most and what is most essential for them. This includes listening to what they are saying not only with words but through their nonverbal communication (e.g., body language, facial expressions, and tone of voice).

4. When you notice indicators of dysregulation in others, such as rapid or shallow breathing, avoidance of eye contact, and shifts in vocal tone (e.g., a quiver in their voice), dedicate time to help support co-regulation.[8]

5. When individuals share challenging experiences, try to resist the urge to provide solutions immediately and instead help guide them toward arriving at their own insights on how to navigate these challenges.

6. Before offering others advice or problem-solving, wait and check in with them to see if they are open to that. Be receptive and respectful of their wishes.

7. Be curious and ask questions aimed at finding out what matters to others and how they feel about their own experiences. After they respond, pause to allow their perspectives to sink in, setting aside your own judgments.

8. Pause or slow down your speech to allow space for others to reflect on what you are sharing. Holding silence can allow time for thoughtful contributions.

9. Take the time to notice, explicitly say, and celebrate what others do well, empowering them and genuinely rejoicing in their successes.

10. Create space in your schedule to ensure that you follow up with others and remain engaged in ongoing conversations.

11. Create space within yourself to hear about others' perspectives and refrain from interrupting when they are speaking.

12. Practice listening generously to others with your undivided attention, much like you would do when watching a sunrise. Just as the sun is fully revealed only after it has risen, so too, a person's complete narrative unfolds when they have finished speaking.

dawn whispers softly:
generous listening is …
watching a sunrise

Hidden Gems (Endnotes)

Preface

1 Following ethical guidelines, subtle changes were made in this description to safeguard my clients' confidentiality and anonymity.
2 The verb *addressing*, as applied to STS, encompasses a wide range of actions, including, but not limited to: coping, mitigating, minimizing, navigating, and overcoming.
3 The concept *beginner's mind* originates from the Buddhist term *shoshin* in Japanese, and "encapsulates the magic of a first-time experience" even in familiar situations (Unkule, 2019, p. 128).

Part I

1 Establishing pure-hearted motivation (Sanskrit; Skt. *śubhāśaya*) signifies affirming the intention to engage with this resource guide with the overarching aspiration of helping others.
2 Driven by the compassionate wish to alleviate suffering, "passion" in this context refers to the concept of *wise passion*. This involves cultivating equanimity with how things are while remaining dedicated to and inspired by how things could be.

Section I

1 The term *trauma* is often used interchangeably to describe: (a) an actual traumatic event, (b) the immediate aftermath of a traumatic event, or (c) the lasting effects/outcomes that follow a traumatic event (Briere & Scott, 2006).

2 An event may be experienced as traumatic "when too much that is too upsetting and too unexpected is experienced too quickly" (Fernando, 2018, p. 37).

3 The term *client* is used to indicate a person with whom you are engaged in a helping relationship. You may substitute another word that better represents your work such as patient, recipient, consumer, or student.

4 Distinguishing between symptoms caused by direct and indirect trauma exposure is a methodological challenge in this field (Sprang & Steckler, 2022).

5 The definitions offered here differ from acute vs. chronic trauma (i.e., wounds) in the field of medicine (Zhou et al., 2022).

6 Scott et al. (2023) further described how these 11 categories relate to the concept of *trauma-informed social media*.

7 The term *interpersonal trauma* refers to traumatic experiences that occur as a result of interactions with others, whereas the term *intrapersonal trauma* involves trauma stemming from internal struggles (e.g., a life-threatening illness; Kira et al., 2022).

8 Relatedly, the term *transgenerational trauma* refers to the effects that traumatic experiences may have not only on those who directly experienced them but also on their children or subsequent generations (Krippner & Barrett, 2019).

9 The PTSD diagnostic criteria presented here are relevant for adults, adolescents, and children older than 6 (e.g., Scheeringa, 2022).

10 Adopting a Buddhist perspective, the focus may transition from labeling cognitions and mood as negative vs. positive to assessing their impact on one's actions in the world, considering them as either unskillful or skillful, respectively (Khong, 2009).

11 In line with DSM-5-TR guidelines, criteria B, C, D, and E have varying prerequisites concerning the number of symptoms necessary to meet each criterion. Specifically, Criteria B and C each require one or more symptoms, whereas criteria D and E each require two or more symptoms (APA, 2022).

12 There is an ongoing debate in the scholarly literature regarding the need to demarcate normal stressors from trauma. This is because viewing trauma as a broad continuum may pathologize normal stressors and pose challenges when operationalizing the term *trauma* for research and clinical practice (Haslam, 2016; Jackson & Haslam, 2022).

13 The term *implicit memory*, in the context of trauma, refers to unconscious memories of sensory experiences associated with the traumatic event. When such memories are not consciously accessible, the individual may not be aware of their influence on sensations, thoughts, emotions, and/or behaviors. This may result in emotional dysregulation and distress triggered by sensory cues that implicitly remind the individual of the traumatic experience (van der Kolk, 2014).

14 The topic of trigger warnings, as a trauma-specific practice, has sparked considerable debate. For example, a study by Jones et al. (2020) did not find evidence that trigger warnings were helpful for individuals who reported a PTSD diagnosis or for those qualified for a likely diagnosis of PTSD. These researchers found evidence that trigger warnings may, counterproductively, reinforce survivors' perception of trauma as a dominant and detrimental aspect of their identity.

15 *Resilience* has been described as the ability to "bounce back" following adversity to pretrauma levels of functioning (e.g., Manyena et al., 2011). Relatedly,

the term *compassion resilience* denotes "the ability to maintain one's physical, emotional, and mental wellbeing, while responding compassionately to people who are suffering" (Compassion Resilience Toolkit, n.d., para. 5).

16 The sequential phases leading up to an organization being considered *trauma informed* have been described as: (a) *trauma aware*, (b) *trauma sensitive*, and (c) *trauma responsive* (Missouri Department of Mental Health, 2014; Trauma-Informed Oregon, 2018).

17 Purkey et al. (2018, p. 170) added a fundamental initial step to SAMHSA's (2014) six principles by including "trauma awareness and acknowledgment" as a necessary first step. Note also that Malchiodi (2022) outlined trauma-informed core principles specifically tailored for expressive arts therapies. These are relevant, given that this resource guide includes practices that incorporate creative art techniques.

18 As far as clients are concerned, trauma-informed care begins with clients' or clients' family members' first point of contact within the caregiving setting (e.g., a receptionist). The following quote exemplifies this notion: "One does not have to be a therapist to be therapeutic" (Ford & Wilson, 2012, as cited in SAMHSA, 2014, p. 11).

19 Alternatively, the organization has an effective referral system in place to help individuals connect with needed trauma screenings, assessments, and/or interventions (SAMHSA, 2014).

20 Stress responses are not necessarily mutually exclusive, and individuals may react with a combination of strategies in response to different types of perceived threats or stressors.

21 "Bottom-up processing refers to the acquisition of and attention to the more automatic, sensory, and contextual characteristics of incoming stimuli, whereas top-down processing describes the more volitional, regulatory, and knowledge-driven mechanisms involved in the enhancement of neural processing of such information" (Stevens & Benjamin, 2018, p. 71).

22 *Feign* is an example of a stress response that engages higher-order thinking by initiating purposeful actions focused on self-preservation. These actions, which can include negotiation and improvisation, are designed to avoid harm and to keep safe (Malchiodi, 2021).

23 The term *mindfulness* is not only a theoretical construct. It encompasses the ongoing practice of cultivating mindfulness and the embodied psychological process of being mindful (Germer, 2005).

24 For further reading on the terms *wisdom* and *compassion,* see Sections III and IV.

25 The polyvagal theory, introduced by Porges (1995), has proposed a revolutionary way in which the body's responses to perceived threat can be understood. According to this theory, the vagus nerve comprises three branches that play crucial roles in regulating the body's "bottom-up" responses to perceived threats: (a) the dorsal vagal complex, (b) the sympathetic nervous system, and (c) the ventral vagal complex, also known as the social engagement system, associated with seeking assistance from others and characterized by connection. The latter-mentioned ventral vagal complex, which is the most evolutionarily sophisticated branch, becomes active during secure social interactions

(which include compassionate interactions), and has a calming effect on defensive responses (Porges, 2011).

26 Although *fight* also signifies facing perceived threat, it signifies doing so aggressively whereas *face* signifies facing perceived threat mindfully.

27 The term *posttraumatic orientation to bodily signals* has been suggested as a comprehensive concept that describes the inclination to interpret bodily sensations as catastrophic after experiencing a traumatic event (Tsur & Talmon, 2023).

28 Additional terms have likewise been used to describe the experience of positive psychological changes following adversity. These include such terms as *adversarial growth, stress-related growth, positive adaptation,* and *perceived benefits.* These terms are employed to encompass generally similar types of positive transformations, although different studies and measurements may highlight distinct aspects of growth concerning each term (Linley & Joseph, 2004).

29 Relevant questions that have been raised regarding PTG, include: (a) whether societal and cultural expectations or pressures for personal development and growth result in individuals feeling an obligation to discover positive aspects in traumatic situations, and (b) whether individuals actually experience personal growth after facing adversity, or alternatively, believe (or want others to believe) that they have grown (Maitlis, 2020). Relatedly, Ho and Cheng (2024) focused on the concept of *illusory growth* (i.e., inaccurate perceptions of PTG).

30 According to Halifax (2018), individuals who embody the purest form of altruism are not seeking validation or acknowledgment from society, nor are they motivated by a desire to enhance their self-esteem. Instead, their altruism symbolically mirrors what Hạnh (2008) figuratively described as the inherent, natural tendency of the right hand to assist the left hand when the latter is injured. Please also note that within this resource guide, the term *altruism* does not encompass what Bachner-Melman and Oakley (2016) described as "pathological altruism:" "The willingness of a person to irrationally place another's perceived needs above his or her own in a way that causes self-harm" (p. 92).

31 Alexander et al. (2021) offered insights on the related concept of *organizational PTG* following organizational trauma. "Organizational trauma can be understood as a particular type of event, one that is necessarily adverse, which can lead to growth if organizations respond effectively" (p. 37).

32 These elements draw inspiration from Tedeschi's (2020) "Five steps for coming out of a crisis stronger" framework, with original adaptations made to suit the specific context of this resource guide.

33 In line with Gross (1998), "emotion regulation . . . refers to attempts to influence which emotions one has, when one has them, and how one experiences or expresses these emotions" (p. 275).

Section II

1 Bride et al. (2023) presented an international expert consensus approach that centered on principles for best practice, designed to mitigate the occurrence and consequences of STS in behavioral health services.

2 While symptoms may persist over an extended period, their transient nature, in line with Buddhist thought, remains unchanged (e.g., Shonin et al., 2014).

3 Sprang et al. (2019) stated that STS may also have consequences beyond the typical symptoms associated with PTSD, such as experiencing moral distress, a decrease in professional self-efficacy, and feeling stigmatized. Gusler et al. (2023) further revealed that "current measures of STS may capture some but not all of the cognitive impacts of indirect trauma exposure" (p. 1).

4 Agapi (2021) stressed that "professionals are urged to avoid seeing clients as causing them harm, regardless of the emotional distress they experience as a result of listening to their stories" (p. 8).

5 Molnar and colleagues (2017) presented a review based primarily on comprehensive literature reviews and meta-analyses, focusing on the prevalence of STS among a wide range of helping professionals including health professionals, mental health professionals, and first responders.

6 Helping professionals should, however, be aware that anticipating such adverse effects may lead to unfavorable outcomes, given the intricate interplay between beliefs and subsequent experiences. For example, while referring to the related concept of *compassion fatigue*, Agapi (2021) described, "during the training I received before starting my job, I was warned of the capacity of my position to cause compassion fatigue. The whole training was built around the idea that one has to be very careful with their involvement with traumatized others. This is in contrast to the Buddhist approach with suffering others" (p. 14). Agapi further mentioned that "the training I received from my job contained repetitions of the idea that engaging with suffering others is harmful and dangerous. During my job, the reality I experienced was based on this belief: hearing stories of traumatic experiences, I experienced empathic overarousal, emotional distress, and physical depletion. The Buddhist mind training I engaged in ulteriorly spoke beautifully of engaging in compassion, and framed it as an opportunity for wellbeing" (p. 14–15).

7 When referring to risk factors associated with STS, it is important to differentiate between correlation and causation. In simpler terms, a risk factor does not necessarily mean that a helping professional will develop STS, it only indicates an increased likelihood of STS developing.

8 Trauma caseload volume, frequency, and ratio refer to the number of trauma cases that helping professionals deal with (volume), how often they encounter such cases (frequency), and the proportion of trauma cases to other types of cases (ratio). These factors can collectively contribute to the risk level associated with professionals' workload in terms of their exposure to trauma-related content. Furthermore, regarding helping professionals' subjective interpretations, Agapi (2021) provided an example: "I stopped thinking that external phenomena can objectively cause me emotional reactions. Instead of believing that listening to a client's story has the power to cause me feelings of discomfort, I started entertaining the idea that my own interpretation and specific focus of attention cause me discomfort" (p. 20).

9 The terms *emotional empathy* and *cognitive empathy* have been referred to as "heart and head" empathy, respectively (i.e., the capacity to resonate with vs. understand others' emotions; Giusti et al., 2021, p. 1).

10 Siegel (1999) introduced the *window of tolerance* framework which is a valuable tool for monitoring negative reactions that may arise following adversity,

including exposure to indirect trauma. In the context of STS, the window of tolerance symbolizes optimal ability to remain regulated when navigating the challenges associated with indirect exposure to trauma. Worth emphasizing is that each helping professional has their own window of tolerance and the specific coping strategies that best help them stay within, and preferably expand, its perimeters.

11 Implementing low-impact debriefing provides a secure way of seeking support from others while minimizing their exposure to traumatic information. As elaborated by Mathieu (2012), this approach comprises four sequential steps that pertain to the individual who is disclosing: (a) increasing self-awareness, (b) providing advance notice to others, (c) waiting for their consent, and (d) limiting disclosure.

12 The notion of an STS champion refers to an individual (or team) within the organization who is committed to fostering positive organizational change concerning STS (Sprang et al., 2023). See the subsection focusing on "Compassion Competence" for further information on workplace champions.

13 Additional terms associated with positive responses to working with individuals who have experienced trauma include: (a) *vicarious resilience* – identified as a parallel process of personal growth that helping professionals may experience as a result of witnessing their clients' resilience (Killian et al., 2017), and (b) *compassion satisfaction* – described as the fulfillment caregivers may derive from effectively helping the individuals in their care (Sacco & Copel, 2018; Stamm, 2010).

Section III

1 *Buddhism* refers to an extensive and multifaceted tradition stretching back more than 2,500 years, encompassing philosophical, psychological, spiritual, and religious aspects. It is also important to recognize that given the many schools of Buddhism, the term *Buddhisms* may be more applicable than *Buddhism* (Harvey, 2013).

2 Wallace (2001, p. 5) eloquently stated, "The cultivation of compassion is like a silken thread that runs through and connects all the pearls of Buddhist meditative practices."

3 See the subsection focusing on "Self-Compassion as Skillful Means" for further reading on the term *skillful means* within contemporary compassion trainings.

4 The term *saṃskāra-duḥkhatā* is a multifaceted term that highlights the inherent unsatisfactoriness that comes from the conditioned nature of existence. For example, deep-rooted mental habits and patterns from one's personal history that affect present and future experiences, often perpetuating cycles of suffering (e.g., Harris, 2014).

5 Recognizing interconnectedness can foster a deeper appreciation of compassion. As Epstein (2001, p. 33) noted, "If people realize that everything is relational, they begin to have compassion for others."

6 The following dialogue is an original translation of the Sanskrit text in the *Vimalakīrti-Nirdeśa-Sūtra* (Study Group on Buddhist Sanskrit Literature, 2006, chapter 4, para. 6–7).

7 The word *world* is a loose translation of the Sanskrit term *saṃsāra* or cyclic existence.

8 The term *great compassion* (Skt., *mahā-karuṇā*) refers to compassion for all sentient beings (Dunne & Manheim, 2023).

9 While taking empathy into account, it, therefore, seems that the compassion of *bodhisattvas* whose levels of emotional empathy hinder their ability to be fully compassionate can be described as sentimental, whereas the compassion of *bodhisattvas* whose levels of cognitive empathy serve as a protective factor can be termed *untainted*.

10 For general knowledge, from a Buddhist standpoint, compassion (Skt. *karuṇā*), is considered alongside the virtuous qualities of loving-kindness or friendliness (Skt. *maitrī*), equanimity or impartiality (Skt. *upekṣā*), and altruistic joy (Skt. *muditā*) – all being components of the *four immeasurables* (Skt. *brahma-vihāra*; Dalai Lama & Chodron, 2017; Kraus & Sears, 2009).

11 Consider the following metaphor for the term *interbeing* by Hạnh (2014). If you gaze deeply into a flower, you can see that within the flower, there is a cloud. Without the cloud, there is no rain, and without the rain, the flower cannot grow. Similarly, the sunlight and the earth are encompassed within the flower. Together, these elements weave the tapestry of the flower's existence and without them, the flower would not have come into being. "A flower can't be by herself alone. A flower can only inter-be with everything else" (Hạnh, 2014, p. 10).

12 Referring back to the concept of no-self (Skt. *anātman*), Gethin (1998) argued that the term *self* should not be entirely eliminated from Buddhist discourse. Gethin further stated that, in line with Buddhist thought, the problem arises not from the term *self* in and of itself, but from our interpretation of the term.

13 Regarding *other-to-self* and *other-to-other* "flows" of compassion, see the "Seeking Refuge" and "Witnessing Compassion Flow" practices, respectively.

14 Self-compassion may thereby be considered "a necessary inclusive step backwards, as it were, prior to enlarging and universalizing the circle of compassion" (Jinpa, 2013, as cited in Anālayo & Dhammadinnā, 2021, p. 1357). Importantly, however, the word "prior" does not imply practicing self-compassion as a stand-alone practice. Instead, this recommendation underscores that the ultimate aim is to universalize the practice of compassion.

15 Nonjudging entails adopting an impartial perspective, a manner of observing others without the influence of implicit biases or personal preferences. It encompasses the practice of acknowledging things "as they are," and refraining from categorizing them as positive or negative (e.g., right vs. wrong or good vs. bad; e.g., Wahbeh et al., 2011).

16 Nussbaum (2003) offered additional insights on judgmental interpretations associated with offering others compassion. These include: (a) *the judgment of seriousness* (i.e., evaluating the severity of the suffering), (b) *the judgment of nondesert* (i.e., assessing whether the suffering is undeserved), (c) *the judgment of shared vulnerabilities* (i.e., evaluating if one has similar vulnerabilities to the individual who is suffering), and (d) *the eudaimonistic judgment* (i.e., assessing whether the individual who is suffering is an important part of one's life).

17 On the other hand, Gilboa and Ben-Shetrit (2009) characterized the capacity for "being with" and "listening to" as "precompassion," suggesting that these

behaviors are foundational elements that precede the development of full compassion in interpersonal interactions. For general knowledge, these authors likewise introduced the term *passive compassion*, describing the capacity to accept behaviors in others that one may perceive as "irregular (e.g., awkward, strange, unconventional)" (p. 255). In Gilboa and Ben-Shetrit's study this was exemplified when children with special needs and those developing typically accepted each other's unique characteristic.

18 Ekman and Ekman (2017) described the related term *global compassion*, representing the overarching goal of alleviating suffering for one and all. Drigas and Papoutsi (2023) further complemented this idea by introducing the all-inclusive term *unity empathy-compassion-love* as the highest level of their pyramid model, culminating in universal love.

19 Sahdra et al. (2023) revealed that the relationship between self- and other-oriented compassion and wellbeing may be moderated by "self-other harmony." This signifies the degree to which an individual's self-compassion and compassion for others are congruent, meaning that an increase in one correlates with an increase in the other (p. 1997).

20 According to Neff (2022), self-compassion can be described as constituting a bipolar continuum that ranges from uncompassionate to compassionate self-responding. Essentially, as per Neff, by being more self-compassionate, individuals move along a continuum away from uncompassionate toward compassionate self-responding.

21 Regarding the term *fierce self-compassion*, Quaglia (2023) discussed the similar concept of *agentic self-compassion* (i.e., agentic relates to the concept of *agency*). In a related vein, Vavrichek (2012) offered perspectives on the term *compassionate assertiveness* which entails assertively expressing one's needs for both personal wellbeing and the wellbeing of others.

22 As cited in Anālayo (2017), a version of this Buddhist text is extant in the *Aṅguttara-Nikāya* as well as in Sanskrit fragments and in what seems to be an *Ekottarika-Āgama* extract.

23 Although Neff and Germer's (2018) mindful self-compassion training focuses specifically on self-compassion, Germer and Neff (2019, p. 12) emphasized that their training "was never meant to be a complete compassion training program." Moreover, they specified that "in our opinion, for compassion to be complete, it should be both inner and outer" (p. 12).

24 There is no specific instruction to direct compassion toward oneself in this meditative practice, as it is understood that those meditating are naturally included within the circle of compassion they offer others. Notably, however, from a Buddhist perspective, even this intrinsic benefit is intricately linked to an altruistic cause (Anālayo, 2019; Anālayo & Dhammadinnā, 2021).

25 Indeed, a square circle does not exist in familiar Euclidean Geometry. However, in Taxicab or Manhattan Geometry, wherein a circle is defined to be all the points that are the same distance away from a given center, a circle is equivalent to a square (e.g., Kemp & Vidakovic, 2023).

26 Similarly, in Vajrayāna Buddhism, "unconditional compassion radiates forth all-inclusively" without mention of *self-compassion* as a stand-alone concept (e.g., Makransky, 2012, p. 1). Note also that this resource does not offer an

in-depth exploration of the Theravāda, Mahāyāna, and Vajrayāna Buddhist traditions, nor does it explore the intricacies of additional Buddhist traditions whose concepts are interwoven throughout (e.g., Zen Buddhism). An in-depth description of these subjects is outside the intended scope of this guide.

27 Dunne and Manheim (2023) offer a related discussion of how, within the context of the contemporary highly individualistic milieu, self-compassion can be considered a skillful means. This perspective is based on the hypothetical assumption that in contemporary times, there is a greater preoccupation with narratives about the self when compared to earlier historical periods.

28 Simmer-Brown (2023) explored the connection between compassion and skillful means, specifically within the Indo-Tibetan Buddhist tradition, offering insights into the relation between compassion and effective action, particularly within the context of secular compassion-based training and research.

29 This also includes reducing the process of self-objectification which may be involved in the practice of self-compassion. As detailed further by Dunne and Manheim (2023), in this context, self-objectification involves treating oneself as an "other" to whom compassion is directed. The act of "othering" oneself, goes against the interconnected and non-dualistic understanding of oneself and others in Buddhist teachings.

30 The word "self" is enclosed in brackets to highlight the concept of no-self (Skt. *anātman*) in Buddhist philosophy. Within the framework of this resource guide, this multifaceted concept primarily promotes the cultivation of a sociocentric mindset, wherein persons (Skt. *pudgala*) recognize their interconnection with others (Samuel, 2015).

Section IV

1 Relatedly, Trzeciak et al. (2019) coined the term *compassionomics* to describe the intersection between compassion and economics.

2 "The capacity to intentionally cultivate compassion may serve as a skillful means to protect against empathy-based stress" (i.e., the term *skillful means* is broadly described as the variety of means that may be used to alleviate suffering in context-sensitive ways; e.g., Quaglia, 2023; Klimecki et al., 2014, as cited in Jennings & Min, 2023, p. 2311).

3 Lanaj et al. (2022) revealed that leaders who offered stakeholders assistance with personal matters were perceived as both more civil and more competent. Leader civility or competence was not linked, however, to leaders' task-related assistance, which, unlike personal support, may be seen as a standard expectation of leaders.

4 Relatedly, Williams and Allen (2015) focused on the term *posttraumatic leadership*. This means that individuals, motivated by their own traumatic experiences (which may include STS), assume leadership roles with the goal of reducing the likelihood of similar challenges reoccurring. Essentially, posttraumatic leadership refers to leaders who channel challenges into positive change.

5 The convergence of these behaviors aligns with the human resource development "soft-hard approach." This approach is consistent both with the human-centered development of employees and the performance-oriented necessities of organizations (Sambrook, 2012, as cited by Shuck et al., 2019).

6 While empathy entails the notion of stepping into someone's shoes, compassion extends beyond that and incorporates action. Building on this distinction, although both empathy and compassion are nouns, it may be more fitting to consider compassion as a verb since it implies compassionate action (e.g., Hạnh, 2006).

7 With respect to helping professionals, Kerig (2018, p. 616) described how professionals working in the juvenile justice system "commonly share feelings of being 'haunted' by the disturbing abuse histories revealed by the youth with whom they work and also by stories youth tell of extreme acts of violence they have perpetrated against others."

8 *Compassionate activism* underscores social action as a central force that can actively help pave the way to a more just and sustainable society (Garavan, 2012). "*Radical compassion* is rooted in mindful, embodied presence, and it is expressed actively through caring that includes all beings" (Brach, 2019, p. xix). Relatedly, the concept of *compassion spheres* extends to the broad-based endeavor of mitigating and relieving suffering, encompassing individuals, communities, societies, and the environment (Harris, 2023).

Part II

1 Reestablishing pure-hearted motivation, (Skt. *śubhāśaya*) signifies reaffirming the intention to engage with this resource guide with the overarching aspiration of helping others.

2 The term *passion* in this context refers to the concept of *wise passion*. This involves cultivating equanimity with how things are while remaining dedicated to and inspired by how things could be.

3 These recommendations draw inspiration from Strycharczyk et al.'s (2021) "Four Cs mental toughness" model, with original adaptations made to suit the specific context of this resource guide.

4 The reframing of a challenge into an opportunity for learning aligns with cognitive restructuring, a technique employed in emotional regulation, as elucidated by McHale (2022).

5 In a similar vein, practicing relevant practices while wrapped in a meditative shawl/scarf can be beneficial. Serving as more than a mere accessory, meditative shawls/scarves can envelop you in a sense of calmness and focus and serve as a cocoon of comfort, shielding you from unnecessary distractions.

6 The Tibetan name for the *bodhisattva* of compassion, Chenrézig (Skt. Avalokiteśvara), can be referred to as the one who looks upon all beings (with the eye of compassion). Accordingly, whether practicing with eyes open or closed, you are invited to channel the compassion that radiates from your practice, "softly and gently, through your eyes, so that your gaze becomes the very gaze of compassion itself, all-pervasive and oceanlike" (Rinpoche, 1992, p. 68).

7 The Buddhist concept of *bodhicitta* (i.e., *bodhi* means "awakening" while *citta* means "heart-mind" and "consciousness"), encapsulates not only a wise and compassionate intention but also the manifestation of wise and compassionate actions aimed at alleviating suffering and promoting wellbeing for all sentient beings (Śāntideva, n.d.).

8 This is an original translation from the *Bodhisattva-Caryā-Avatāra* by Śāntideva (late 7th to mid-8th century CE; Goodman, 2016). The title of this Sanskrit text signifies "Undertaking the way to awakening" or "Entering the (bodhisattva's) way to awakening" (Akira, 2024, para. 1; Śāntideva, n.d., p. xxx; Vaidya, 1960, chapter 3, verse 27, p. 43). See Appendix C for Sanskrit pronunciation guidelines.

Foundational Practices

1 Attachment theory is a psychological framework that explores the emotional bonds formed between individuals, and their impact on human development. *Attachment priming* is a related term that refers to a psychological phenomenon in which exposure to certain stimuli reactivates and influences an individual's attachment system (Condon & Makransky, 2020a, 2023).

2 This practice draws inspiration from Condon and Makransky's (2020a, 2020b) "Receptive mode" practice, with original adaptations made to suit the specific context of this resource guide.

3 A soft gaze can be characterized as a state of openness and receptivity to possibilities, as it implies a relaxed, open view that takes in everything without focusing on any one thing in particular.

4 Dupasquier et al. (2018) further found evidence that self-compassion training can effectively reduce the positive association between perceived risks of distress disclosure (i.e., disclosure of personally distressing information) and fear of receiving compassion. This suggests that engaging in self-compassion practices can help counterbalance the maladaptive relation between the perceived risk of disclosing STS and the fear of receiving compassion from others. In a related context, Gilbert et al. (2011) not only discussed the topic of fear of receiving compassion from others but also explored the topics of fear of affiliative emotions in general, fear of compassion for others, and fear of self-compassion.

5 Throughout this resource guide, practices that have a self-to-self orientation are intentionally interwoven throughout rather than grouped together. The aim is not to isolate them as stand-alone practices but to emphasize their association with additional "flows" of compassion.

6 In Sanskrit, *āna* means the incoming breath, while *apāna* means the outgoing breath. Combined with the word *smṛti,* which literally means "memory" or "calling to mind," and is commonly translated as "mindfulness," the full term *ānāpāna-smṛti* can signify "mindfulness of breathing" (e.g., Bhikkhu, 1980). Significantly, Goenka (1990) underscored that *smṛti* encompasses being mindful of one's bodily sensations; and Freese (2023) stated that the practice of *vipaśyanā* as taught by Goenka, "contains a robust somatic theory and practice that could be applied to recognizing and responding to trauma" (p. 463).

7 "Compassion is often seen as grounded in mindfulness: the capacity to sustain moment-by-moment focused awareness of – and openness to – one's internal experience and immediate environment, without judgment and with acceptance" (Briere, 2012, p. 267). Relevantly, Rand (2004) stated that practicing mindfulness enables helping professionals to recognize that their emotions

(including STS-related emotions) originate within their own bodies rather than being externally projected onto them by their clients.

8 A related metacognitive technique known as "urge surfing" (Bowen et al., 2021), can involve helping professionals applying mindfulness skills when they experience the urge to engage in unhelpful STS-related coping strategies. In line with this technique, such urges can be mindfully observed and considered rather than suppressed or reflexively acted upon, as they gradually increase in intensity, reach a peak, and eventually subside.

9 In this practice, as in most others in this resource guide, you are invited to breathe in and out through your nostrils, keeping your mouth gently closed (e.g., Allen, 2015).

10 Relatedly, Mitra and Greenberg (2016) highlighted a "path for contemplative practice that proceeds from mindfulness and self-compassion to the practice of cultivation of broader, generalized compassion with and for others" (p. 413).

11 This practice draws inspiration from Halifax's (2018) "Strong back, soft front" practice, with original adaptations made to suit the specific context of this resource guide.

12 Additional grounding ideas involve connecting with nature through the five senses. For example, consider hugging a tree, watching a sunrise, smelling a flower, listening to birds chirping, or savoring the taste of freshly picked fruit.

13 Yoga has been found to be effective in reducing occupational stress in healthcare workers. For example, based on a systematic review and meta-analysis of randomized controlled trials, Zhang et al. (2021) recommended that organizations consider implementing yoga into workplace wellness programs.

14 *Añjali-mudrā* is a hand gesture made by drawing the palms together in front of the heart, with fingers aligned vertically and thumbs pointed backward. It is used to enhance composure and a sense of harmony (Le Page & Le Page, 2013).

15 Following are a few more helpful tips for group members to take into consideration when practicing this yoga posture. Participants can be invited to: (a) focus their gaze in front of them on something stable to help keep their balance, (b) avoid pressing their raised foot into their knee (this means that they should place their raised foot either above or below the knee of their standing leg), (c) align their hips while holding the posture, (d) point the foot of their standing leg straight ahead, and the foot of their raised leg down toward the ground, (e) actively engage their core as this can provide increased steadiness (f) feel free to use a wall to help keep their balance, or leave their standing foot partially on the ground for balance, and (g) pay attention to all the micro-movements that the sole of their standing foot is making in order to help them maintain their balance.

16 To access detailed instructions for the multiple variations of the double tree posture, please search for instructions online. Also, given that this activity involves physical contact, participants' consent is necessary.

17 Recommended basic materials for preparing a "compassion pole" include a relatively large wooden post, paints, paintbrushes, and wood preservative. Alternatively, if preferred, a smaller wooden post can be used, with the "compassion pole" "planted" in a plant pot indoors.

18 In this context, the Sanskrit word *dharma* can be loosely translated to the "teaching" of the redwood tree.

19 Creating such a library of positive memories to revisit in challenging times can help create neural pathways that counterbalance the brain's innate negativity bias. Negativity bias describes the human tendency to assign greater importance to negative events in comparison to positive or neutral ones. This inclination stems from the evolutionary and neurological hard-wiring of our brains, which prioritize vigilance toward negative events for survival purposes (Norris, 2021).

Practices for Addressing Secondary Traumatic Stress (STS)

1 Aligned with Buddhist thought and in the context of secondary traumatic stress (STS), wisdom and compassion can be likened to two wings of a bird working in tandem to steer the wise and compassionate resolution of repercussions arising from indirect exposure to trauma (e.g., Siegel & Germer, 2012).

2 Senthil and Britto (2022) explained why *trāṭaka* is considered a cleansing technique, based on two classical Sanskrit scriptures – the *Gheraṇḍa-Saṃhitā* and the *Haṭha-Yoga-Pradīpikā*.

3 Make sure to follow safety precautions when practicing candlelight gazing. Alternatively, you may use a digital candle.

4 The term *third eye* refers to the area known as the *ājñā-cakra*, which symbolizes intuition and intellect and is metaphorically situated in the center of the forehead, approximately midway between the eyebrows (Singh, 2015).

5 Inviting group members to sit in a circle, which is relevant for additional group practices as well, is considered a trauma-informed recommendation since it promotes a sense of safety and inclusivity. This seating arrangement ensures that everyone is within each other's view, and can help participants feel more welcomed, connected, and supported (Spence, 2021).

6 This practice draws inspiration from Brach's (2019) "RAIN" practice, with original adaptations made to suit the specific context of this resource guide.

7 This self-reflection prompt is in line with Glennon et al. (2019) who referred to real-time self-care strategies as strategies that helping professionals can utilize while they are actively caregiving.

8 This practice draws inspiration from Neff and Germer's (2018) "Self-compassion break" practice, with original adaptations made to suit the specific context of this resource guide.

9 This practice draws inspiration from the ACT (2021) program, with original adaptations made to suit the specific context of this resource guide.

10 Within the limbic system, the amygdala plays a role in shaping our preferences and aversions, as well as in how our emotions guide our behaviors and influence the intensity of our memories (Ferry, 2017).

11 *Interoception*, the process of perceiving and monitoring somatic sensations, holds significant relevance in the context of self-compassion. This is because it enables individuals to connect distressing sensations to self-compassionate, goal-oriented actions aimed at restoring their sense of homeostasis (e.g., Paulus et al., 2009). Furthermore, by fostering a deeper understanding of their own

bodily cues, individuals may become better equipped to extend compassion outward as they recognize and respond to somatic distress signals of those around them.

12 Relevantly, the Buddhist practice of *lojong* ("mind-training" in Tibetan) employs a collection of concise slogans. These contemplative tools are designed to cultivate and reinforce qualities like compassion, serving as constant reminders throughout the day. The following *lojong* slogan refers to setting morning and evening intentions: "Two activities: one at the beginning, one at the end" (Chödrön, 2017a, p. 82).

13 For example, Doty (n.d.) recommended beginning each day by reciting the qualities that comprise the "Alphabet of the heart" mnemonic (i.e., **C**ompassion, **D**ignity, **E**quanimity, **F**orgiveness, **G**ratitude, **H**umility, **I**ntegrity, **J**ustice, **K**indness, and **L**ove). Embodying these ten qualities can assist helping professionals fortify their emotional wellbeing, potentially indirectly bolstering their capacity to navigate STS-related challenges.

14 This practice draws inspiration from Brown's (2017) "Permission slip" practice, with original adaptations made to suit the specific context of this resource guide.

15 The "Yes-And" approach, rooted in improvisational theater, emphasizes both agreement and contribution. Within the context of this resource guide, this technique can help you foster mindfulness and lead to compassionate problem-solving (e.g., Benjamin & Kline, 2019).

16 This is one of the reasons why mindfulness practices often highlight the importance of focusing on bodily sensations as a means to enhance awareness. Becoming aware of the subtle shifts in bodily sensations and their impermanent nature linked to a specific thought can eventually lead to the thought's dereification. More generally, reification occurs when abstract concepts are conceptualized or treated as concrete entities. By contrast, dereification refers to the extent to which thoughts and feelings are interpreted as subjective mental processes rather than as concrete entities (Lutz et al., 2015).

17 See the section focusing on "Guidance for Group Leaders" for added information regarding appreciative feedback.

18 While your body can differentiate between self-initiated touch and touch from others (Boehme et al., 2019), in both cases, it naturally responds to physical gestures of warmth and care (Hayashi et al., 2022).

19 While engaging in this practice, consider also how your physical boundaries are a reminder of your interconnectedness with others. Even though this may sound counterintuitive, it is so, as the "skin does not isolate us from our surroundings but rather immerses us in reciprocal relations" (Rosenthal & Vanderbeke, 2015, p. 2). Nieuwenhuis (2019, p. 2) further illuminated that due to its permeability, "the skin . . . blurs the boundaries of the body with what (and who) resides outside of it." Thus, metaphorically nurturing this shared interface through practicing *karuṇā-mudrā* can symbolize a collective, compassionate embrace.

20 According to attachment theory, variations in adult attachment styles stem from the attachments established in infancy and early childhood with primary caregivers. Individuals with insecure attachments might resist receiving compassion from others or practicing self-compassion, fearing it could trigger recollections

of unsatisfying relationships and intensify feelings of loneliness (Gilbert et al., 2011).

21 See the section focusing on "Guidance for Group Leaders" for added information regarding appreciative feedback.

22 If participants are sitting on cushions on the ground during the group sharing session, a suggested practice is for both the speaker and the listeners to place their hands on the ground after each participant shares, as a symbolic gesture that promotes a sense of grounding. This recommendation, adapted from the authentic movement technique, can also be integrated into the sharing sessions of other group practices (Adler, 2002).

23 This practice draws inspiration from Neff and Germer's (2018) "In for me, out for you" practice, with original adaptations made to suit the specific context of this resource guide.

24 "For it is in the giving that we receive" – Saint Francis of Assisi.

25 This initial step aligns with the principles of *shikantaza*, a Buddhist meditation technique focused on objectless awareness (Martínková & Wang, 2022).

26 Bhalla and DiCuirci (2023) equate altruistic self-care with "Me time" for mothers – a pause from maternal responsibilities that serves as a positive contribution to family wellbeing.

27 See the section focusing on "Guidance for Group Leaders" for added information regarding appreciative feedback.

28 This practice draws inspiration from Neff and Germer's (2018) "Compassionate letter to myself" practice, with original adaptations made to suit the specific context of this resource guide.

29 Rereading involves repeatedly engaging with the text. Through revisiting the message, previously unnoticed aspects may come to light, allowing for deeper contemplation.

30 See the section focusing on "Guidance for Group Leaders" for added information regarding appreciative feedback.

31 Journaling picture prompts are visual stimuli, often in the form of images or photographs, designed to inspire and guide the process of journaling. Relatedly, a visual journal entails incorporating artistic elements, including sketches and doodles, into the journaling process (e.g., Gibson, 2018).

32 See the section focusing on "Guidance for Group Leaders" for added information regarding appreciative feedback.

33 This practice draws inspiration from Rook's (2016) "How to create a stress-reducing playlist" practice, with original adaptations made to suit the specific context of this resource guide.

34 In the context of listening to music with lyrics rather than instrumental music, hermeneutic contamination implies that the words inherently possess their own meanings, which can influence your personal interpretations and feelings about the music (Theodore, 2020).

35 This practice draws inspiration from Worline and Dutton's (2017, p. 209) associated reflection prompt, with original adaptations made to suit the specific context of this resource guide.

36 This practice draws inspiration from Broderick's (2021) "Mindful listening" activity, with original adaptations made to suit the specific context of this resource guide.

37 *Loving-kindness*, referred to as *maitrī* in Sanskrit, signifies friendliness and the wish for all beings to experience happiness and its causes (e.g., Hao et al., 2021; Shonin et al., 2015).

38 Regarding happiness, Hạnh (2002a) taught that limiting our capacity for happiness arises when we attach ourselves to a specific notion of what happiness should be. When we release preconceived notions about happiness, we create space to discover happiness within the existing conditions of our here and now.

39 For example, Agapi (2021) highlighted that "the practice of inhalation of negativity, and subsequently reliable release from this negativity proved to me that I can empathize with my clients without any negative side effects" (Agapi, 2021, p. 26).

40 *Voluntary reciprocal altruism* refers to a form of altruism whereby individuals engage in mutually beneficial actions voluntarily (Landry, 2006).

41 *Kintsugi*, the art of golden repair, embodies the essence of *wabi sabi*, a Japanese aesthetic philosophy that centers on finding beauty in imperfection (e.g., Dobkin, 2022).

42 This part of the activity can be conducted under the guidance of an experienced quilter.

43 This practice draws inspiration from the "Just like me" and "Moving from me to we" practices by Tan (2018) and Salzberg (2013), respectively. Original adaptations were made to suit the specific context of this resource guide.

44 In line with Śāntideva (n.d.), the traditional Buddhist practice of "equalizing and exchanging oneself with others," encourages practitioners to reflect on the idea that while "I am one, others are infinite" (p. xix). Consequently, the wellbeing of others can be seen as carrying more weight than that of a single person.

45 This practice draws inspiration from Levine's (2010) "Pendulation" technique, with original adaptations made to suit the specific context of this resource guide.

46 Hạnh (2014) similarly advised pausing to compassionately acknowledge suffering without trying to deny it or push it away. Internally saying such mindful phrases as "Breathing in, I know suffering is there," and "Breathing out, I say hello to my suffering" (p. 15) is, therefore, likewise recommended; as is mindfully observing any shifts that may occur as you face, rather than ignore, distressing experiences.

47 Equanimity can lead to the "calm experience of compassion" (Condon & Feldman Barrett, 2013, as cited in Weber, 2017, p. 152) – "So that when faced with a situation, regardless of pleasant, unpleasant or indeed neutral, one is best able to cultivate compassion on the basis of this quality" (i.e., equanimity; p. 152).

48 This practice draws inspiration from the "Authentic movement" technique (Adler, 2002), with original adaptations made to suit the specific context of this resource guide.

49 In a traditional authentic movement session, participants are encouraged to attentively follow their inner urges to move, allowing these impulses to unfold spontaneously without any form of directive. This adaptation of the technique creates a safe and supportive environment specifically designed to explore STS and nonSTS-related sensations.

50 Musicant (1994, p. 97) suggested that "after being seen by another, one begins to see oneself." In this spirit, "movers" may begin to cultivate an *inner witness* (Barkai, 2022) which in the context of this practice can serve as an STS-related self-compassionate ally.

51 As previously mentioned, Bhalla and DiCuirci (2023) equate altruistic self-care with "Me time" for mothers – a pause from maternal responsibilities that serves as a positive contribution to family wellbeing.

52 Unlike traditional *brainstorming* where ideas are verbally discussed, *brainwriting* is a technique for generating ideas and solutions to a problem in which ideas are first written down (Heslin, 2009).

53 Self-affirmations, comprising statements that validate one's inherent value, worth, or capabilities, have been shown to increase self-compassion and prosocial behaviors (Lindsay & Creswell, 2014).

54 In the context of STS, it is important for helping professionals to integrate altruistic self-care practices into their daily work routines to maintain their wellbeing and effectiveness (e.g., taking a brief meditative break). Additionally, it is recommended that workplaces actively support such practices by creating a culture that encourages regular altruistic self-care activities and provides the necessary resources and time to facilitate them (e.g., Cassie & DuBose, 2023).

55 This practice draws inspiration from the "Compassion Resilience Toolkit" (n.d.) framework, with original adaptations made to suit the specific context of this resource guide.

56 While this practice has a self-and-other orientation, it serves as a catalyst for the subsequent flow of compassion from others to self.

57 This practice draws inspiration from Rubin's (2002, p. 26) invitation titled "Will the real SMART goals please stand up?" with original adaptations made to suit the specific context of this resource guide.

58 Requesting compassionate support aligns with the *tend-and-befriend* response, which involves seeking social support as a strategy for dealing with stress (e.g., forming social bonds and seeking compassionate assistance; Taylor et al., 2000).

59 These listening recommendations are also relevant for becoming more attuned to notice compassionate interactions within the workplace, as they can help cultivate a receptive state of mind and a heightened sensitivity to the subtleties of human interaction (e.g., Rakel, 2018).

60 This practice draws inspiration from Li et al.'s (2017) "INSPIRE" framework, with original adaptations made to suit the specific context of this resource guide.

61 This practice draws inspiration from Lyman's (1981) "Think-pair-square-share" practice, with original adaptations made to suit the specific context of this resource guide.

62 Gratitude can also be extended toward oneself as well as extended to encompass situations, activities, and events (Tachon et al., 2022).

63 This practice draws inspiration from Altman's (2014) "GLAD" technique, with original adaptations made to suit the specific context of this resource guide.

Practices for Promoting Vicarious Posttraumatic Growth (VPTG)

1 Intentional smiling can elicit comparable brain activity to that of spontaneous smiling. For example, the activation of feedback pathways from facial expression muscles to the brain can physiologically enhance positive emotions (Beamish et al., 2019).

2 Inspired by the idea that a smile can be referred to as "mouth yoga," this haiku, focusing on a flower practicing yoga, is placed here to uplift the spirits of the endnote section – just in case the endnotes go unnoticed:)

> dew-kissed petals bow
> in a garden yoga class:
> flower *āsana*

In modern yoga discourse, the Sanskrit word *āsana* refers to a yoga "posture."

3 This practice draws inspiration from Tedeschi and Calhoun's (1996) "Posttraumatic Growth Inventory," with original adaptations made to suit the specific context of this resource guide.

4 This practice draws inspiration from Campbell's (2008) "Hero's journey" framework, with original adaptations made to suit the specific context of this resource guide.

5 To reiterate, VPTG encompasses positive changes related to the following five factors: (a) personal strength, (b) spiritual growth, (c) new possibilities, (d) appreciation of life, and (e) improved relationships (Kalaitzaki et al., 2022; Tedeschi & Calhoun, 2004).

6 As defined in Part I of this resource guide, PTSD is a stress-related mental health disorder that may emerge after experiencing one or more traumatic events (APA, 2022). In contrast, PTG represents the potential for transformative positive psychological changes that can arise following one or more traumatic events (Tedeschi & Calhoun, 2004).

7 This practice draws inspiration from Hanson's (2013, 2020) "HEAL" practice, with original adaptations made to suit the specific context of this resource guide.

8 To reiterate, you may experience VPTG through positive psychological changes in the following five domains: (a) personal strength, (b) spiritual growth, (c) new possibilities, (d) appreciation of life, and (e) improved relationships (Tedeschi & Calhoun, 2004).

9 The Dalai Lama distinguished between compassion and loving-kindness in the following way: "Just as compassion is the wish that all sentient beings be free of suffering, loving-kindness is the wish that all may enjoy happiness" (2001, p. 96).

10 Alternatively, you might wish to consider imagining that you are emanating wishes of loving-kindness in all directions without following the previously outlined progressive steps (Wallace, 2004). Interestingly, in line with the Buddhist concept of no-self, Anālayo (2019) pointed out that the inclusion of "oneself" in this traditional loving-kindness meditation may have originated from a potential misspelling in a classical Buddhist text known as the *Visuddhi-Magga*. This discrepancy arises from variations in the spelling of the terms *sabbatthatāya*

or *sabbattatāya*, with the former suggesting "in every way" and the latter implying "to all, as to oneself."

11 In line with Zahavi (2019) and Garfield (2019), although the first-person plural pronoun "we" is used here, treating third persons as you would treat yourself or those in your second-person circle, is recommended.

12 In line with the broadening circles of the "VPTG-wish chain method," the broaden-and-build theoretical model posits that positive emotions can expand individuals' modes of thinking and behavior which, in turn, can enhance their resources. This is so, as positive emotions can enhance the likelihood of individuals exploring and experimenting with new skills, relationships, and activities. Furthermore, the broaden-and-build model proposes that such personal resources are cumulative, meaning that they can be drawn upon in the future to help individuals cope with new challenges and ultimately thrive (Fredrickson, 1998).

13 While I see two hearts, I also recognize that within the two, there is one (i.e., the heart within the figure). Unity that prevails beneath the surface of apparent divisions aligns with the Buddhist concept of nonduality (Skt. *advaya*; Loy, 2019).

Guidance for Group Leaders

1 The Sanskrit word *saṅgha* signifies "gathering," "assembly," "association" or "community." Interestingly, as cited by Volkan (2013, p. 50), the Tibetan word for *saṅgha*, "*gedun*," signifies "to strive after virtue."

Appendices

1 For research purposes, supplementing a collection of relevant validated quantitative assessments with pre- and post-in-depth qualitative interviews would provide a comprehensive and personalized perspective regarding helping professionals' experiences with this training program. Moreover, including physiological as well as neurophysiological measurement tools to evaluate the impacts of this training program would align with recommendations by Kirby (2017).

2 For this version of the scale, the STSS DSM-5 (Bride, 2013) underwent the following changes: (a) the items were reordered according to their respective domains, (b) the time frame was changed to the past month instead of the past week to align with posttraumatic stress disorder (PTSD) DSM-5-TR diagnostic criteria, (c) item number 5 was removed as it did not align with PTSD DSM-5-TR diagnostic criteria, and (d) the items were rephrased in the present tense to assist helping professionals in recognizing that STS-related challenges are a current reality for which they can take compassionate action, rather than something that has already happened and thereby cannot be changed (American Psychiatric Association [APA], 2022).

3 Domain scores range as follows: Intrusion reactions (5–25), avoidance reactions (2–10), negative cognition and mood reactions (7–35), and hyperarousal and reactivity reactions (6–30).

4 Online synchronous training sessions typically follow a structured format. Based on Knox and Franco (2023), this format can comprise several key components: check-in, introduction to the topic of the session, personal and group-context practices, sharing sessions in pairs and/or small groups (e.g., using Zoom breakout rooms), larger group sharing session, and closing.

5 In emergency situations requiring immediate action, pausing may not be suitable. In such cases, prompt responses may be essential to ensure safety and address urgent needs effectively.

6 Regarding objectivity, consider also that our understanding of the world is inherently filtered through our perceptions, meaning that we cannot truly know that which is external to us in its unmediated form, separate from our perception of it. The latter statement by Vasubandhu, an influential philosophical Buddhist thinker (late 4th to early 5th century CE), is further discussed by Tzohar (2019).

7 In this context, mirroring entails the process of reiterating an expressed idea, usually by paraphrasing it in your own words. Occasionally, it may also involve repeating the speaker's exact words or a significant portion thereof (Ferrara, 1994).

8 Co-regulation, as understood through the lens of the polyvagal theory, refers to the interpersonal process whereby individuals positively influence each other's autonomic nervous states in order to achieve a balanced state of autonomic nervous system functioning (Dana, 2020). Parenthetically, *co-regulation* is one of the polyvagal theory's three organizing principles alongside *hierarchy* and *neuroception* – as detailed further by D'Angelo (2022).

INDEX